Acknowledgements

The present book was made possible by the efforts of the entire scientific community of nuclear medicine and radiopharmacy that in last 30 years has pursued the research in the field of molecular imaging. The authors in particular want to mention the outstanding contribution of great scientists as Michael Phelps and Markus Schwaiger to the present development of PET imaging.

Stefano Fanti owes thanks again to all his colleagues, and in particular to Dr. Mario Marengo, whose vision in planning Bologna's PET site was determinant for every result obtained, Dr. Stefano Boschi for patiently providing all the required tracers with great professionality, and to Dr. Paolo Castellucci, Dr. Cristina Nanni, and Dr. Arturo Chiti for their invaluable capabilities and friendship.

Mohsen Farsad wishes to record, with appreciation, the support and commitment offered by the staff of nuclear medicine of Bolzano Hospital and want to thank the following individuals who have assisted him in various ways: Dr. Patrizia Pernter, Dr. Alessandro Imondi, Dr. Federica Ferro, and especially Dr. Luzian Osele. Finally thanks are extended to Rosanna who graciously encouraged him to continue working on realization of this atlas.

Luigi Mansi dedicates his contribution to Nagia, his wife, and to his son David, to further stimulate the realization of his dream: become *one of us*, a molecular imager searching for the keys opening the mind and the eyes to the knowledge.

Stefano Fanti – Mohsen Farsad – Luigi Mansi

PET-CT Beyond FDG

A Quick Guide to Image Interpretation

Stefano Fanti – Mohsen Farsad – Luigi Mansi

PET-CT Beyond FDG A Quick Guide to Image Interpretation

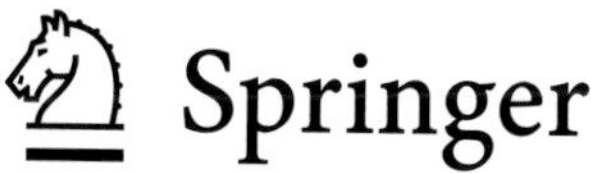

Stefano Fanti, Prof.
University of Bologna
Policlinico S.Orsola-Malpighi
Medicina Nucleare
PAD 30-Via Massarenti 9
40138 Bologna
Italy
stefano.fanti@aosp.bo.it

Luigi Mansi, Prof. Dr.
Università Napoli
Ist. Scienze Radiologiche
Piazza Miraglia, 2
80138 Napoli
Italy
luigi.mansi@unina2.it

Mohsen Farsad, Dr.
Assistant Director
Central Hospital Bozen
Nuclear Medicine
Via Boehler 5
39100 Bolzano
Italy
mohsen.farsad@asbz.it

ISBN: 978-3-540-93908-5 e-ISBN: 978-3-540-93909-2

DOI: 10.1007/978-3-540-93909-2

Library of Congress Control Number: 2009934508

Cover design: eStudio Calamar, Spain

Printed on acid-free paper

Springer is part & Springer Science + Business Media (www.springer.com)

Contents

Contributors

Vincenzo Allegri U.O. Medicina Nucleare – Centro PET, Policlinico S.Orsola-Malpighi, Bologna, Italy

Valentina Ambrosini U.O. Medicina Nucleare – Centro PET, Policlinico S.Orsola-Malpighi – Università di Bologna, Bologna, Italy

Catherine Beckers Division of Nuclear Medicine, University Hospital of Liège, Liège, Belgium

Ambrose J. Beer Nuclearmedizinische Klinik, Technische Universität München, München, Germany

Adrienne H. Brouwers Department of Nuclear Medicine and Molecular Imaging, University of Groningen and University Medical Center Groningen, Groningen, The Netherlands

Andreas Buck Nuclearmedizinische Klinik, Technische Universität München, München, Germany

Paolo Castellucci U.O. Medicina Nucleare – Centro PET, Policlinico S.Orsola-Malpighi, Bologna, Italy

Franca Chierichetti U.O. Medicina Nucleare – Centro PET, P.O. Castelfranco Veneto (ULSS 8 Regione Veneto), Castelfranco Veneto (TV), Italy

Vincenzo Cuccurullo U.O.C. Medicina Nucleare, Seconda Università di Napoli, Napoli, Italy

Erik F.J. de Vries Department of Nuclear Medicine and Molecular Imaging, University Medical Center Groningen, University of Groningen, Groningen, The Netherlands

Rudi A.J.O. Dierckx Department of Nuclear Medicine and Molecular Imaging, University of Groningen and University Medical Center Groningen, Groningen, The Netherlands

Philip H. Elsinga Department of Nuclear Medicine and Molecular Imaging, University of Groningen and University Medical Center Groningen, Groningen, The Netherlands

Stefano Fanti University of Bologna, Policlinico S.Orsola-Malpighi, Medicina Nucleare, Bologna, Italy

Mohsen Farsad Assistant Director, Central Hospital Bozen, Nuclear Medicine, Bolzano, Italy

Andor W.J.M. Glaudemans Department of Nuclear Medicine and Molecular Imaging, University Medical Center Groningen, University of Groningen, Groningen, The Netherlands

Tove J. Gronroos Turku PET Centre, University of Turku, Turku, Finland

Ken Herrmann Nuclearmedizinische Klinik, Technische Universität München, München, Germany

Rodney J. Hicks Centre for Molecular Imaging, Peter MacCallum Cancer Centre, Melbourne, Victoria, Australia

Geke A.P. Hospers Department of Medical Oncology, University Medical Center Groningen, University of Groningen, Groningen, The Netherlands

Roland Hustinx Division of Nuclear Medicine, University Hospital of Liège, Liège, Belgium

Jae Min Jeong Department of Nuclear Medicine, Seoul National University College of Medicine, Seoul, Korea

Keon Wook Kang Department of Nuclear Medicine, Seoul National University College of Medicine, Seoul, Korea

Klaas P. Koopmans Department of Nuclear Medicine and Molecular Imaging, University of Groningen and University Medical Center Groningen, Groningen, The Netherlands

Luigi Mansi Università Napoli, Ist. Scienze Radiologiche, Italy

Heikki Minn Turku PET Centre and Department of Oncology and Radiotherapy, Turku University Hospital, Turku, Finland

GianCarlo Montini U.O. Medicina Nucleare – Centro PET, Policlinico S.Orsola-Malpighi, Bologna, Italy

Cristina Nanni U.O. Medicina Nucleare – Centro PET, Policlinico S.Orsola-Malpighi, Bologna, Italy

Gabriele Popperl Klinik für Nuklearmedizin, Katharinenhospital, Stuttgart, Germany

Pier Francesco Rambaldi U.O.C. Medicina Nucleare, Seconda Università di Napoli, Napoli, Italy

Caroline P. Schroder Department of Medical Oncology, University Medical Center Groningen, University of Groningen, Groningen, The Netherlands

Chapter 1 Importance of Radiotracers Other than FDG in Oncology

Luigi Mansi, Pier Francesco Rambaldi, and Vincenzo Cuccurullo

Diagnostic imaging is based on two different approaches acting as two separate "monocular visions": (a) morphostructural imaging, analyzing anatomy (structure and morphology) and using pathology as the golden standard; (b) functional imaging, analyzing physiology (function) and using pathophysiology as a reference to define the disease.

Traditionally, when multiple diagnostic contributions are available, the final diagnosis is achieved through a visual comparison of the different studies. The computer revolution, permitting work on digital matrixes, has created the option to "fuse" images together. In this way, it is possible to overlap two different images, separately acquired, in a new "fused" image, including both morphostructural and functional information, for a patient.

A major improvement in fusion imaging is the advent of the so-called "hybrid machines", i.e., of scanners having the capacity to produce two studies simultaneously. Today, while Positron Emission Tomography-Magnetic Resonance (PET-MR) is still in the prototype phase, the Single Photon Emission Tomography – Computed Tomography (SPET-CT) is already in clinical practice. But among hybrid machines, the leading position is certainly occupied by PET-CT, by now a primary tool in the whole diagnostic scenario.

It has to be pointed out that when a PET-CT is used, while the CT information remains the same, the PET component can give various diagnostic contributions, depending on the radiotracer used.

At present, more than 95% of PET studies worldwide are performed in oncologic patients, using F-18 Fluorodeoxyglucose (FDG). But, despite its high diagnostic accuracy in determining the pivotal role in the restaging (and staging) of the neoplasm, FDG is handicapped by false negative and positive results, creating limitations in the differential diagnosis of cancer. Moreover, PET- FDG shares with all the other diagnostic techniques the inability to answer all the questions of the oncologist, the surgeon, and the radiotherapist. It cannot function alone, either in the diagnostic field, or in giving all the information connected with prognosis and pursue a "tailored strategy" for each patient. Therefore, despite its primary role, there is a wide range of indications in oncologic patients that other radiotracers may be useful, and in this chapter we shall try to understand them.

How to Improve Diagnostic Accuracy with PET–FDG

False Negative and False Positive Results of PET-FDG

In oncology, the results concerning neoplastic lesions not detected by the procedure are called false negative results of FDG. Conversely, false positive results are those connected with benign lesions, showing FDG uptake.

It has to be pointed out that false negative and false positive results can also be the consequence of pitfalls and artifacts. For a deeper understanding of these problems we suggest a reading of the *Atlas of PET-CT: A Quick Guide to Image Interpretation (Springer, 2009).*

A hybrid PET-CT scanner permits higher accuracy with respect to PET alone, because of the added morphostructural information and the anatomical location of the FDG activity allowed by CT. This advantage is particularly significant in evaluating areas with a complex anatomy, e.g. the head and neck, or partially "covered" by the emunctory system, e.g. along the ureteral course; a major diagnostic improvement is obtained in the case of small lesions, such as the evaluation of a lymph node neoplastic involvement. Despite using PET-CT, false negative and false positive results are, however, present. An improvement in sensitivity and specificity with the use of PET radiotracers other than FDG, can therefore significantly increase overall diagnostic accuracy.

With respect to methodology, many causes can affect glucose kinetics, creating difficulties in FDG utilization. The major problem is high glucose serum levels, as observed, in particular, in diabetes; but many other conditions can determine an unfavorable physiological and/or para – physiological distribution, creating pitfalls and artifacts decreasing PET-FDG accuracy. For example, it is well known that determining a nonspecific FDG uptake requires correct timing for a reliable evaluation of patients who have undergone surgery, radiotherapy, or chemotherapy. Therefore, the availability of radiotracers not affected by conditions such as high glucose levels, inflammation, altered permeability or vascularity, can help in finding a rationale to choose an alternative to FDG. Thus, a more effective clinical value can be reached, for example, in diabetic patients, or when the clinical history of the patient suggests that the analysis obtained by using FDG is not reliable.

How to Increase Sensitivity with Respect to FDG

False negative results of PET-FDG are mainly due to lesions that are too small to be PET's spatial resolution, which is usually above 5 mm. It has to be pointed out that the positive indicators as FDG, i.e., radiotracers with a higher uptake in lesions than in the surrounding normal tissue, can also occasionally detect lesions that are less than the spatial resolution value. As the image is the result of differences in concentration, the detectability of the lesion depends mainly on the lesion/background (L/B) ratio. To use a simile, it is easier to see an ant on white marble on a sunny day than a black cat on a dark night. As a result, as demonstrated by bone scans, it is possible to detect lesions "many months before" they attain the theoretically minimum detectable size. This favorable condition, creating a premise for an early diagnosis, happens when a high L/B ratio is achieved. It depends more on the uptake mechanism of the radiotracer than on the PET scanner. With respect to FDG, a higher L/B can be achieved by different radiotracers allowing a higher tumor uptake and/or a lower background activity.

Radiotracers Allowing a Higher Tumors Uptake with Respect to FDG

Independent of the size, not all tumors present a higher FDG uptake with respect to normal tissues. Therefore, false negative results can be observed even in patients with tumors of 1 cm or more, characterized by a normal or reduced glucose metabolism. It can happen under many conditions, in differentiated types of tumors, in the presence of slow tumor growth, and in cystic and/or mucinous lesions. For example, many false negative results are observed in patients with prostate cancer or well-differentiated neuroendocrine tumors. In the following chapters of this Atlas, the ability of radiotracers such as choline, somatostatin analogues, acetate, DOPA and tryptophan to significantly improve sensitivity in these patients is demonstrated. However, it is interesting to note that, despite the low sensitivity in patients with well-differentiated tumors, FDG plays an important prognostic role in the follow up of these subjects. For example, in the follow up of patients affected with neuroendocrine tumors and thyroid carcinomas, the presence of FDG uptake, which is an expression of de-differentiation, is a negative prognostic factor.

Another possibility of increasing overall sensitivity with respect to FDG is the use of radiotracers allowing a higher L/B ratio on the basis of a more favorable uptake mechanism. An example (see Chap. 5) is the detection of bone metastases, where a mismatch can be observed between FDG, concentrating on the pathological skeletal content, and F-18 fluoride, becoming part of the mineral bone matrix. As a consequence, radio-fluoride can detect a higher number of skeletal metastases in patients affected by tumors, metastasizing through a neoplastic involvement determining early osteobastic response (as it frequently happens in prostate, breast and lung cancer). Conversely, FDG can detect a higher number of malignant lesions in patients with myeloma because of the late involvement of a periosteal reaction in the subjects. Therefore, radio-fluoride can find a clinical indication during follow up (and/or staging) of patients with cancer with a high prevalence of bone metastases, when there is an early osteoblastic reaction. Moreover, in some cases, the complementary information provided by fluoride about FDG can be utilized to better evaluate the skeletal involvement to adjacent malignant lesions.

Radiotracers Allowing a Lower Background with Respect to FDG

Analysis of the normal FDG distribution in humans shows that the highest uptake is at the level of the brain, the only organ to use glucose exclusively as carburant. Therefore, although PET-FDG is born evaluate brain diseases, the high activity in the normal gray matter creates difficulties in tumor detection. Therefore, although an important role in dementia and in prognostic evaluation of primary cancer, PET-FDG cannot be considered a reliable procedure in detecting brain metastases. Moreover, despite the added value of CT (or MRI) in precisely localizing FDG uptake and anatomical structures, diagnosis of recurrence can be difficult both because of the possible presence of faint nonspecific uptakes and the confusion caused by normal tissue, due to the partial volume effect. To avoid these limitations, the use of radiotracers with a minimal uptake in the normal brain has been proposed. The best results achievable for a clinical use are provided by radio-amino-acids such as methyonine (see Chap. 4) and thyrosine (Chap. 6). An alternative to better evaluate brain tumors may be the use of radio- choline (Chap. 3) and acetate (Chap. 8).

In the case of whole body analysis, difficulties in evaluating lesions at the level of the head and neck have been significantly reduced by the primary complementary role of CT in improving overall accuracy. Thoracic analysis is characterized by a quite unpredictable myocardial uptake while there is no pulmonary activity. Therefore, this is an area typically characterized by low background FDG, in general easily analyzable with the help of CT. This favorable condition proves more advantageous when a respiratory gating is available. While lesion detection is in general easy for FDG at the level of the limbs, as demonstrated by the high sensitivity in the diagnosis of melanomas, the analysis at the level of the abdomen and pelvis is more complex. Difficulties in liver tumor detection are caused mainly by pathophysiology, being high the sensitivity in detecting hepatic metastases and low accuracy in the diagnosis of liver cancer. As previously described, one of the most critical problems for FDG is detecting tumors localized in areas partially occupied by a nonspecific uptake, as those adjacent and/or interlaced with the emunctory systems. Therefore, a major diagnostic problem can be, for example, diagnosing prostate cancer, where the low accuracy depends both on a high background and on a low FDG tumor uptake, resulting in an unfavorable T/B ratio. In this scenario, a significant improvement can be obtained by radiotracers such as radio-choline or acetate, characterized by an uptake mechanism dependent on an aerobic metabolism less related to malignancy or growth rate with respect to FDG. This ability is an advantage in detecting recurrence or lymphnode metastases. Conversely, the possible uptake by benign lesions limits the diagnosis of primary cancer. To demonstrate the effect of radiochemistry and pharmacokinetics, it is interesting to compare different choline radiotracer pharmacokinetics, as reported in Chap. 3. While no C-11 choline is present in the urine, activity in the bladder can be observed after F-18 choline administration, because of a different excretion or as consequence of an in vivo de-fluorination. It means that a lower background can be observed using the former rather than the latter. Less significant is the role of radiotracers other than FDG in intestinal tumors. CT plays a major role in improving FDG accuracy in the differential diagnosis of recurrent bowel cancer.

How to Increase Specificity with Respect to FDG

As in the case of sensitivity, the morphostructural contribution of CT plays a major role in decreasing the false positive results of FDG. Similarly, the achievement of a higher L/B ratio can improve specificity with respect to FDG, because of an easier and more reliable analysis. False positive results of FDG are mainly due to the presence of active inflammation, but they can also be dependent on many physiological, para-physiological and pathological conditions such as active scar, fractures, benign thyroid diseases, active brown fat, muscular stress, posttherapeutic response and others (See *Atlas of PET-CT: A quick guide to Image Interpretation* (Springer, 2009)).

The following chapters describe a major improvement in specificity with respect to FDG, which can be achieved using radiotracers with an uptake mechanism that does not determine an increased concentration in inflammation. It happens, for example, with the use of amino-acids or DNA precursors, such as F-18 thymidine (FLT). It has to be pointed out, however, that even with alternative PET radiotracers, false negative and positive results are present. For example, many false positives can be detected in the diagnosis of primary prostate cancer with the use of acetate or choline. Similarly, F-18 fluoride permits a higher sensitivity in detecting bone metastases in patients with prostate, lung and breast cancer, but in the presence of a low specificity, due to the large number of benign pathological conditions characterized by increased osteoblastic activity.

Therefore, the choice of an alternative radiotracer should be based on a deep and strong knowledge of the pathophysiological premises of their uptake mechanism. The following chapters describe why, when and how to use these radio-compounds to further improve the pivotal role of FDG in oncology. As a deeper analysis is to be found in the respective chapters, only the major ideas are given here.

Why and When to Use Different Radiotracers with Respect to FDG in Oncology: To Improve its Diagnostic Accuracy

As mentioned earlier, the first justification for choosing radiotracers others than FDG is improving accuracy. This result can be achieved in different ways, depending on the clinical situation.

Brain cancer. To improve diagnostic accuracy in brain cancer, the main strategy is to use radiocompounds not concentrated in the normal brain. The ideal radiotracer could also have a specific uptake mechanism, permitting a differential diagnosis between benign and malignant lesions. At present, the main category of tracers already in clinical practice is that of amino-acids, having as clinical prototype methionine and thyrosine. Amino-acids present an increased uptake in tumors, but not in the normal brain and in inflammatory lesions. Therefore they can improve accuracy with respect to FDG (and CT and MRI) in the diagnosis of tumor recurrence, acting both on sensitivity and specificity. Conversely, because of their presence in both benign and malignant tumors, they are not reliable for a prognostic evaluation. A less significant clinical interest is seen with the use of radio-choline and acetate.

Whole body cancer. To improve the diagnostic accuracy of FDG in patients with whole body cancer, one of the main strategies is to choose radiocompounds concentrating through an uptake mechanism present in the differentiated tumors.

a. A favorable result can be obtained using radiotracers concentrating through an oxygen dependent mechanism. This is typical of the differentiated tumors with a substantially conserved regular vascular support and a not significant neo-angiogenesis. This rationale has been used for proposing radiotracers such as acetate and choline, both defining an increased metabolic activity not depending on anaerobiosis. Because of the lack of vesical concentration, the use of these radiocompounds has found clinical value in tumors such as prostate cancer, finding a possible clinical role also in hepatomas, renal cancer and brain tumors.
b. A more specific approach is utilizing the peculiar characteristics of some tumors. A very effective clinical application is the use of somatostin analogues in neuroendocrine tumors, or the use of cathecolamine analogues in pheocromocytoma and other tumors showing increased metabolism. Similarly, a higher accuracy in restaging differentiated thyroid cancer is obtained with I-124 iodide, which has the advantage of also permitting a more rigorous quantitative evaluation of the corresponding gamma emitters.
c. As previously described, an increased sensitivity in detecting bone metastases can be obtained with F-18 fluoride. It has to be pointed out that this radiotracer presents a nonspecific, although sensitive, uptake mechanism, i.e., increased osteoblastic activity. A better accuracy is permitted by the simultaneous CT acquisition, acting mainly through a significant reduction of false positive results.

Why and When to Use Different Radiotracers with Respect to FDG: To Answer Different Questions

In modern medicine, tumor detection is certainly the major request of the clinician, but it does not provide all the information needed for a diagnostic and therapeutic strategy "tailored" for each single patient. Therefore, a wide field of applications for radiotracers other than FDG is available, to give more information, and answer many questions not answered by FDG, especially those connected with prognosis and therapy.

Some of the most interesting possibilities already available in the clinical field in humans are considered here, with a deeper analysis of the clinical aspects in "specific" chapters.

Prognostic information. A promising approach to add a relevant clinical improvement to FDG in prognostic evaluation and in better defining the tumor response is related to the use of radiocompounds tracing the growth rate. The best proposal, already in clinical practice, is linked to the use of radiolabeled thymidine (see Chap. 9), a marker of the DNA multiplication rate. This information, although nonspecific, is different from that obtained by FDG, because it is not significantly influenced by anaerobiosis and the presence of inflammatory cells. FLT could also be important in the near future for a reliable evaluation of tumor response. In fact, FDG plays a significant role in this field, but with an uptake mechanism not strictly related to the growth rate. Although its contribution will certainly remain important for this application, FLT could occupy a clinical role in better defining an early response.

Hypoxia. The presence or absence of hypoxia is relevant in predicting therapeutic efficacy. These data can create an important diagnostic premise, mainly in the evaluation of patients undergoing radiotherapy.

Receptor state. It is well known that the presence of receptors is crucial, both in defining prognosis and in better deciding a therapeutic strategy. In this sense, clinical improvement can be obtained, for example, using radiocompounds tracing hormone receptors (estradiol and androgens) or somatostatin receptors in neuroendocrine tumors.

Cathecolamine and serotonine precursors. This is a limited but very important field of clinical interest, not only in oncology. In fact, despite the presence of reliable radiotracers labeled with gamma emitters, the use of PET in patients with pathological conditions such as pheocromocytoma and neuroendocrine tumors, and with non-oncologic cardiac or neurological diseases, could give a significant impulse for a better definition of therapeutic strategies.

Angiogenesis. One of the most important frontiers in oncology is to acquire all information on tumor angiogenesis in the patient. The availability of radiocompounds tracing this target can make a major contribution, more than mere diagnosis, to the prognostic evaluation and the definition and monitoring of the best therapeutic strategies.

Relationship between diagnosis and therapy. Historically, the major success of radionuclide therapy has been (and continues to be) obtained in patients with differentiated thyroid cancer. In these subjects, a whole body diagnosis using a gamma emitter, such as I-131 or I-123, permits the recruitment of pretherapeutic patients who will benefit from an effective radionuclide therapy. In this field, a positron emitter such as I-124 could permit the accurate calculation of dosimetry, and the lowest dose to be administered. Similarly, useful information can be obtained from patients undergoing radionuclide therapy using other radiocompounds such as somatostain analogues, cathecolamine precursors, and bone seeking indicators.

In conclusion, although FDG will be the workhorse of clinical PET for many years, today nuclear medicine can already offer the oncologist, the surgeon, and the radiotherapist many other weapons effective in destroying the big killer: cancer.

To better define the role of these new acquisitions in clinical practice, the deep involvement of pioneers working in Institutions having a scientific background, based not only on imaging, but also on radiochemistry, physiology, pharmacology, molecular biology and clinics, will be important. But to reach the goal three other protagonists are mandatory: (1) the Industry, that has to invest in the production and distribution of new radiotracers already available for clinical practice; (2) the nuclear physician, who has to optimize the use of these new powerful instruments; and (3) the clinician, who has to understand the real relevance of these procedures in clinical practice.

The objective of the authors of this Atlas is to contribute their best efforts in the stimulating new areas of clinical development of nuclear medicine.

Chapter 2 Considerations About PET Isotopes

Luigi Mansi, Vincenzo Cuccurullo,
and Pier Francesco Rambaldi

Nuclear Medicine and Molecular Imaging

Human beings, like all living organisms, are made of bio-molecules. Health can be considered as the expression of homeostasis, i.e., the ability of a system to regulate its internal environment, thereby tending to maintain a stable and "normal" condition. In this sense, the real essence of life is the phenomenon in which multiple dynamic equilibrium and regulation mechanisms are needed to make homeostasis possible. Many diseases result from disturbances in homeostasis and are characterized by a condition known as homeostatic imbalance, where a molecular system goes out of equilibrium.

Based on this premise, one of the most effective approaches to diagnose and treat diseases is to follow bio-molecular kinetics in the normal state (physiology) and in illness (pathophysiology). This can become a reality when *tracers* for that specific molecule are available. To follow the bio-molecular kinetics, without interfering with the native molecule, tracers need to be detected by an outside scanner to become a diagnostic tool.

We call this *Molecular Imaging*, a new term that has to be well understood to avoid confusion. If we want to *image* a normal or altered *molecular system*, i.e., an environment where specific molecules are connected through a dynamic interaction, we do not have to modify it. In other words, a molecular process can be studied, without being disturbed, using *tracing molecules*, the number of which will be relatively low when compared to the total number of native molecules involved in the system. Interference and/or effects on the kinetics that are to be analyzed can be avoided by using *tracing molecules*. Starting from this premise, it is possible to obtain a *true* molecular imaging today, in the large majority of the systems (and/or diseases),only by nuclear medicine (NM) and optical imaging (OI). In fact, only NM and OI can produce images with pico/nanomolar amounts of tracers, while CT and MRI need micro/millimoles, too high to permit a rigorous and harmless functional evaluation.

Although it plays a pivotal role in basic research, OI is not yet ready for clinical use because of its incapability to analyze deep structures. Therefore, molecular imaging in humans can be almost identified with NM today.

It is important to note that NM is born and can exist only as Molecular Imaging or therapy. For example,since the 40s, Iodine-131 has been a diagnostic (and therapeutic) tool in patients with thyroid diseases because of its *molecular* uptake mechanism. Today's molecular imaging of thyroid can be identified with the old thyroid scintigraphy because radioiodine's concentration in normal and differentiated malignant cells has become a matter of importance for the molecular biologist; in fact, through the *molecular thyroid scintigraphy*, it is possible to demonstrate the *in vivo* presence of the iodine symporter gene both in normal and in neoplastic cells.

Therefore, NM is and has ever been Molecular Imaging; if this term sounds new, born in the third millennium, it is only because we have recently entered the Genome era, with gene and bio-molecules at the center of the diagnostic universe; a further impulse to the diffusion of this term has been given by the incredible technological evolution: it is possible today to study bio-phenomena with a very high spatial and temporal resolution, enabling to detect and characterize lesions sub-millimeters (in animal imaging). The best instrument to image bio-molecules in humans is PET–CT, which gives standard morpho-structural information with CT and a variegated spectrum of functional solutions through the PET scanner.

As described in the previous chapter, although F-18 Fluorodeoxyglucose (FDG) in oncology represents, at present, more than 95% of clinical indications, there is a wide field of new applications, both for FDG in the non-oncologic area and, using other radiotracers, FDG in oncology.

The goal of this Atlas being the presentation of the capabilities of positron emitter radiotracers other than FDG in the oncologic clinical practice, the following chapters provide a wider discussion of each specific radio-compound, analyzing general problems and common issues.

Radiotracers, Radioisotopes, and "*in vivo*" Distribution of Radioactivity

A radiotracer is a radio-compound, constituted by a radionuclide (radioisotope) labeling a *vector* molecule (cell), determining the *in vivo* distribution. In the radio-compound, the radionuclide acts as a label permitting the detection of the tracer by an external scanner. From a theoretical point of view, all *imaged* radioactivity would correspond only to the radiotracer and its distribution would be dependent only on specific uptake mechanisms.

Practically, after *in vivo* administration, radioactivity can image both the injected radiotracer (with a distribution determined by specific and nonspecific mechanisms, or by its presence in the vascular pool or in the emunctories) and other radiochemical forms such as metabolites, complexes, and free radionuclides.

The goal of this chapter is to discuss the main issues regarding PET radiotracers from the radiochemical and pharmacological points of view.

Radioisotopes: Most Diffuse Positron Emitters

The most diffuse positron emitters are those that can be produced with a small cyclotron. In this series are included Carbon-11 (C-11), Nitrogen (N-13), Oxygen (O-15), and Fluorine (F-18). While the first three permit radiolabeling through an isotopic radiochemical substitution of atoms present in the large majority of bio-molecules, F-18 is a halogen, i.e.,it can substitute hydrogen by halogenation. Leaving the deeper analysis of radiochemistry and radio-pharmacology to other books and specific papers, this work focuses on the half life (HL) of positron emitters which is the primary physical characteristic to be known before their *in vivo* use in humans. In fact, to reliably use a radiotracer, we have to first consider the total time needed for the various steps such as radiochemistry, quality control, time of arrival of the dose to the patient, and pharmacokinetics after the administration of the radiotracer. It is clear that too short an HL can create problems in its clinical use.

Positron Emitters with a Short Half-Life: C-11, N-13, 0–15

Among the four radio-nuclides presented above, because of its very short HL, tracers labeled with O-15 (HL: 2.03 min) cannot be used in the absence of a cyclotron adjacent to the scanner's room. To permit a reliable utilization of C-11 (HL: 20.4 m) and N-13 (HL: 9.98 m) radio-compounds, the cyclotron should be positioned preferably in the same place where the PET scanner is located. Moreover, because of their fast decay, C-11, N-13, and O-15 radio-compounds have to be produced very rapidly and in high amounts, therefore requiring the *in loco* presence of expert radio-chemists and of a well organized complex structure.

A further problem of the clinical use of short lived positron emitters is connected with the *in vivo* pharmacokinetic of the corresponding radiotracers. In this sense, to use C-11, N-13, and O-15 radiocompounds, the following are necessary: the availability of high amounts of radioactivity and, preferably, of a PET scanner allowing a high count rate, and also a very fast or a very slow achievement of a satisfactory tumor/background ratio. As a consequence, radiotracers labeled with C-11, N-13, or O-15 are almost exclusively used today by institutions which own a cyclotron. In these secondary PET centers, the utilization of these radiotracers, but for N-13 ammonia, which is very easily produced, is mainly limited to groups including professional radio-chemists, who also stimulate research of/with new radiotracers.

As a consequence, the diffusion of radio-compounds labeled with C-11, N-13, or O-15 is not too wide at present. In particular, the interest evinced by industries for the distribution of the easiest and cheapest radio-compound strongly stimulated the development of a radiochemistry based on F-18, generators products, and other radio-nuclides with a slower decay. In fact, these radioisotopes permit to produce, distribute, and reliably use a large number of radiotracers other than FDG in PET centers without cyclotrons which are the majority. A routine use of C-11, N-13, and O-15 radiotracers,on the other hand, is feasible only for well organized, complex PET centers. The use of the radiotracers is therefore mainly of interest for research purposes.

Radio-Fluorine (F-18)

F-18 is today the most diffuse positron emitter. The main reason being its favorable HL, which is 109.8 min, and this in turn gives the advantages of radioprotection (not being too long), of technical and methodological issues, and of the possibility of a long travel transport. In fact, radio-fluorinated compounds can be produced by cyclotrons located at a distance of 3 hours and more from the PET scanner; therefore they are utilizable by a high number of PET centers spread over a wide territory. This condition, together with the unique possibility of labeling the glucose tracer, deoxy-glucose, gave F-18 a fundamental role in the diffusion of PET. The advantages described above stimulated radio-chemists and industries to develop new syntheses using this radionuclide. The number of F-18 radiotracers available for clinical use in humans is increasing each day, frequently substituting radio-compounds previously labeled with C-11. Some examples are reported in the following chapters of this Atlas. From the radiopharmaceutical point of view, it has to be remembered that the possibility of an in vivo de-fluorination of F-18 radiotracers determining the production of metabolites and of free fluorine have to be considered in a rigorous pharmacokinetic evaluation.

Radio-Iodine (I-124)

Historically, starting from old experiences based on I-131 and I-125, radio-iodination has a pivotal position in radiochemistry. At present, there is a wide use of the pure gamma emitter I-123 for diagnostic purposes. The positron emitter isotope I-124 is characterized by a very long HL (6019.2 minutes, almost 5 days). This condition is advantageous for the worldwide shipment of high amounts of radioactivity, ready for use. Conversely, as negative consequence, dosimetry (for the patient, the personnel, the relatives and the environment) can reach unjustified values when compared with the I-123 corresponding radiotracers, permitting, however, to achieve satisfactory clinical results. Another major disadvantage is the expense and danger involved in the treatment of radioactive wastes. Moreover, although radiochemistry of radioiodine makes the synthesis of a large series of radiotracers, of targets such as antibodies, peptides, and many other molecules, possible, the *in vivo* presence of a significant de-iodination can create problems both in dosimetry and in rigorous pharmacokinetic analysis. As consequence, the only diffuse and the one already used in clinical practice, the compound labeled with I-124, is the simplest and that is iodide. Also in competition with I-123 and I-131, on the basis of being most cost/effective, I-124 had better clinical diagnostic value for patients with thyroid cancer; it helps both in permitting a rigorous pretherapeutic individual dosimetry and in the follow up.

Radio-Copper (Cu-64)

Copper by 64 (Cu-64) is a positron emitter produced in a large majority by reactors today, although the development of syntheses by cyclotrons have already been available. From the physical point of view, Cu-64 is characterized by the simultaneous emission of positron and beta minus radiations, with an HL of 12.8 h. Therefore, tracers labeled with this radionuclide can be used, clearly at different dosages, both for diagnostic and therapeutic purposes. This prerogative created significant interest in developing new radio-compounds, with the main focus on those used for radionuclide therapies also. Examples of radiotracers ready for clinical practice in humans are presented in the following chapters of this Atlas.

Radio-Gallium (Ga-68)

The pivotal role in the development of medicine carried out by generators and, in particular, by the Mo-99/Tc-99m system is well known to nuclear physicians. This technology is, since many years, available also for positron emitters, mainly with reference to the Ge-68/Ga-68 generator. Germanium 68 has an HL of 271 days, permitting a relatively cheap routine availability of positron emitters for many days, without needing a cyclotron. Gallium - 68 has a favorable HL of 68.0 min and is very promising and already in clinical use. The main utilization is in labeling peptides and, among them, somatostatin analogues. A strong and stable radiochemical bond is obtained through chelation. It has to be pointed out that a similar radiochemistry is utilized for labeling the same molecules using gamma emitters, as Indium-111, or beta minus emitters, as Yttrium-90 or Lutetium-177. With respect to In-111 radio-compounds, radiotracers labeled with Ga-68 permit a higher diagnostic accuracy mainly because of the use of the PET technique. The similarity with the corresponding radiochemical forms labeled Y-90 and Lu-177, used for radionuclide therapy, stimulated the clinical use of Ga-68 radiotracers for the recruitment of patients to be treated; moreover, it is possible to calculate the dosimetry pretherapeutically, permitting a better definition of the dose to be administered. It has to be pointed out, as a minor limitation, that for a rigorous dosimetry, Ga-68 is characterized by a relatively too short HL to calculate the pharmacokinetic analysis of the *in vivo* distribution up to 24–48 h and longer.

It has to be reported that some researchers, on the basis of some similarities with the Tc-99m radiochemistry, are working on the possible use of Ga-68 for labeling instant kits. At present, this is more a perspective, but it is already evident that there is keen interest in developing the highest number of radiochemical syntheses involving Ga-68.

General Considerations About Radiotracers

Although radio-compounds can trace bio-molecules, following their functional pathways, the pharmacokinetics of these compounds do not completely overlap as they are conditioned by radio-labeling. In other words, the same molecule can present some differences in the *in vivo* distribution, if labeled with different radio-nuclides, with different activities of the same radionuclide, with a different specific activity (i.e., with a different amount of the vector molecule). The reason, as already explained above, is that after the *in vivo* administration, the image is the resultant of a radioactivity's distribution which is dependent not only on the injected radiotracer (specific and nonspecific uptake, presence in the vascular pool or in the emunctories), but also on all the other *in vivo* produced radiochemical forms such as, metabolites, complexes, and free radionuclide.

This is a major risk in using "new" radiotracers in clinical practice. A reliable use can be obtained only when the "*molecular imager*" has a deep and wide knowledge of patho–physiological premises; he/she has to learn uptake and distribution mechanisms determined by physiology, para-physiological conditions, pathological events; he/she has to know normal patterns, pitfalls and artifacts; he/she has to predict the behavior in benign and malignant diseases.

Therefore, a thorough but fascinating study is required to become an expert in PET–CT. In particular, it is necessary to learn the functional premises, pathophysiology, radiochemistry, and pharmacology to avoid the major mistake, that is, to think that PET – CT is simply indicating a colored spot on an anatomical structure.

In this Atlas, we want to open your mind to the widening field of the clinical use of PET outside the FDG kingdom. In this Atlas, you will learn that, to detect prostate cancer it is better to choose a radiotracer, which is not eliminated through the urine, to detect brain recurrence an amino-acid is better than FDG because of the lack of uptake by normal cells, and to diagnose differentiated neuroendocrine tumors, radiopeptides have a higher accuracy than FDG. You will also understand that it is possible to acquire important prognostic information, connected to the growing rate, through radiolabeled thymidine, or that you can decide a better therapeutic strategy for women with breast cancer, starting from the knowledge of *in vivo* distribution of estrogen receptors. In this scenario, you will understand how oncologists, surgeons, radiotherapists, and all the other clinicians can acquire further advantage in addition to the pivotal role already played by FDG. The first area of interest can be found in fields where FDG has limitations because of the presence of false negative or false positive results. But a further relevant indication for the use of PET radiotracers other than FDG is the former's incapability, shared with all the diagnostic procedures, to answer alone all the possible questions concerning diagnosis, prognosis, and those connected with the therapy.

We conclude this chapter with a final major remark: as far as PET–CT is concerned, while CT always gives the same morpho-structural information, it is PET that permits this hybrid machine to declare its primacy in Molecular Imaging in humans.

Chapter 3 Choline PET-CT

Mohsen Farsad, Vincenzo Allegri,
and Paolo Castellucci

Radiolabeled Choline (labeled to ^{11}C or ^{18}F) is one of the most applied and promising PET tracers for cancer imaging. Choline is a substrate for the synthesis of phosphatidylcholine, which is a major phospholipid in the cell membrane. It has been hypothesized that uptake of radiolabeled Choline reflects proliferative activity by estimating membrane lipid synthesis. However, the exact uptake mechanism has to be established.

Choline was first labeled to ^{11}Carbon for cancer imaging in 1997. ^{11}C-Choline is cleared very rapidly from the blood, and optimal tumor-to-background contrast is reached within 5–7 min after administration of tracer. This allows for imaging as early as 3–5 min after tracer injection and provides images of good diagnostic quality. Physiologically increased tracer uptake is noted in salivary glands, liver, kidney parenchyma and pancreas and faint uptake in spleen, bone marrow and muscles. Bowel activity is variable and occasionally urinary bladder activity can be observed. ^{11}Carbon has, however, a short half-life time (20 min) and must be used rapidly after production; it requires a local cyclotron and is therefore not a widely available option.

For these reasons, F-labeled Choline tracers like Fluoro-ethyl-choline (FEC) and Fluoromethl-dimethyl-hydroxyethylammonium (FCH) were proposed. Both compounds show similar properties (rapid blood clearance and uptake in prostate tissue) with minor differences (later peak uptake for FEC). The main contrast with ^{11}C-Choline is the early urinary appearance of ^{18}F-Choline, probably caused by incomplete tubular reabsorption.

Although Choline PET has been used for identification of various tumor tissues, the main application field of Choline PET is prostate Imaging. PET imaging has been proposed for early detection of primary prostate cancer, for staging of tumor and identification of nodal involvement, and finally for detection of tumor recurrence.

Choline uptake seems to be similar in patients with benign prostatic diseases (prostatitis, prostatic hypertrophy) and proven prostate cancer. This finding, in addition to the limited spatial resolution of PET-CT devices, clearly represents the major limits for the use of this tracer for identification of primary tumor. Despite a tendency towards a higher uptake of Choline in prostate cancer foci, taking all preliminary results into account, Choline PET cannot be recommended for diagnosing primary prostate cancer.

With regard to prostate staging, Choline PET imaging seems not to be accurate enough to be proposed for evaluation of extracapsular extension, seminal vesicle involvement, and detection of lymph node micrometastases. This is mainly due to the limited spatial resolution of PET-CT devices. However, Choline PET may have a role in selected cases: in patients with high-risk prostate cancer, it may assist the clinicians in the decision of aborting surgical treatment in presence of lymph node or distant metastasis. In addition, Choline PET imaging could be helpful by showing lymph node metastasis outside the generally recommended surgery regions, which could have an impact on extent of lymphadenectomy and on survival after radical prostatectomy. However, at present, the use of Choline PET imaging in predicting stage at presentation cannot be recommended for a routine clinical use.

Choline PET imaging plays a more relevant role in the detection of prostate cancer relapse. Choline PET shows higher specificity and consequently higher accuracy compared to all conventional imaging methods together for detection of prostate cancer recurrence. Choline PET imaging, supplying a whole body tomography exam, has the major advantage of detecting local and distant metastasis within a single session with a good accuracy.

However, patient referral criteria still have to be defined. At present, no definite data exist with regard to the thresholds of serum PSA level under which radiolabeled Choline should not be used. Moreover, the influence of medication (e.g., testosterone deprivation) and PSA kinetics on PET-CT detection rate has to be clarified. Despite these limitations, the use of PET-CT with Choline in patients with biochemical failure has shown a significantly better detection rate, when compared to CT or bone scan.

Therefore, in absence of general patient referral criteria for Choline PET Imaging in detection of prostate cancer recurrence, it seems reasonable to use PET imaging in individual cases, where a satisfactory sensitivity is to be expected and imaging findings will have a therapeutic relevance. In particular, patients with high risk of distant metastases or those susceptible to surgery and/or radiation therapy could benefit the most from early identification of the site of recurrence.

Besides prostate cancer imaging, Choline PET has also been used for other minor aims. The minimal background activity of ^{11}C-Choline in the pelvis, due to the low level of excretion via the urinary tract has permitted the use of this tracer in various tumors of urogenital tract other than prostate cancer (bladder and uterine cancer). Diagnostic accuracy of Choline PET for detection of residual bladder cancer after TURB seems to be comparable to CT, but Choline PET appears to be superior to CT for the evaluation of potential additional lymph node metastases. However, only few studies are present in literature on this issue and there is, therefore, a weak rationale for Choline PET imaging in these cancers.

Radiolabeled Choline also seems to be a suitable PET tracer for brain tumor imaging. Choline PET shows a low accumulation in normal brain tissue and allows for the detection of brain tumors with a high tumor/background ratio. Choline PET has been applied successfully for characterization of brain lesions and seems to be in conjunction to MR imaging as an accurate diagnostic tool for identification and detection of high-grade gliomas and meningiomas. On the other hand, Choline PET does not allow one to differentiate low-grade gliomas from nonneoplastic lesions. Despite these good preliminary results, in the absence of data from large series of patients, the clinical role of Choline PET for the evaluation of brain tumors is not fully established, and MET PET remains the metabolic tracer of choice for brain tumor imaging.

Choline PET was also used for identification of myelomatous lesions. Choline PET appeared to be more sensitive than FDG PET for the detection of bony myelomatous lesions, and surprisingly, the SUVmax turned out higher with Choline compared to FDG. However, these data have to be confirmed in a larger series of patients.

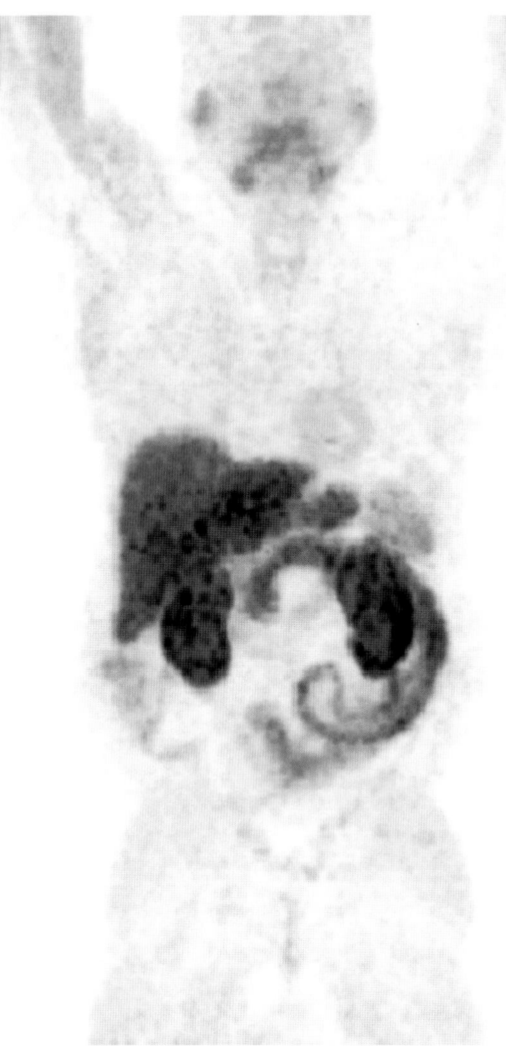

^{11}C-Choline

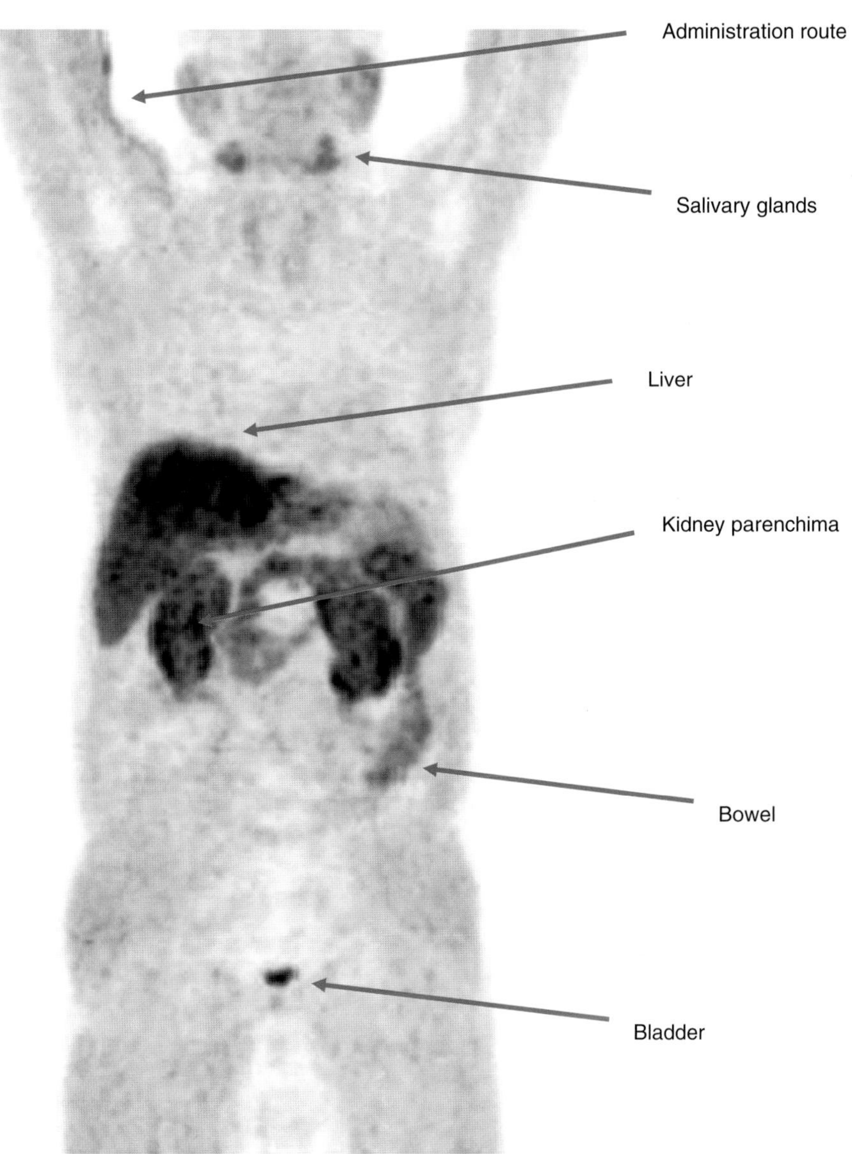

^{11}C-choline finding

Physiologic ^{11}C-choline uptake.

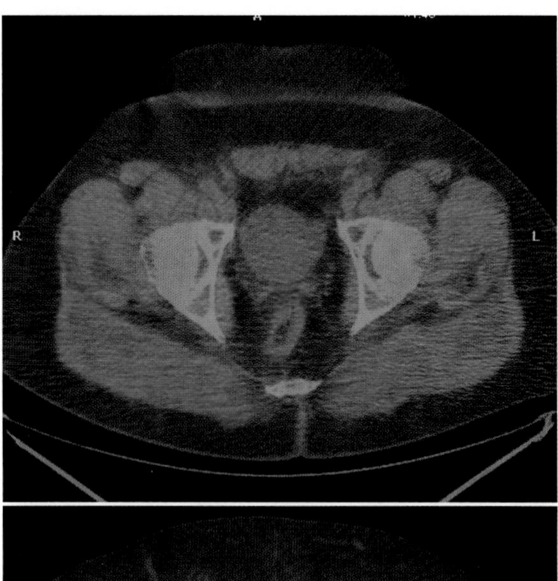

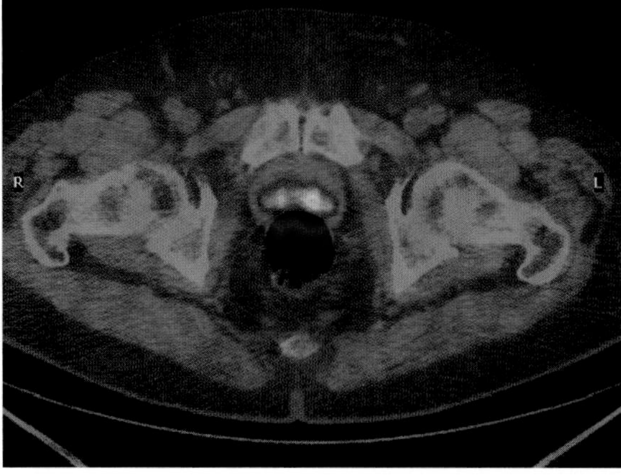

Teaching point

Urinary excretion of ^{11}C-choline may increase over time, and has to be taken into account especially if the scan is acquired more than 5 min after injection.

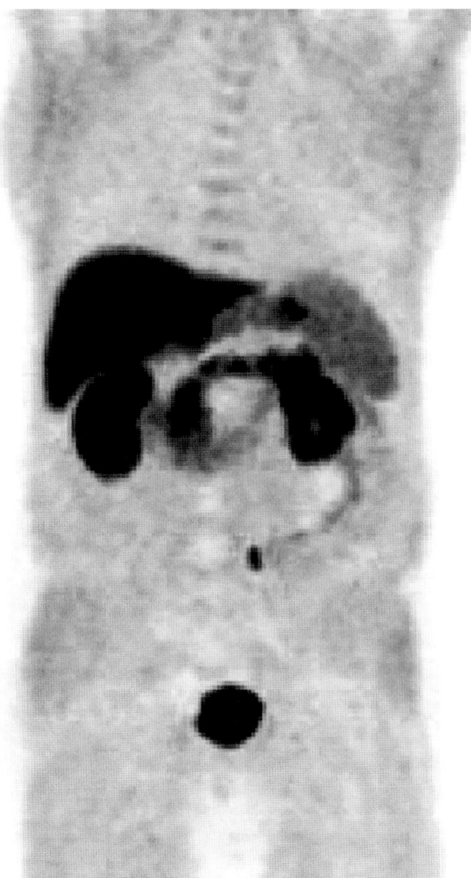

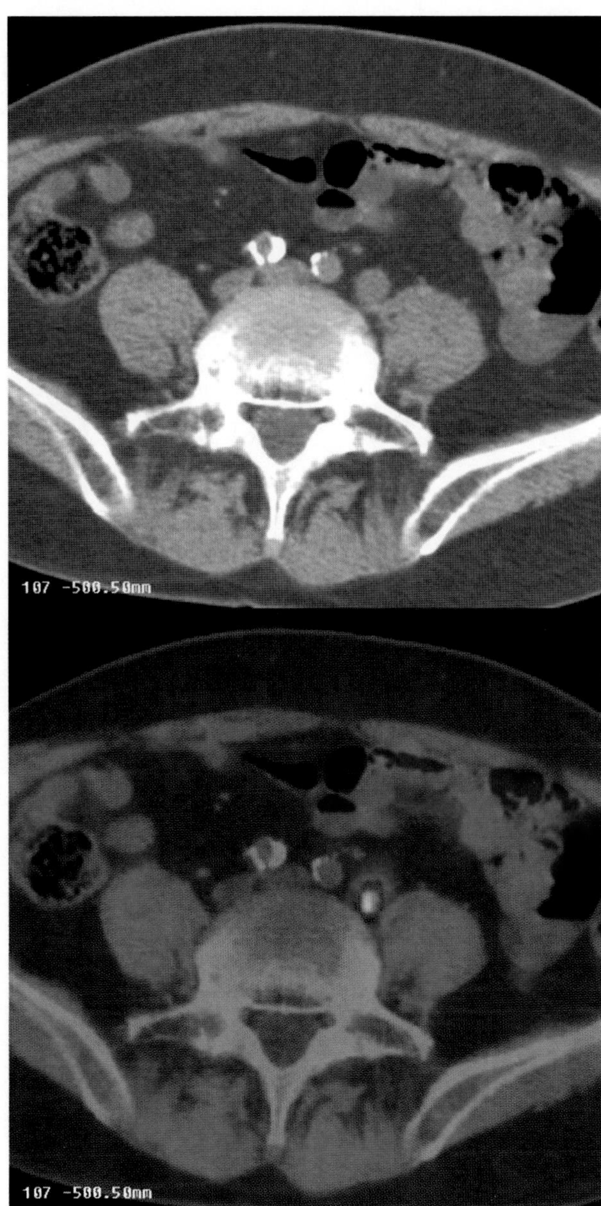

^{11}C-choline finding

Pathologic increased ^{11}C-choline uptake in iliac lymph node.

Male 71 years

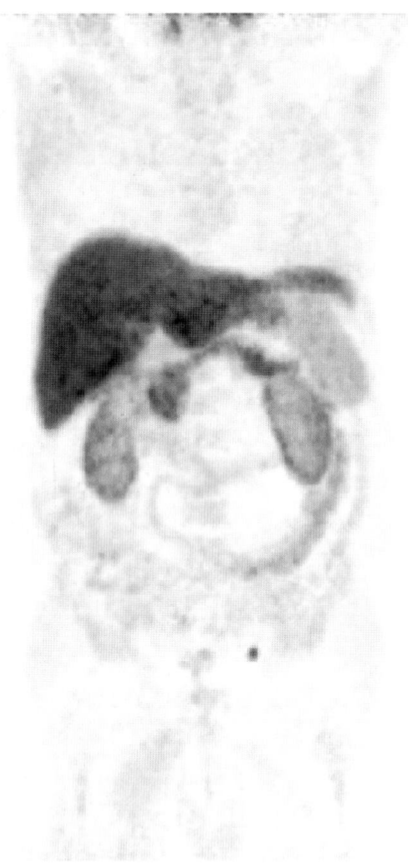

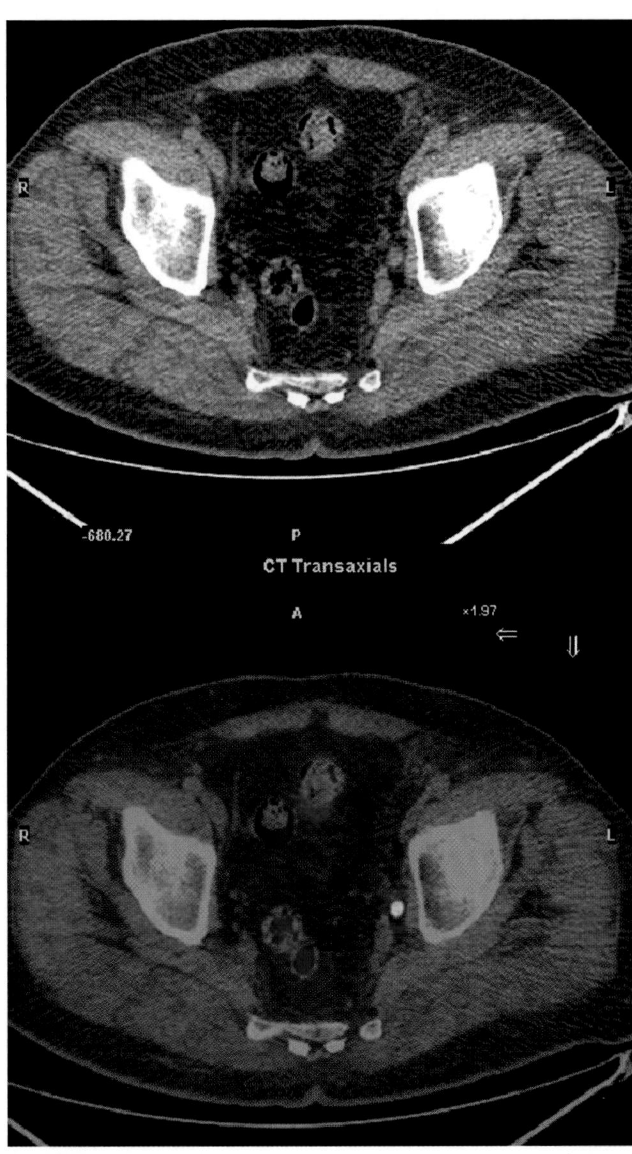

^{11}C-choline finding

Pathologic uptake in pelvic lymph node

Teaching point

Patient PSA was 1.3 but with a short doubling time (<3 months).

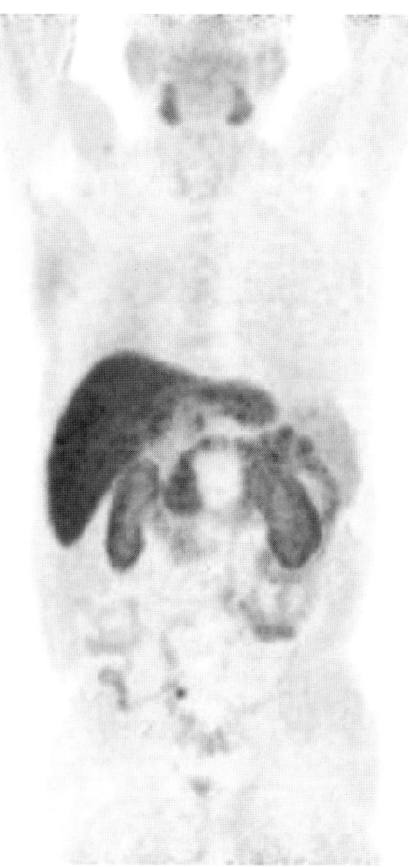

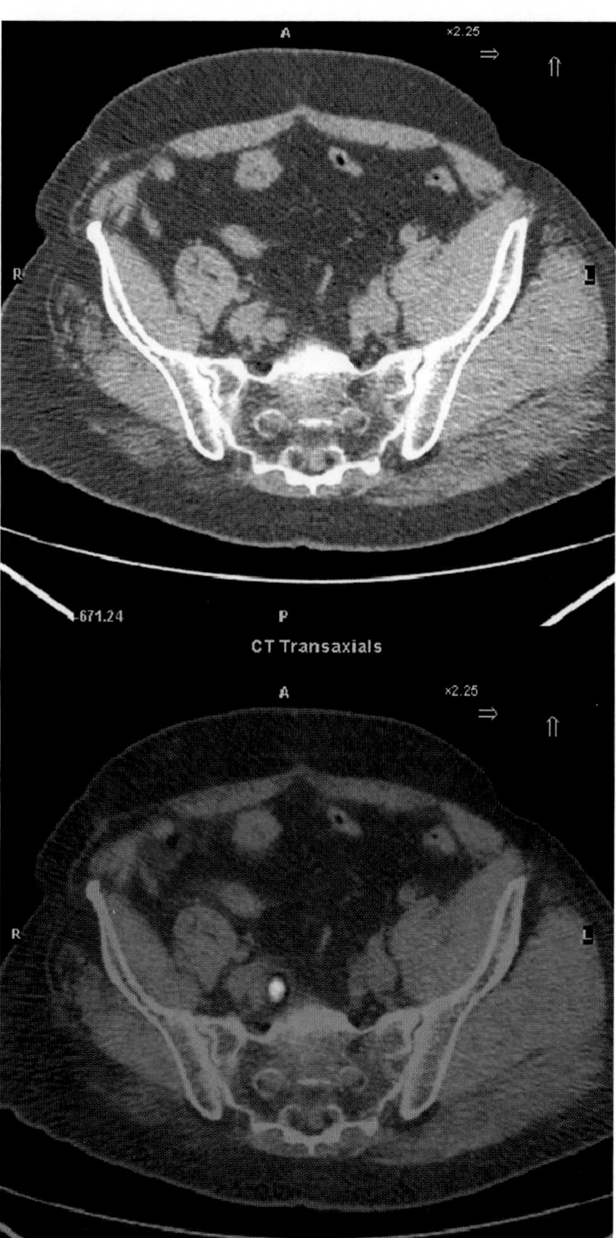

^{11}C-choline finding

Pathologic uptake in presacral lymph node

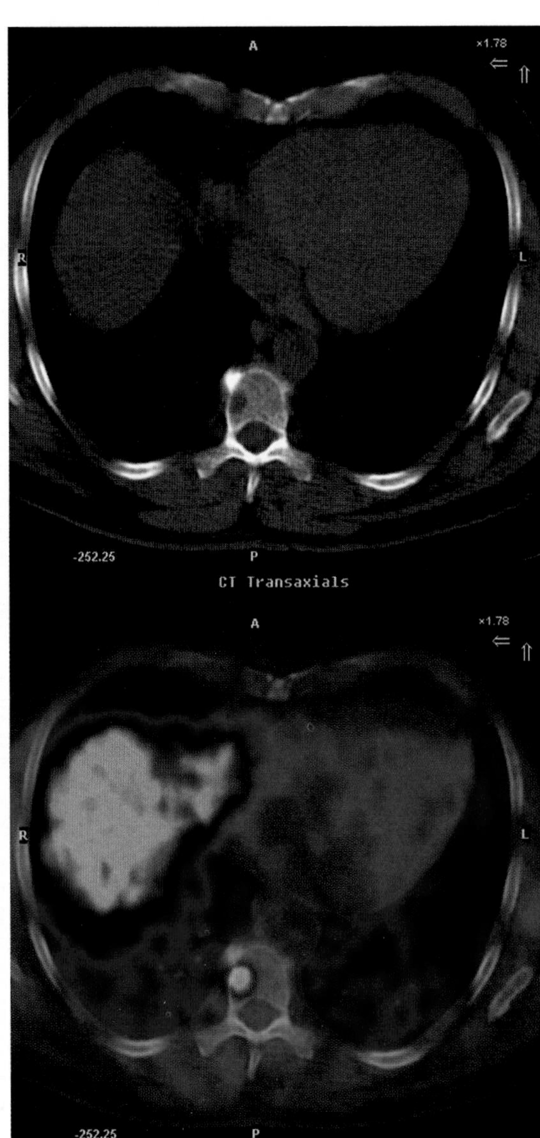

^{11}C-choline finding

Pathologic uptake in bone lesions with different radiological characteristics.

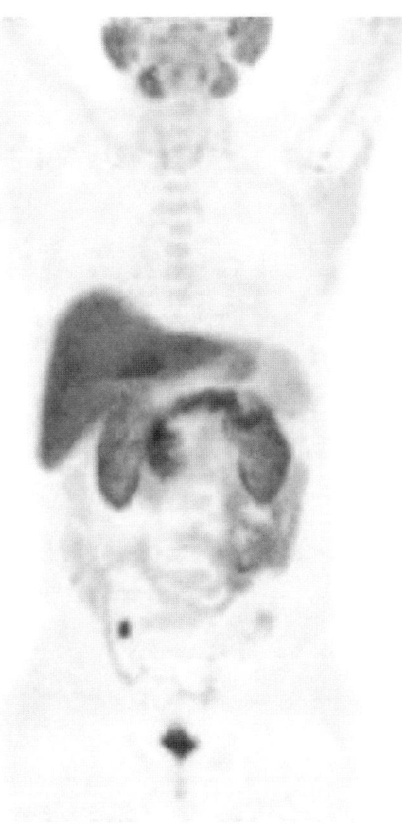

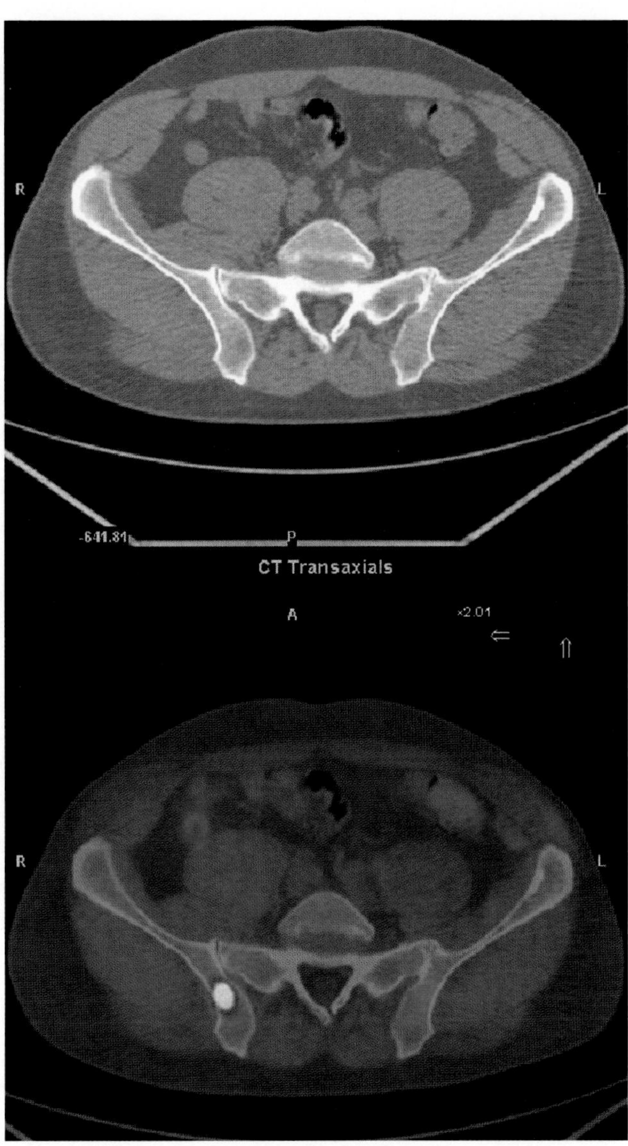

■ ^{11}C-choline finding

Pathologic uptake at bone level.

Teaching point

CT and bone scintigraphy were negative; choline PET-CT may reveal bone lesions before other imaging methods.

Case 9 Prostate Cancer: Staging

Male 71 year

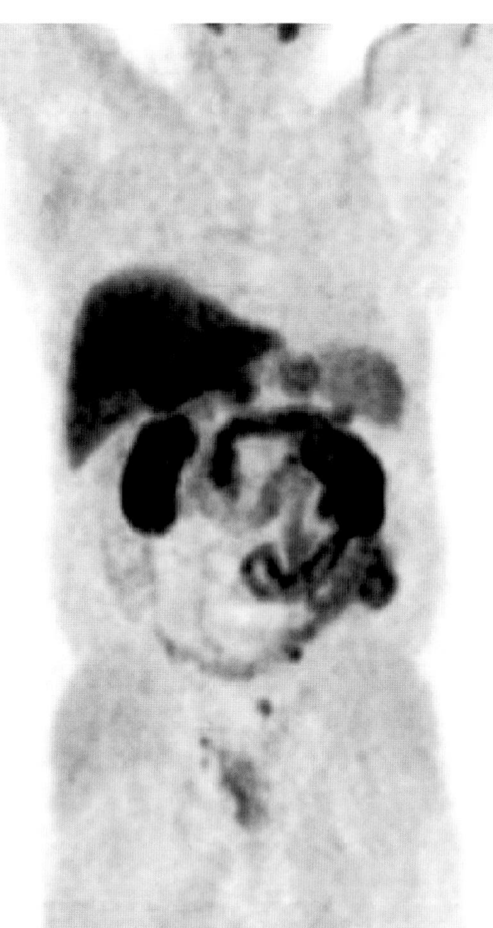

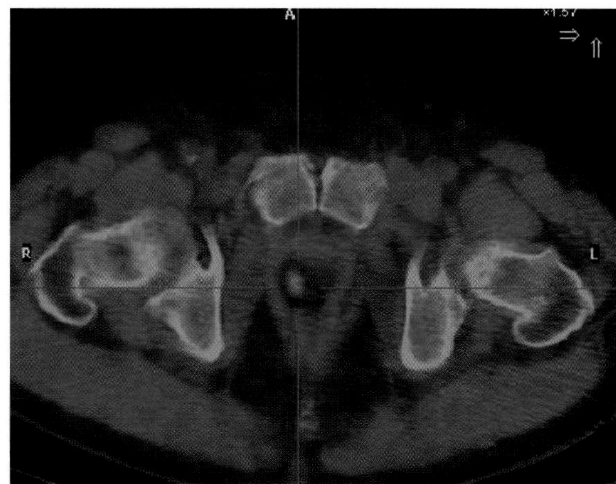

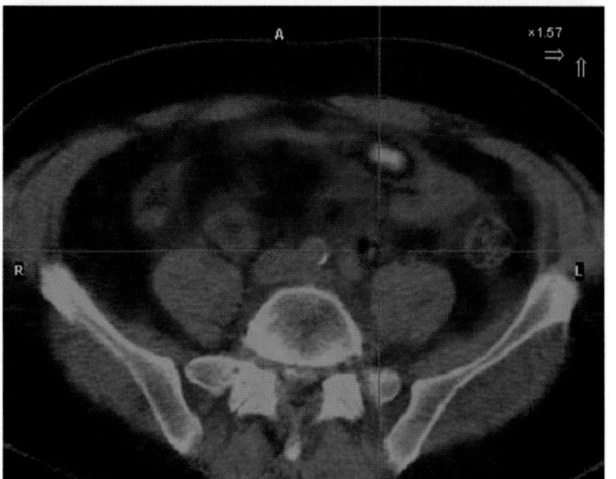

^{11}C-choline finding

Pathologic uptake at primary tumor and at two lymph nodes.

Teaching point

Choline PET-CT is not routinely used for staging purposes.

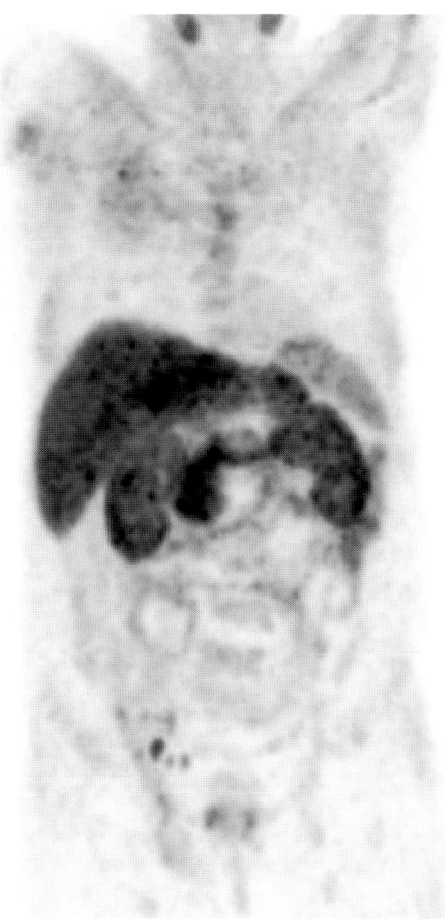

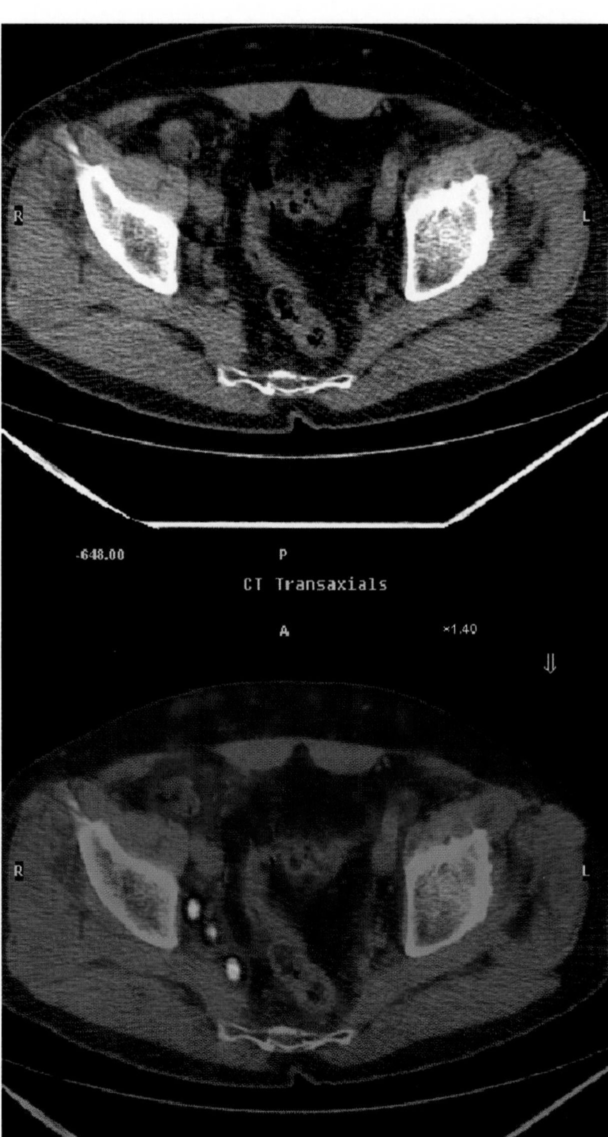

^{11}C-choline finding

Pathologic uptake at several obturatory lymph nodes.

Teaching point

Choline PET-CT may occasionally be useful for staging purposes in patients at high risk of nodal spread, to guide a correct surgical approach.

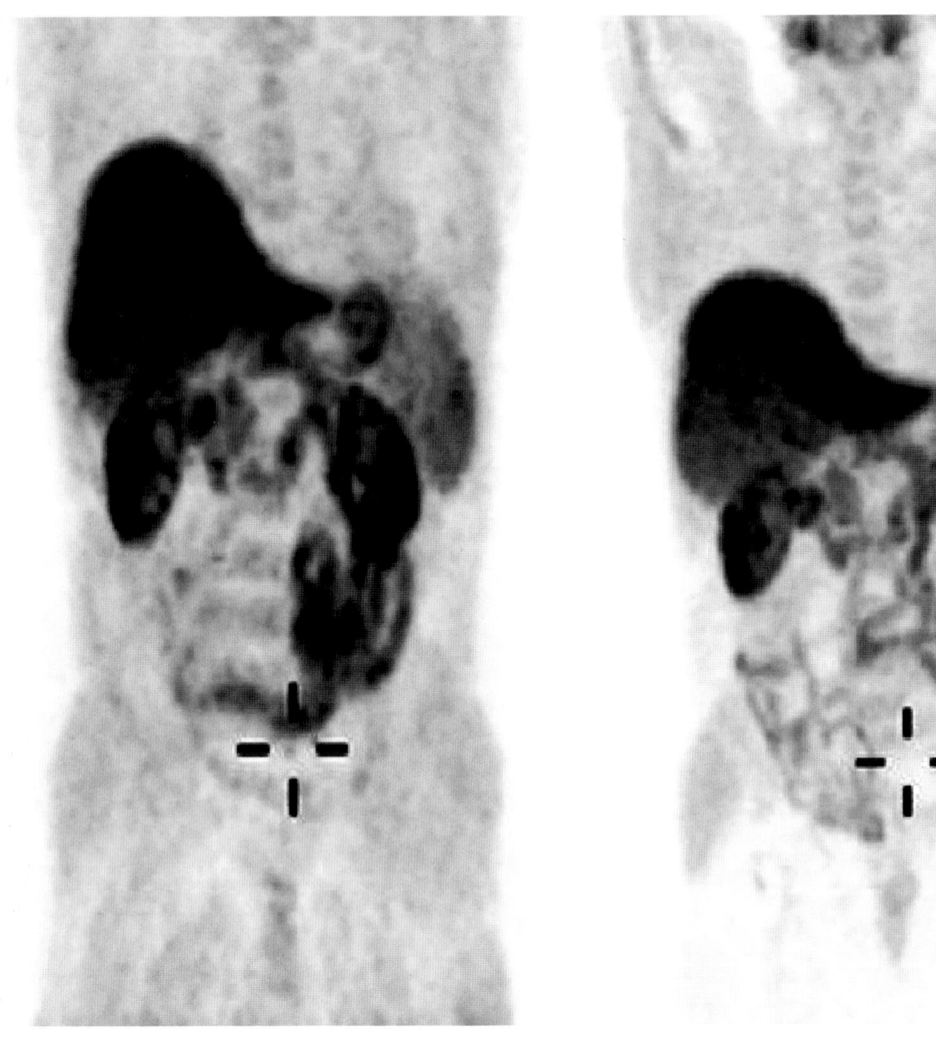

^{11}C-choline finding

Before treatment pathologic uptake at one presacral lymph nodes, no uptake after therapy.

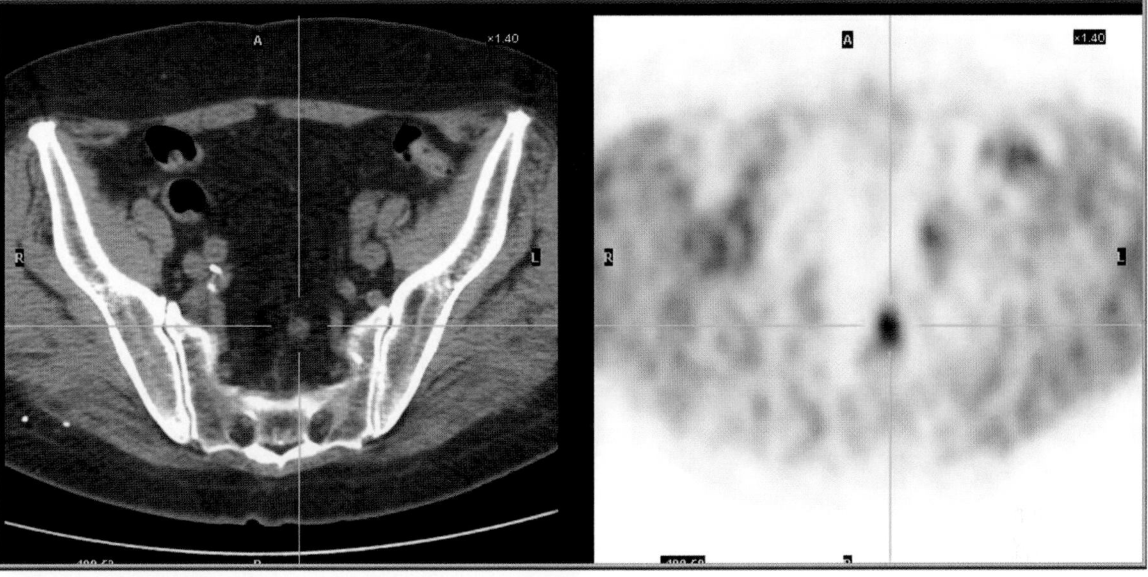

Before

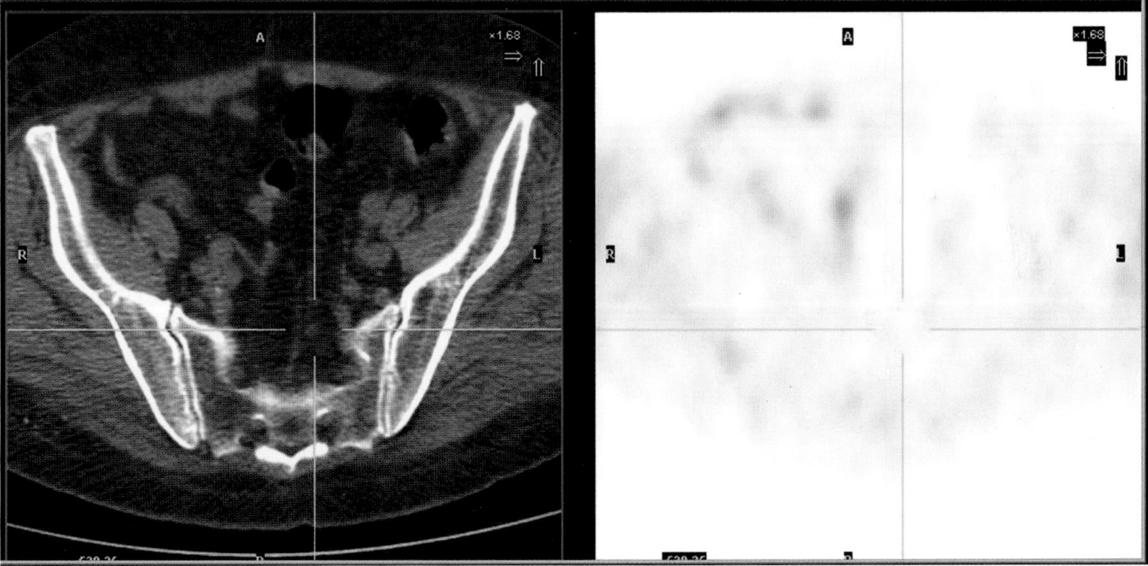

After

Teaching point

Choline PET-CT is not routinely used for evaluating response to therapy, but may be useful in selected cases.

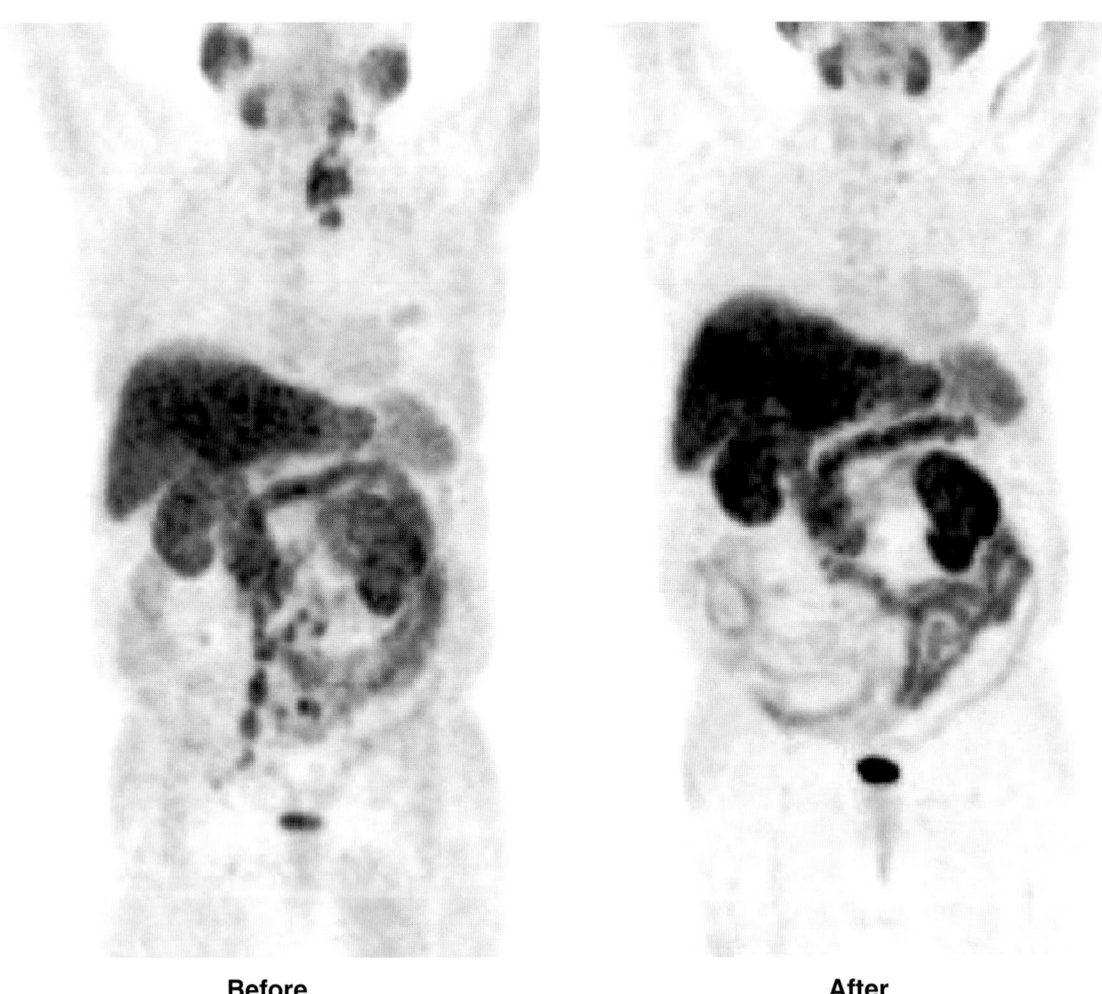

^{11}C-choline finding

Before treatment pathologic uptake at several sites, minor uptake after therapy.

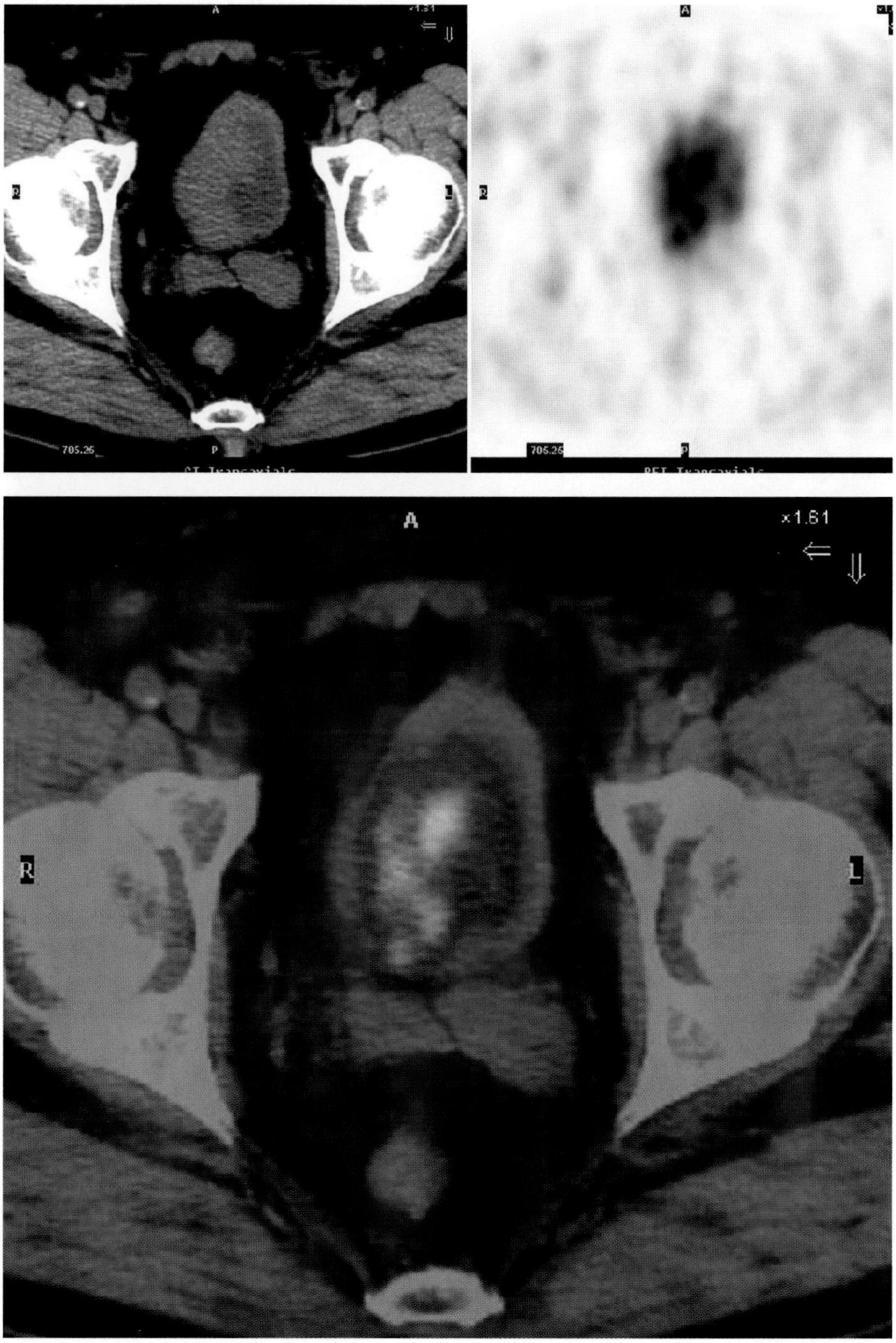

^{11}C-choline finding

Pathologic uptake in primary bladder tumor.

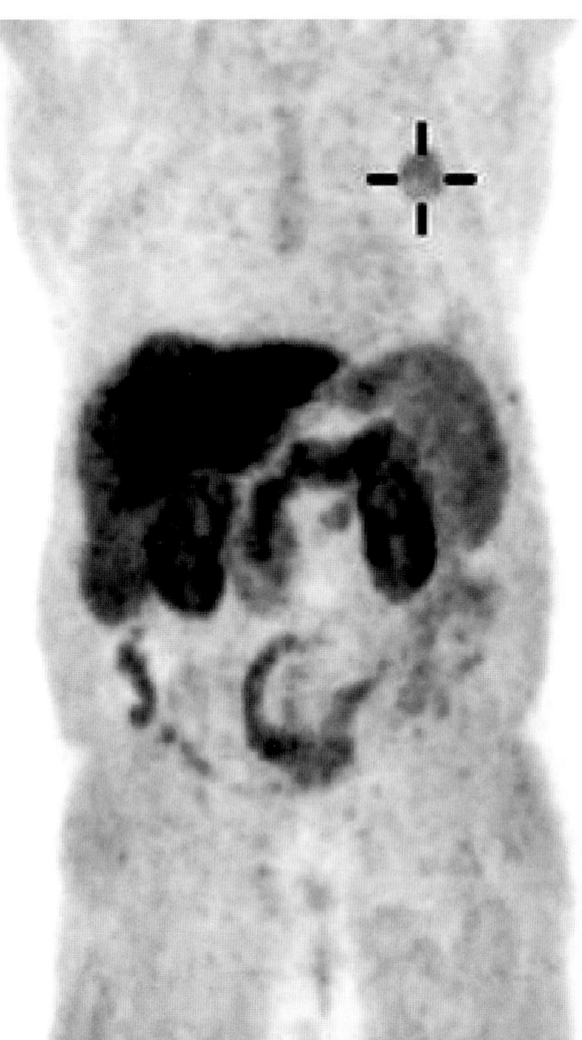

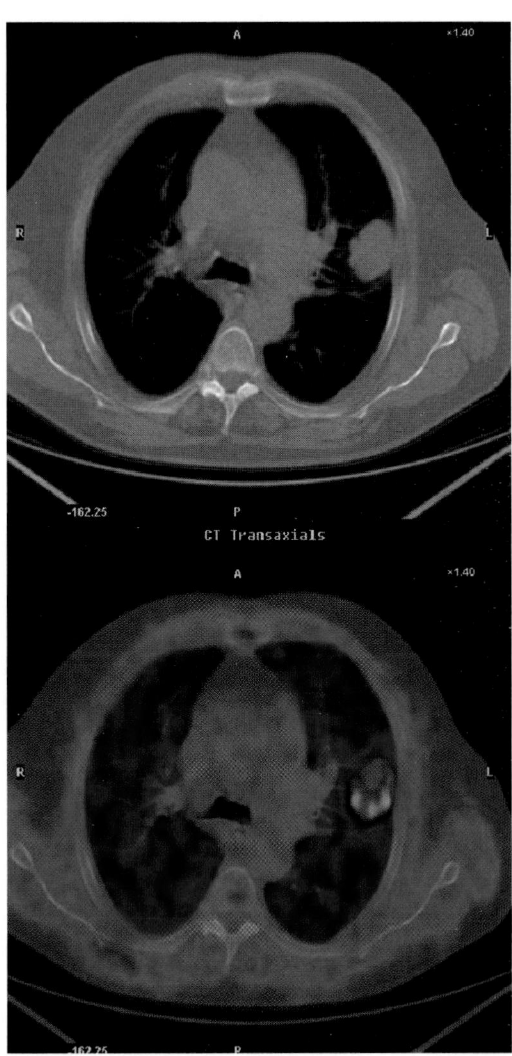

¹¹C-choline finding

Pathologic uptake at pulmonary primary lesion.

Teaching point

Choline PET-CT may occasionally be useful for other tumors when FDG PET-CT is known to lack sensitivity.

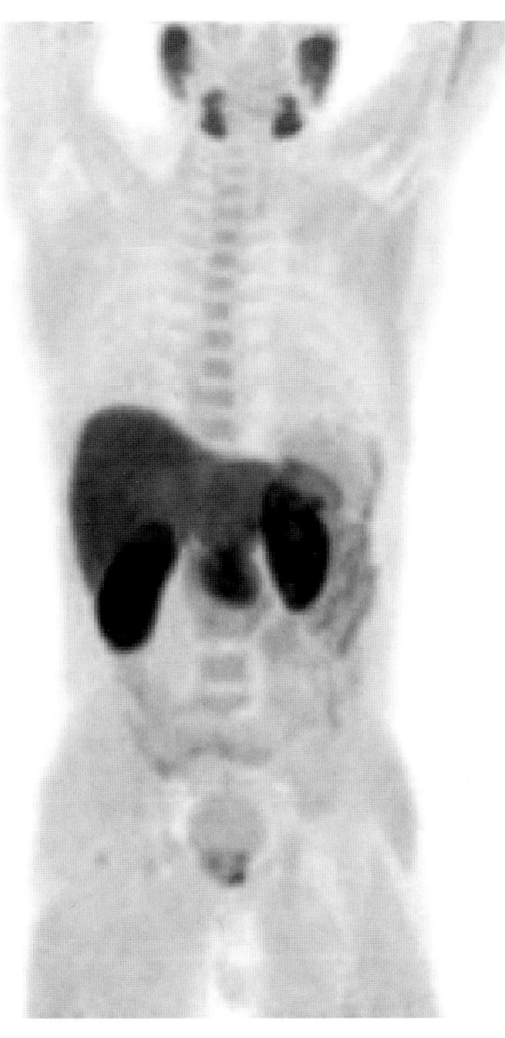

^{18}F-Choline

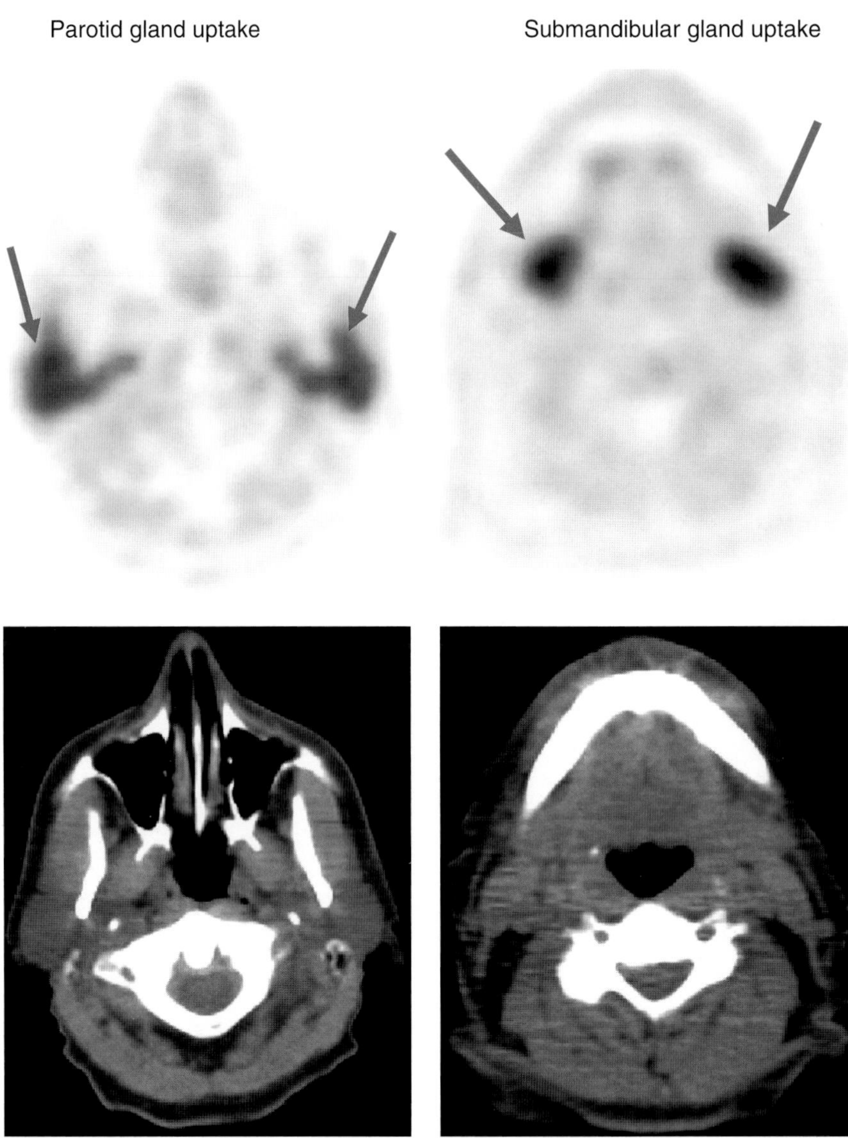

■ ^{18}F-choline finding

Physiologic ^{18}F-choline uptake in the salivary glands.

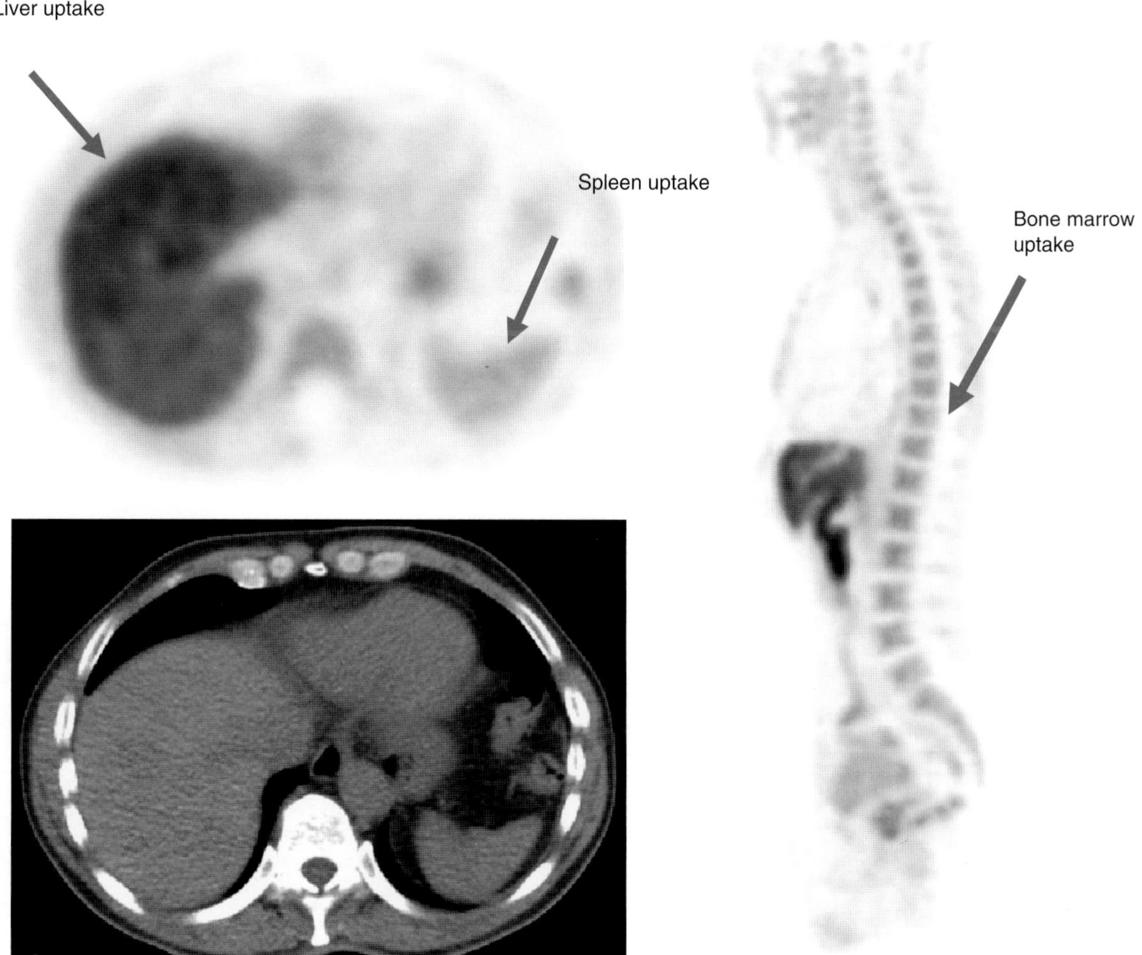

^{18}F-choline finding

Physiologic ^{18}F-choline uptake in the liver, spleen, and in the bone marrow.

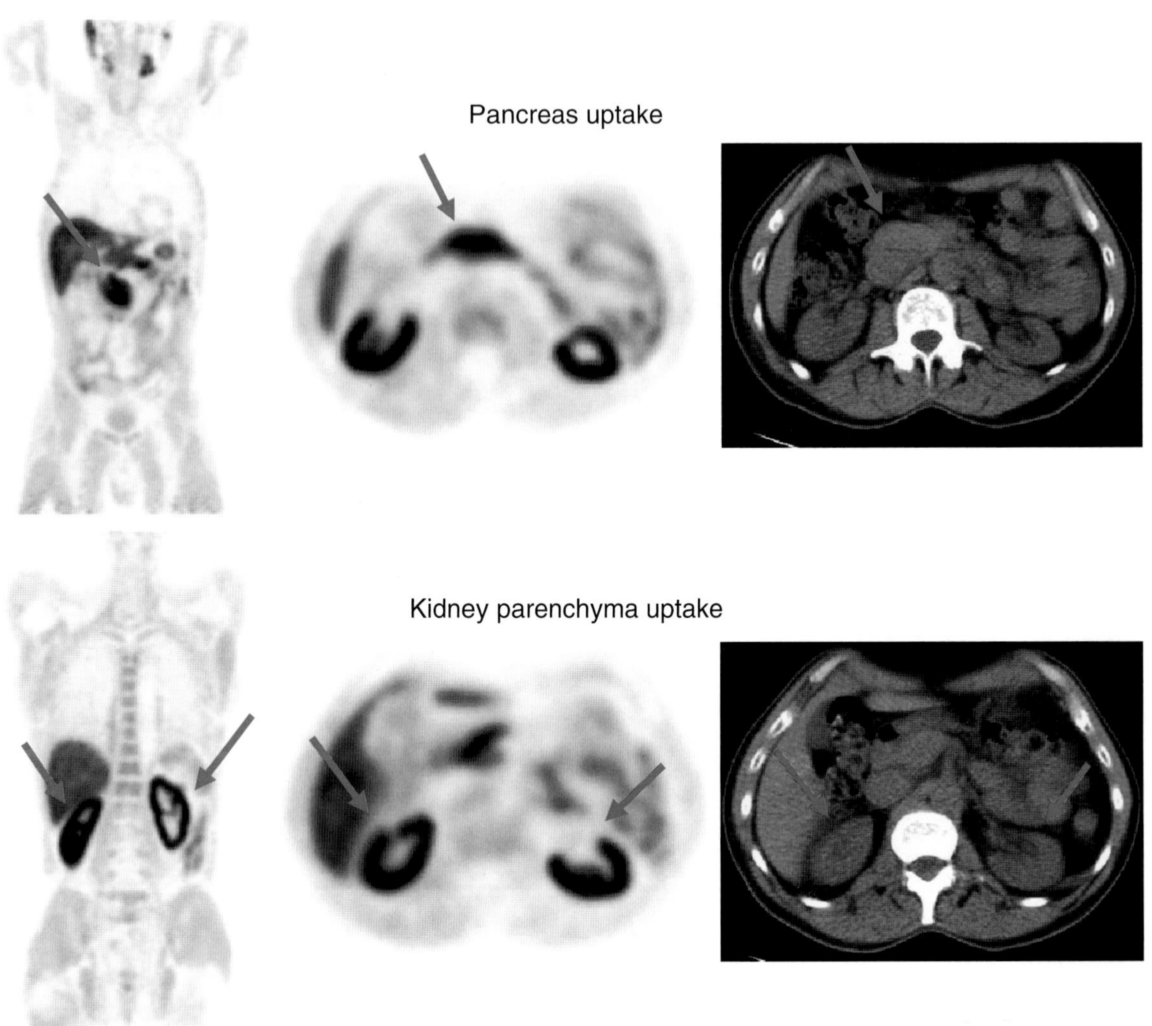

^{18}F-choline finding

Physiologic ^{18}F-choline uptake in the pancreas and in kidneys parenchyma.

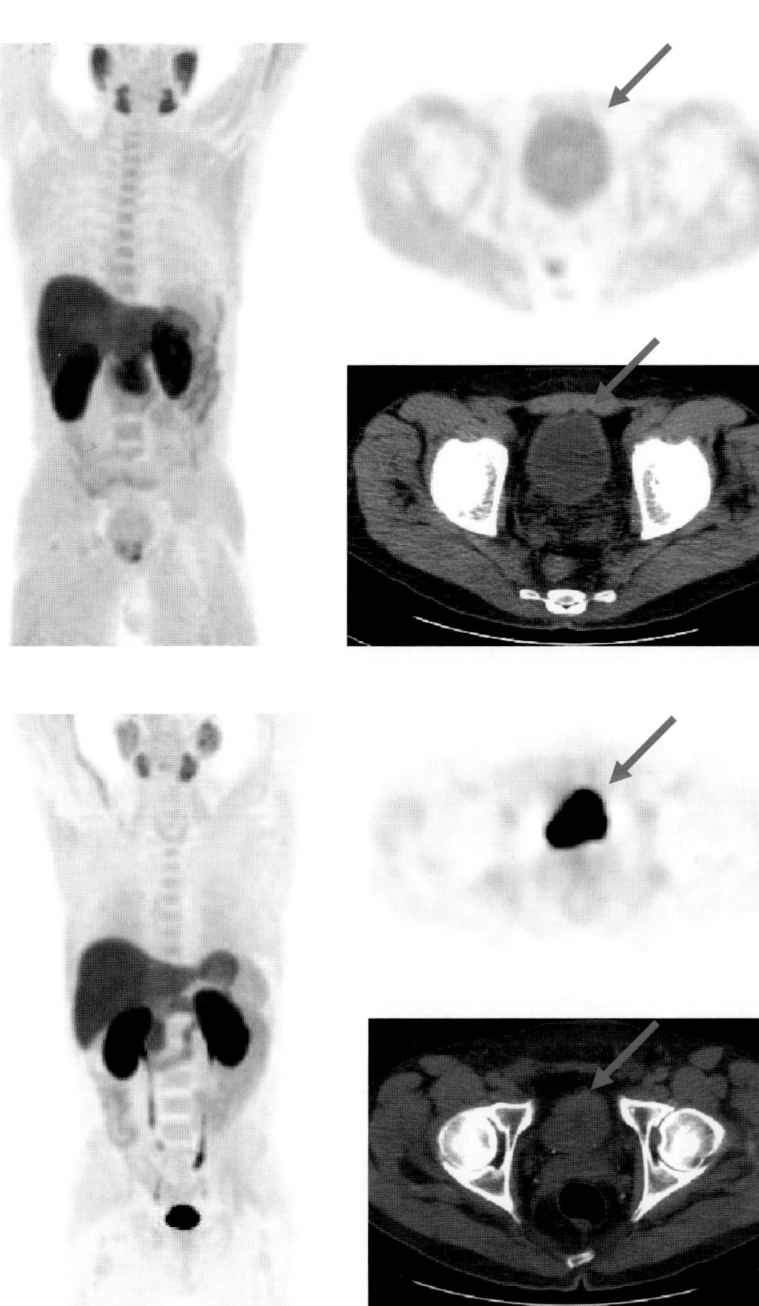

Teaching point

Urinary excretion of ^{18}F-choline may cause difficulties in evaluating pathologic uptake in prostate bed. Patients should be well-hydrated and be invited to void before scanning.

Male 65 years

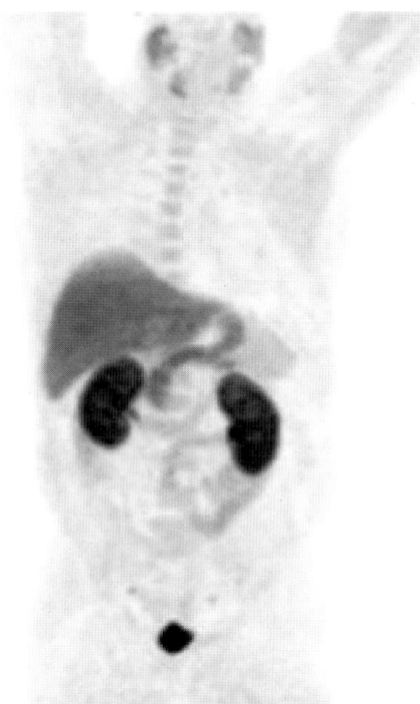

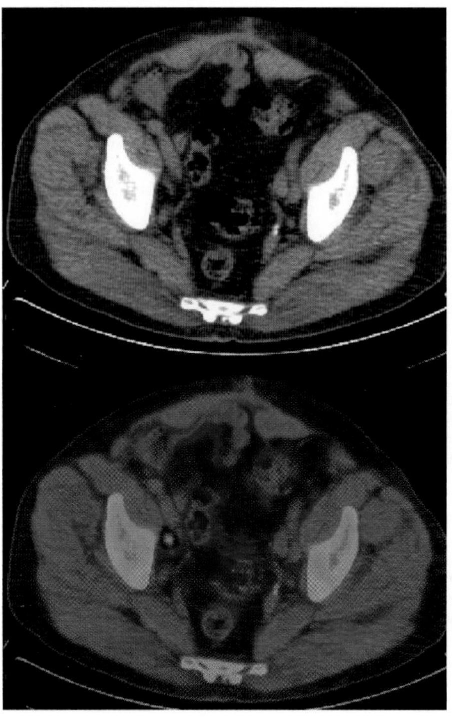

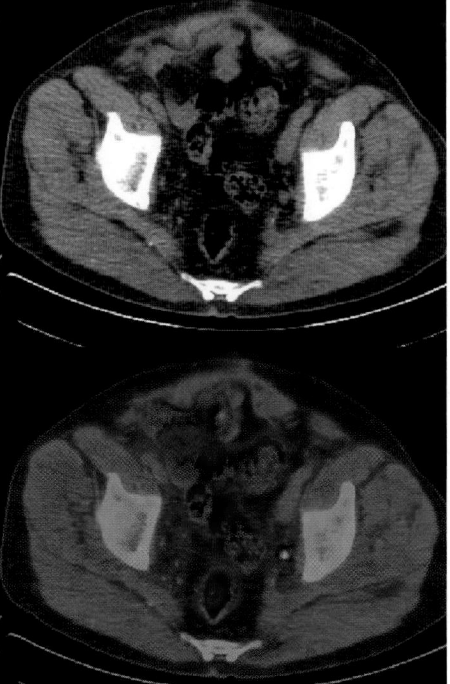

^{18}F-choline finding

Pathologic increased ^{18}F-choline uptake in pelvic lymph nodes.

Teaching point

^{18}F-choline PET-CT allows to identify secondary lymph nodes not easily detectable on conventional CT scan (<10 mm).

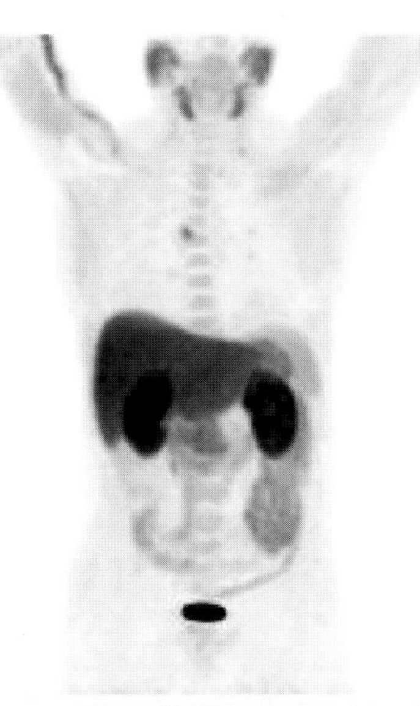

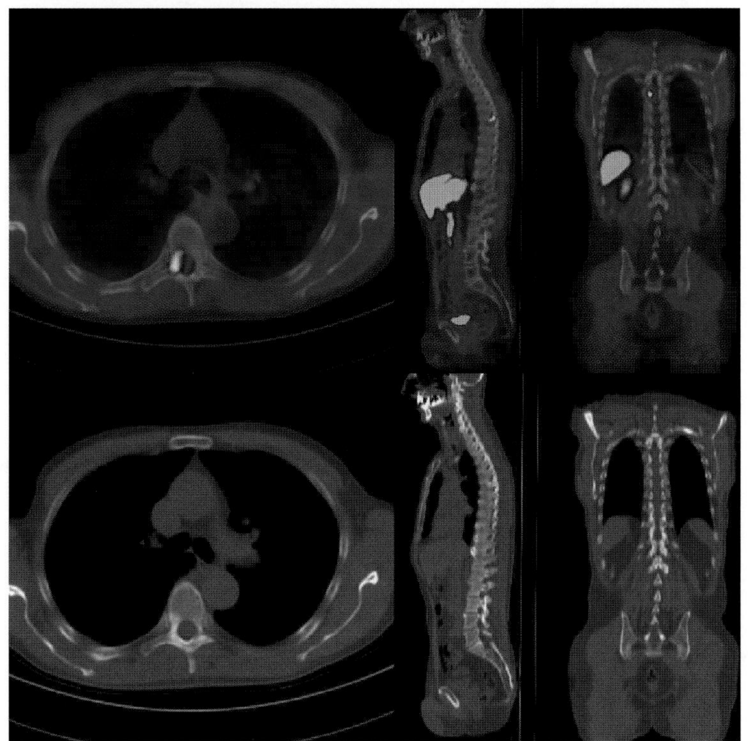

^{18}F-choline finding

Pathologic increased ^{18}F-choline uptake in right vertebral pedicle of D5.

Teaching point

^{18}F-choline PET-CT allows to identify secondary lesions that are not easily detectable on conventional bone scan.

Male 63 years

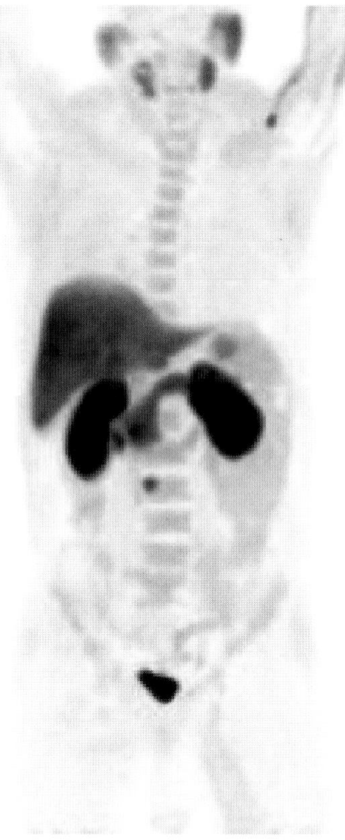

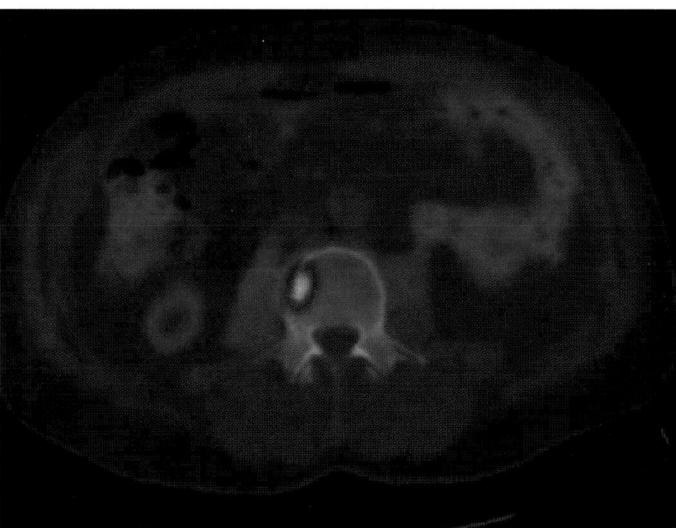

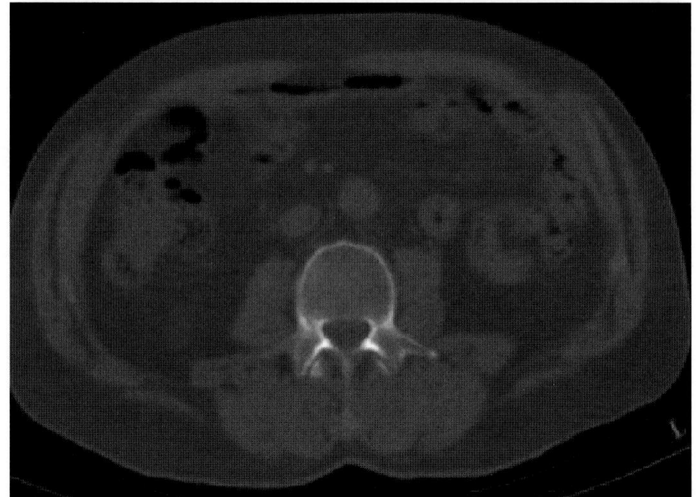

^{18}F-choline finding

Pathologic increased ^{18}F-choline uptake in the body of a lumbar vertebra.

Teaching point

^{18}F-choline PET-CT allows to detect early stage bone metastasis.

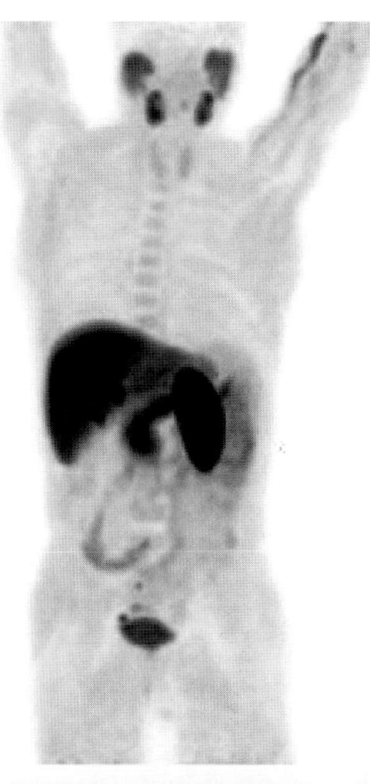

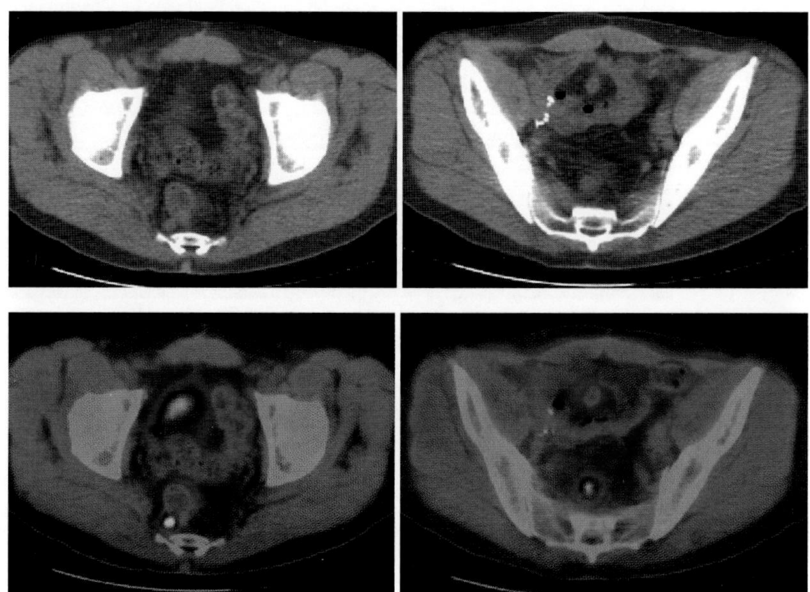

^{18}F-choline finding

Increased ^{18}F-choline uptake in presacral lymph nodes.

Teaching point

^{18}F-choline PET-CT allows to identify secondary lymph node lesions in regions that are usually not included in limited pelvic lymph node dissection.

Male 69 years

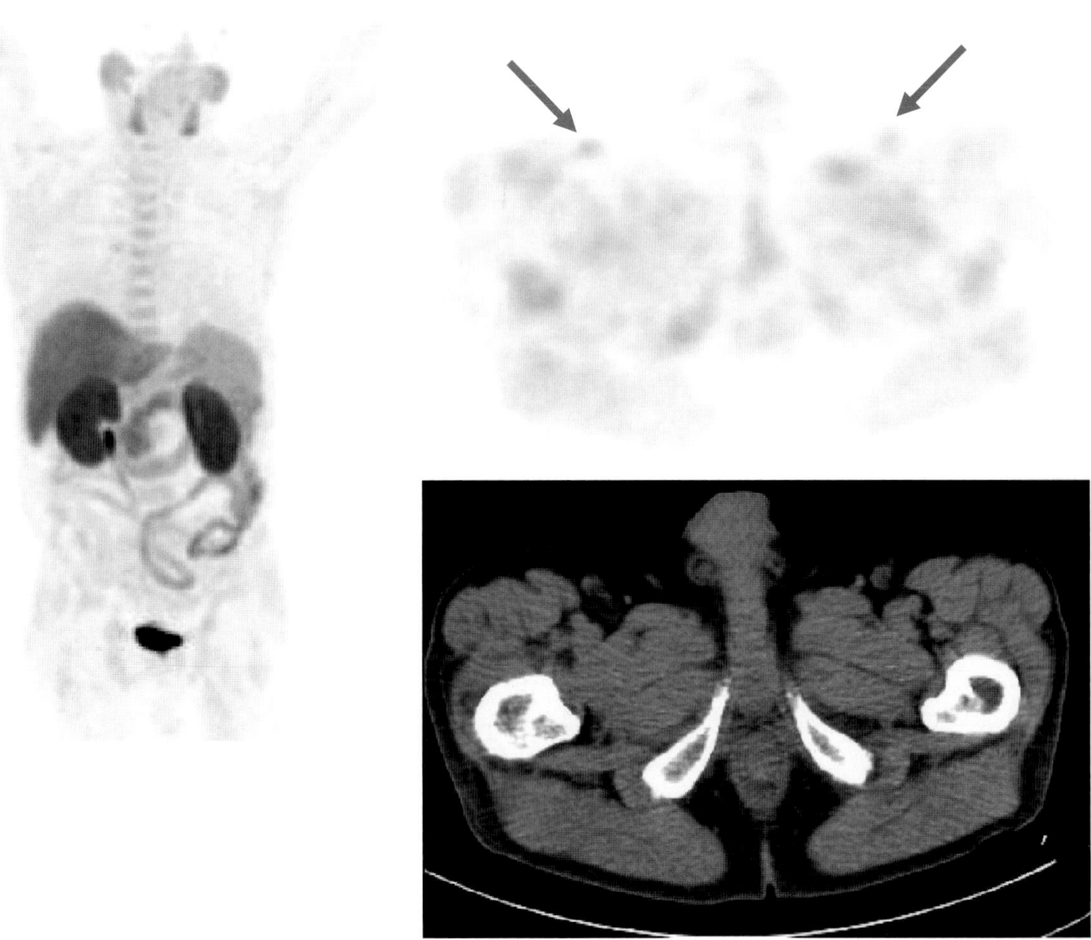

^{18}F-choline finding

Morphologically reactive inguinal lymph nodes visible on low-dose CT show mild ^{18}F-choline uptake.

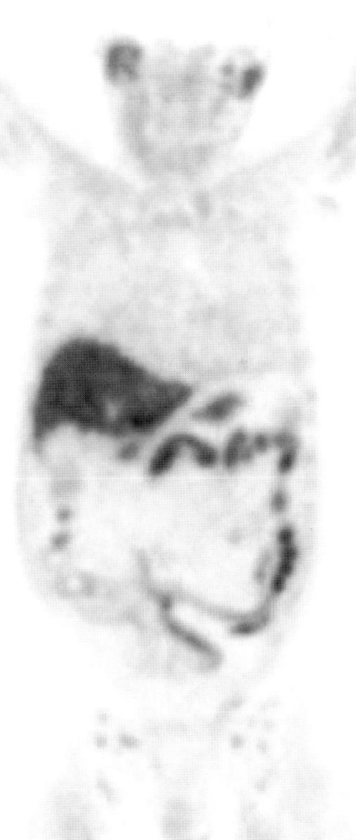

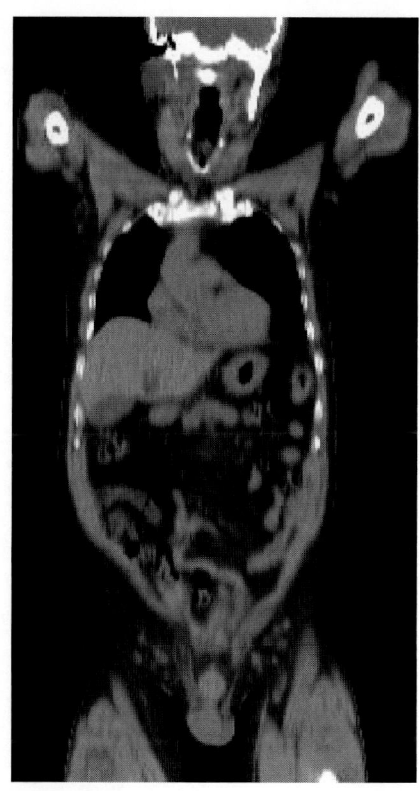

Teaching point

Mild ^{18}F-choline uptake can occur in reactive inguinal lymph nodes and should not be interpreted falsely as secondary uptake.

Male 66 years

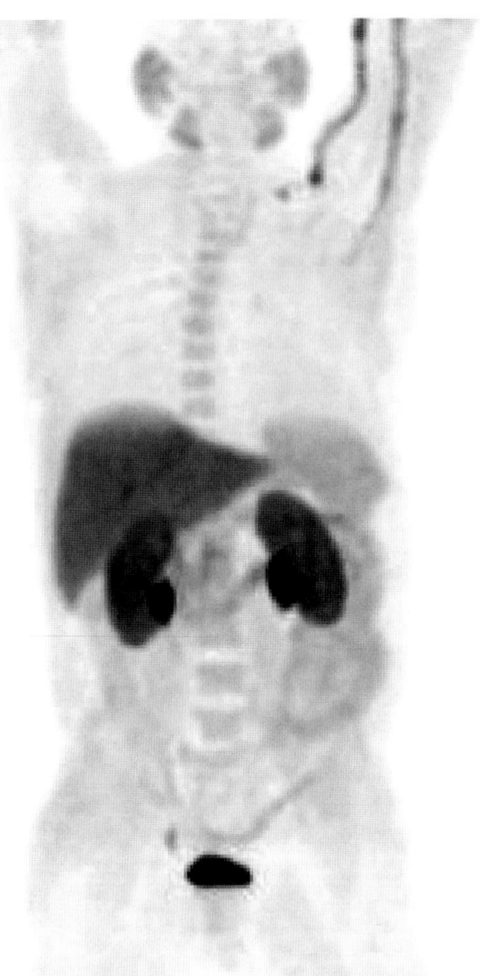

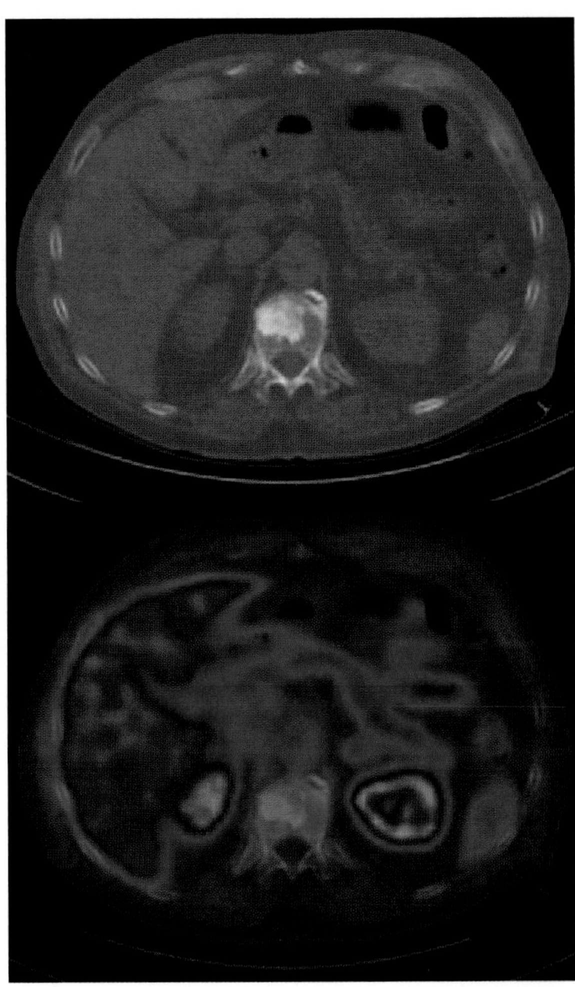

^{18}F-choline finding

Sclerotic secondary bone lesions visible on low-dose CT without ^{18}F-choline uptake.

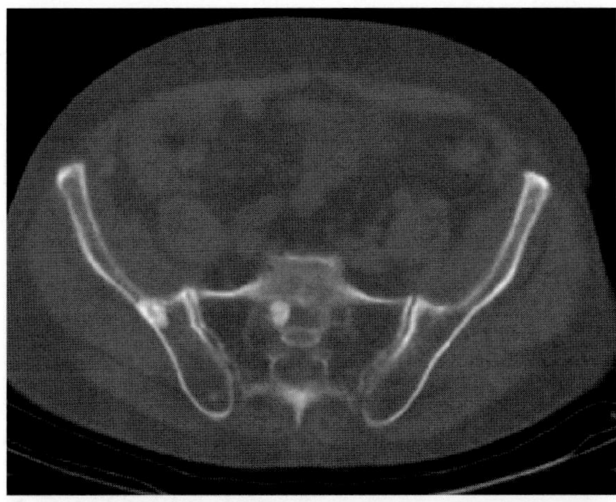

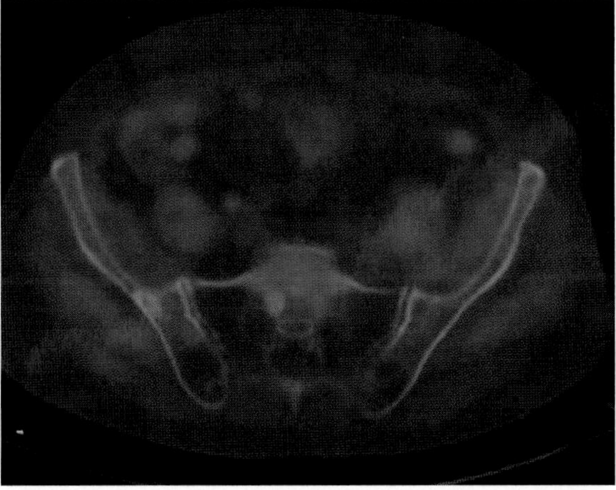

Teaching point

Hormonal responsive lesions of prostate cancer may not show ^{18}F-choline uptake.

Male 75 years

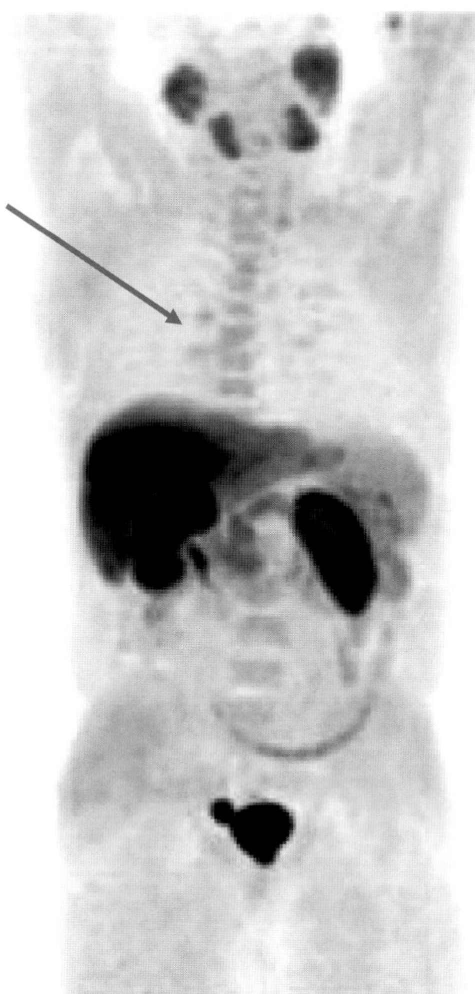

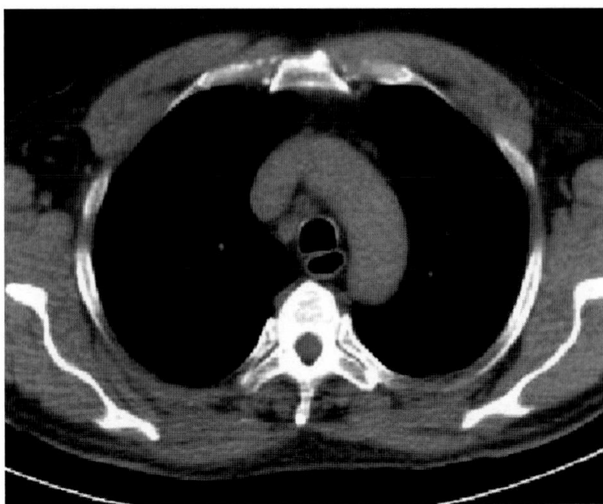

^{18}F-choline finding

Mild increased ^{18}F-choline uptake in hilar and mediastinal region.

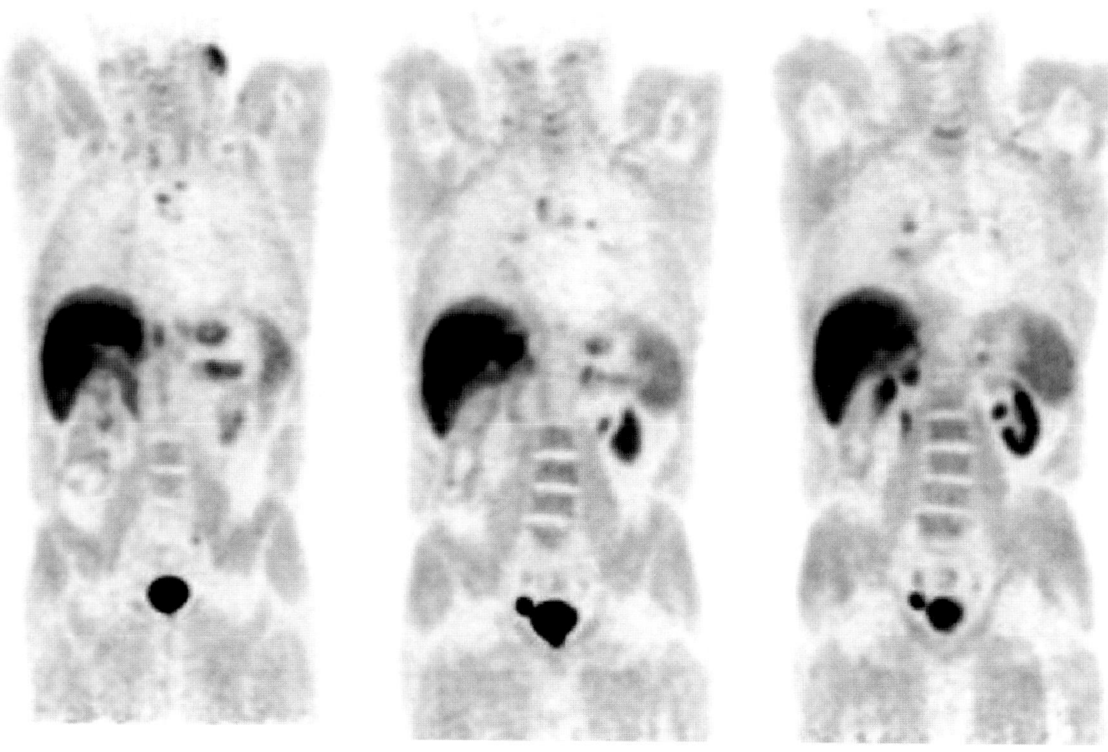

Teaching point

Mild ^{18}F-choline uptake in hilar and mediastinal regions can be often identified on PET-CT images, which is due to inflammatory changes.

Male 69 years

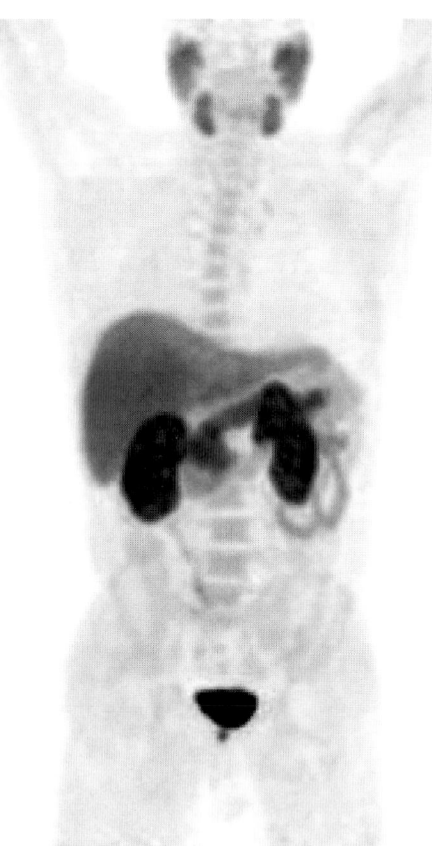

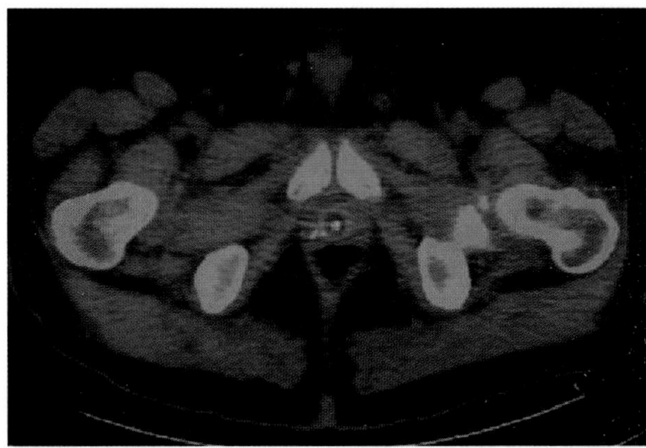

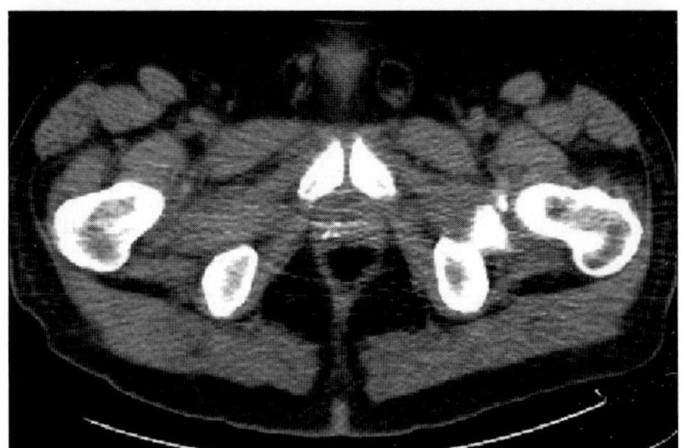

^{18}F-choline finding

Central focal ^{18}F-choline uptake immediately under the bladder.

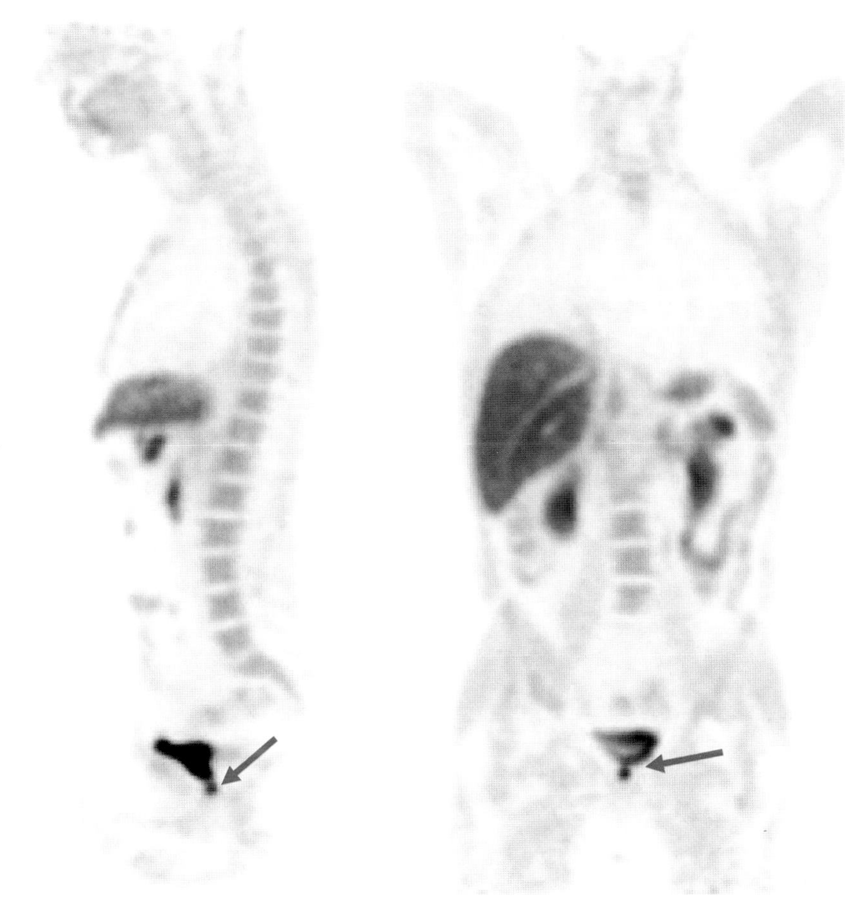

Teaching point

Focal ^{18}F-choline uptake below the bladder, due to residual urethral uptake, should not be misinterpreted as local recurrence.

Chapter 4 Methionine PET-CT

Cristina Nanni, Valentina Ambrosini, and Stefano Fanti

^{11}C-Methionine (^{11}C-METH) is an aminoacidic PET tracer whose main employment regards the diagnosis of central nervous system tumors. Methionine is, in fact, one of the five essential amino acids that can be involved in different metabolic pathways at a cellular level. The main destiny of this molecule is the proteic synthesis within ribosomes, but it can also be converted to enter the citric-acid cycle (to produce energy) and as a cofactor for transferring monocarbon units.

The uptake mechanism of ^{11}C-METH within brain tumors is still uncertain, but the most probable theories are based on the combination of a passive diffusion through the damaged brain blood barrier (BBB) and an active tumor uptake mediated by a carrier due to an increased proteic synthesis (related to the active proliferation).

One of the great advantages of using ^{11}C-METH for the diagnosis of brain tumors is the very low background that is found in healthy brain. Normal brain tissue, in fact, recognizes only glucose as metabolic substrate and therefore does not present any significant ^{11}C-METH uptake. On the other hand, brain tumors present an increased tracer uptake, and therefore the tumor-to-background ratio is really favorable, making the ^{11}C-METH PET quite easy to read and interpret.

From a practical point of view, a PET-CT with ^{11}C-METH is easy and fast to perform. Usually 370–740 MBq of tracer are injected intravenously and, because of the short half-life of ^{11}C-labeled molecules (20 min), the uptake time ranges from only 20 to 30 min. Then, a segmental static image acquisition is performed on brain for 10–15 min. No fasting is usually required and no collateral effects have never been described.

The role of ^{11}C-METH PET-CT in clinical practice is limited to those patients with brain tumors with an inconclusive MRI (or CT). It is well-known, in fact, that after treatment (surgery, chemotherapy or radiotherapy) para-physiological phenomena like fibrosis, necrosis or edema may occur as a consequence of therapy. Those phenomena may present with morphological characteristics very similar to a disease relapse, making the interpretation of conventional imaging equivocal. However, the early identification of disease relapse may be very important in the clinical history of those patients, since an early second line therapy can improve their survival.

Since fibrosis, necrosis or edema are not cellular proliferating processes, they do not present any significant increase in the tracer uptake and so a differential diagnosis between disease relapse (positive ^{11}C-METH PET) and benign response to therapy (negative ^{11}C-METH PET) can be done with a very good accuracy.

This good reliability of PET is based on the fact that the tracer uptake is not present in enhancing necrosis, is not influenced by corticosteroid therapy (that can be administrated for reducing edema), and is proportional to the grade of the disease (even low-grade brain tumors are positive). The false positive results are due to recognizable clinical events (very recent biopsy, acute inflammations, hematoma, acute stroke with reperfusion) causing an aspecific leakage of the tracer within the intercellular space related to a vascular damage or an increased vascular permeability (Methionine is a very small molecule). It is important to point out that ^{11}C-METH PET presents less false positive (post RT inflammation is negative at ^{11}C-METH PET) and less false negative results compared to 18F-FDG brain PET.

The main limitation of this technique is the spatial resolution (approximately 5 mm) and the low availability of the tracer. In fact, the short half-life of ^{11}C prevents the distribution of tracer on the territory and requires a cyclotron-based PET center with particular skills on ^{11}C-based molecules.

Despite the main clinical application of ^{11}C-METH PET-CT in brain tumors with regard to the diagnosis of disease relapse of low- and high-grade tumors, this exam has been used for other minor aims. In fact, studies from literature have proved that ^{11}C-METH PET-CT can be successfully used for guiding the tumor biopsy by indicating the most active area inside the mass and can be used as a prognostic index, since its uptake is proportional to the malignancy of the tumor and its cellular proliferative index. In fact, the proportionality between tracer uptake and tumor grade may be used to show early, a change in tumor grade without requiring any invasive procedure. This is not always possible with MRI as many high-grade tumors do not have any significant enhancement. The tumor grade is a prognostic index, and therefore a correlation between ^{11}C-METH uptake and survival was found. Patients with hypermetabolic tumors have a significantly worse prognosis, while patients with hypo or isometabolic tumors have a better life expectation.

Furthermore, ^{11}C-METH PET-CT may also be used for the early diagnosis of a response to both chemo and radiation therapies.

The role of ^{11}C-METH PET for the diagnosis of unbiopsied brain masses is controversial. Few studies are present in literature since the major part of brain masses, despite being negative at ^{11}C-METH PET, are biopsied for histopathological confirmation anyway. There is, therefore, a weak rationale for the execution of the exam in newlydiagnosed brain masses.

A possible advantage of ^{11}C-METH PET in the early evaluation of brain tumors relies on the fact that MRI may fail to identify tumor infiltrated margins, and this could be a disadvantage during tumor resection, resulting in a margin to be indiscriminately added to radiotherapy treatment volumes to account for these infiltrating cells. As this margin includes normal brain, the total dose used has to be reduced to reduce the risk of radiation necrosis. As a consequence, gliomas recur within the treatment volume in the majority of patients. Though other PET tracers were tried for the diagnostics of brain tumors (in particular 18F-FDG and ^{11}C-Choline), ^{11}C-METH turned out to be the most accurate and is therefore recognized now as the PET tracer of choice in this field.

Besides brain tumors, other minor applications of ^{11}C-METH PET-CT were analyzed in literature with equivocal results. A possible role of this tracer was found in the diagnosis of hyperparathyroidism, and this field deserves a particular explanation in consideration of the good preliminary results, despite not being a routine clinical application as yet.

The principle of ^{11}C-METH uptake in hyperfunctioning parathyroids relies on the fact that this tracer is an aminoacid that can be incorporated into parathormone, which is largely produced in those glands. The advantages over MIBI-SPECT are, of course, the lower dose delivered to the patient, the much higher anatomical detail given by the CT (which is very important for the correct localization of the hyperfunctioning glands that should be surgically removed), the higher spatial resolution compared to conventional scintigraphy, and the much shorter time needed to complete the entire procedure. According to recent literature, it was preliminary proved that ^{11}C-METH PET-CT is accurate both for primary and secondary hyperparathyroidism, with a true positive rate of approximately 85%. Of course, further studies are needed to confirm these preliminary encouraging data.

Other clinical applications of ^{11}C-METH PET were explored in the past years. Some interesting published protocols were designed on the theory that ^{11}C-METH does not present any significant uptake in enlarged inflammatory lymph nodes (or at least a much lower uptake compared to the standard FDG), and this was thought to be somehow useful for the staging of mediastinal lymph nodes in patients affected by lung cancer before surgery. The low ^{11}C-METH uptake in post radiotherapy inflammation suggested some protocols in oncological patients (mainly affected by sarcomas or head and neck cancer) for the early evaluation of post radiotherapy response to treatment, in order to identify a possible contribution of this tracer to reduce false positive results obtained with FDG.

Furthermore, the normal increased uptake of ^{11}C-METH in salivary glands and pancreas suggested some groups to evaluate it as a tracer for the functional evaluation of those glands.

All these studies gave equivocal results remaining purely speculative, and no clinical applications were recognized for ^{11}C-METH PET, besides the evaluation of central nervous system tumors and a minor application in hyperparathyroidism.

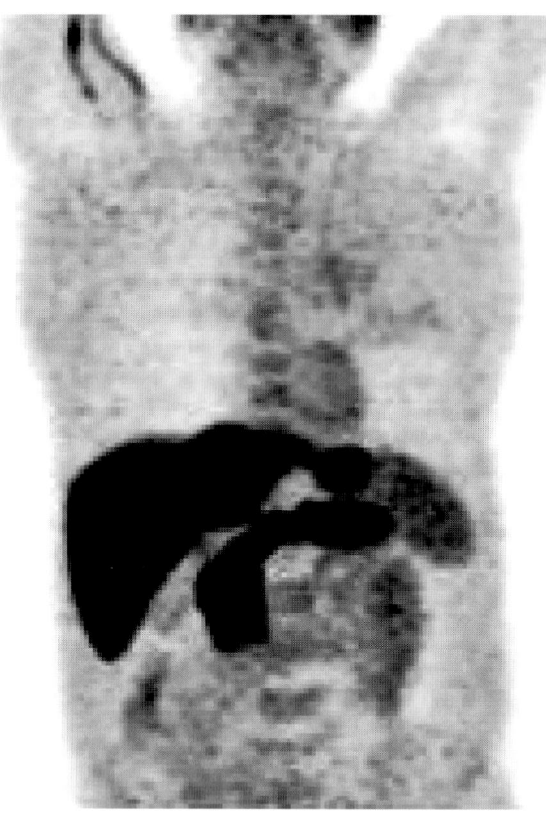

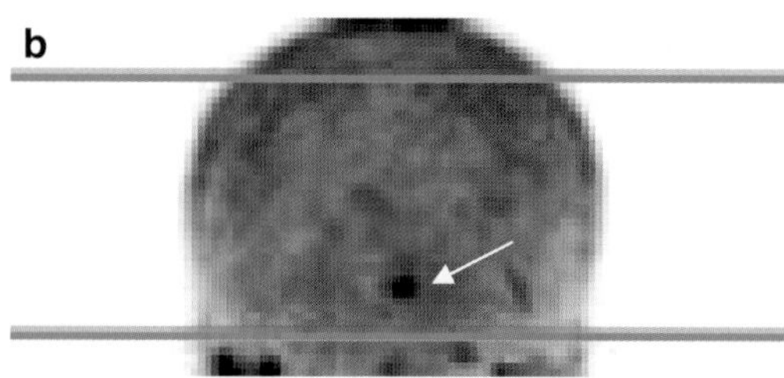

^{11}C-Methionine finding

Physiological biodistribution of ^{11}C-METH: (a) total body; (b) brain.

Teaching point

(a) Note the normal increased uptake in the liver and pancreas associated to a lower uptake in the spleen.
(b) The brain does not present any significant uptake of the tracer except for the pituitary gland (*white arrow*).

MR

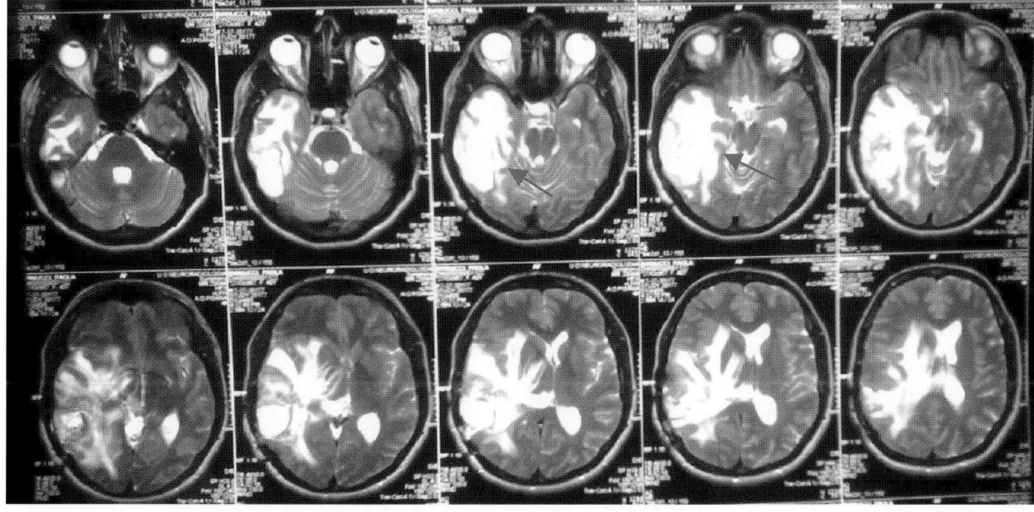

^{11}C-METH PET

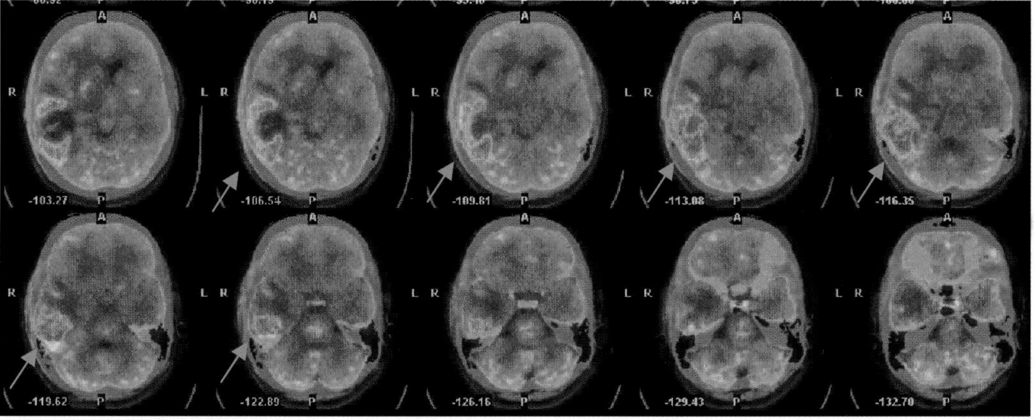

^{11}C-Methionine finding

At MR gliosis and edema.
^{11}C-METH PET highlights an area of increased uptake consistent with disease relapse, close to the margin of surgical resection.

Teaching point

After treatment (surgery, chemotherapy, or radiotherapy), paraphysiological phenomena like fibrosis, necrosis, or edema may occur as a consequence of therapy. Those phenomena may be similar to a disease relapse, making the interpretation of conventional imaging equivocal. ^{11}C-METH PET helps in identifying disease relapse in case of unclear conventional imaging, leading to an early therapy onset.

MR

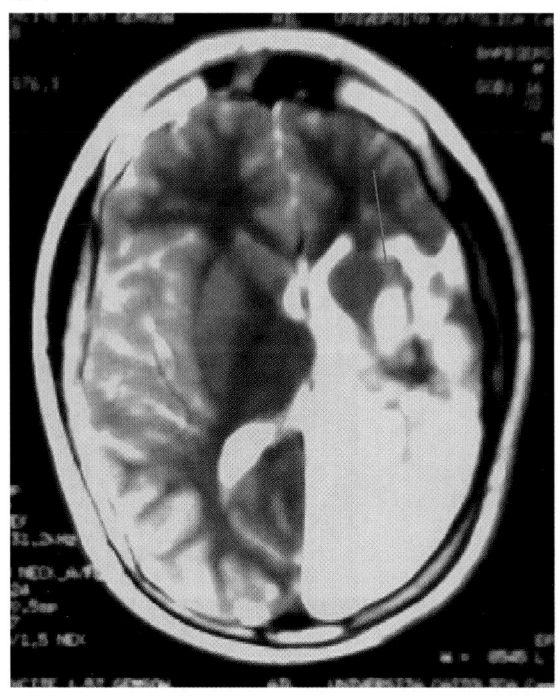

^{11}C-METH PET

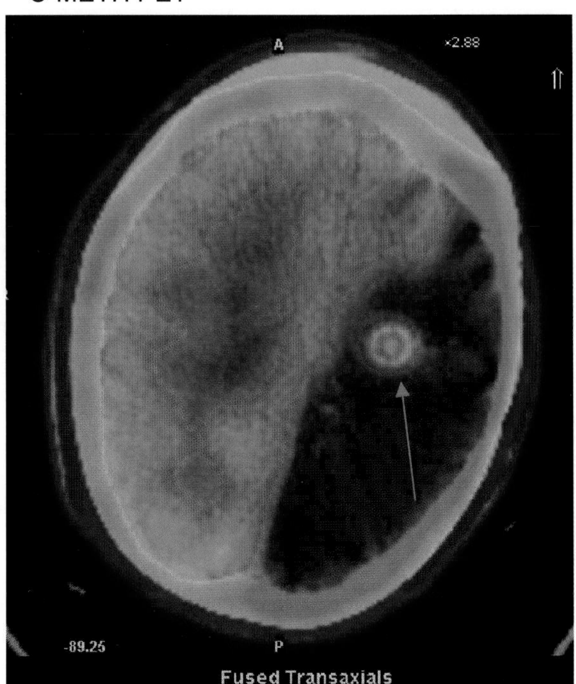

^{11}C-Methionine finding

PET demonstrates an area of focal increased uptake showing a disease relapse that was unrecognized at MR.

Teaching point

Sometimes a small area of disease relapse may be somehow hidden within paraphysiological reactions to surgery and radiotherapy. MR pathological findings may appear, therefore, uniform in morphology but combined begign and malignant processes may be present at the same time.

MR

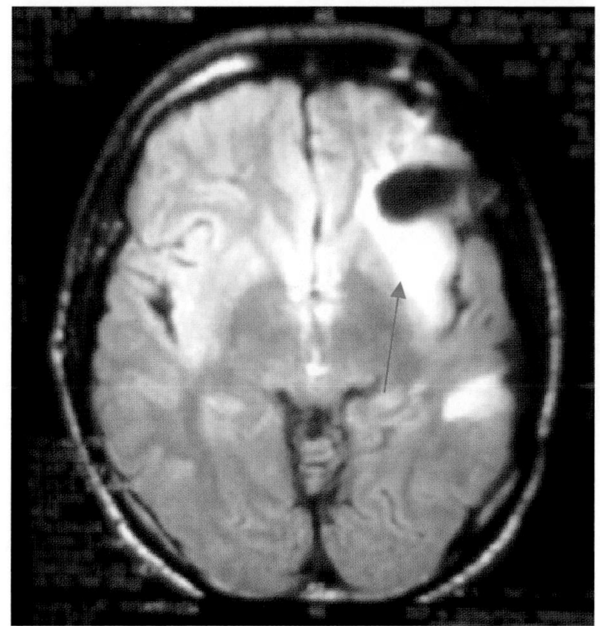

^{11}C-METH PET

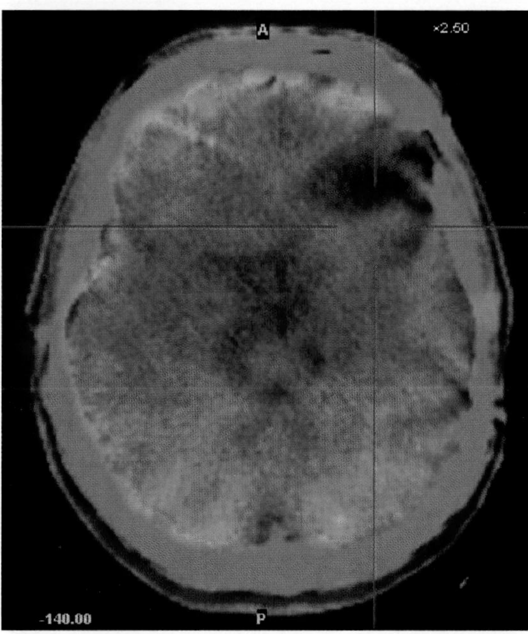

^{11}C-Methionine finding

PET is negative demonstrating posttherapy benign changes.

Teaching point

Since fibrosis, necrosis, or edema are not cellular proliferating processes, they do not present any significant increase in the tracer uptake and so a differential diagnosis between disease relapse (positive ^{11}C-METH PET) and benign response to therapy (negative ^{11}C-METH PET) can be done with a very good accuracy.

MR

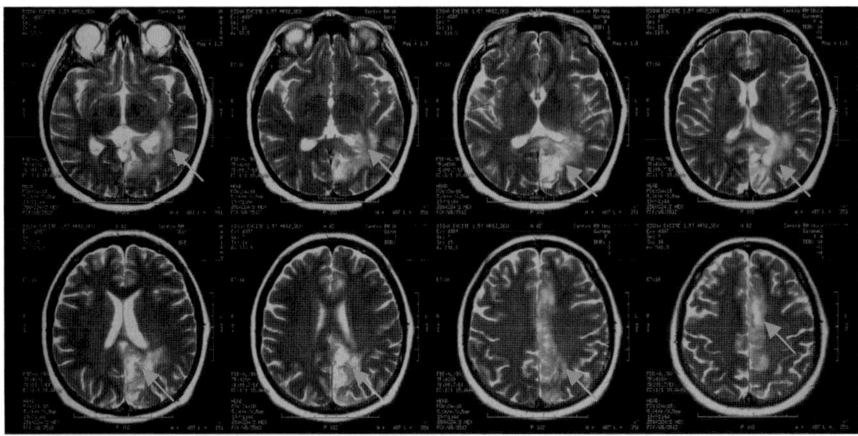

^{11}C-METH PET

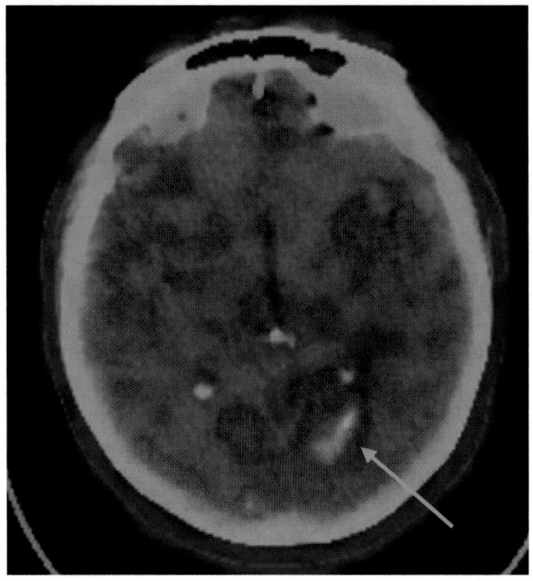

^{11}C-Methionine finding

PET demonstrates an area of persistent increased uptake showing an incomplete response to therapy.

Teaching point

An early identification of persistent active disease may lead to a prolonged chemotherapy, in order to better control the unresectable disease.

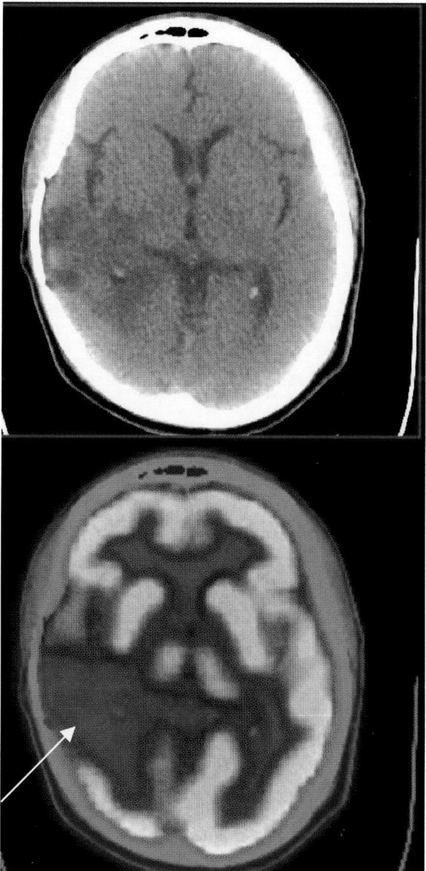

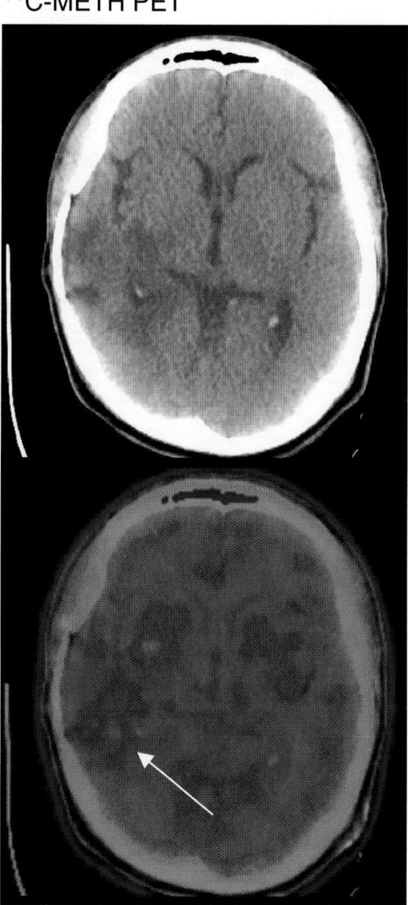

PET finding

^{18}F-FDG PET fails to demonstrate disease relapse because of the increased normal brain uptake. ^{11}C-METH PET highlights an area of mild increased uptake, which is consistent with disease relapse.

Teaching point

^{11}C-METH PET is more sensitive than FDG for the identification of disease relapse because of the better contrast resolution of images. Normal brain, in fact, does not present a significantly increased tracer uptake since amino acids are not a metabolic substrate of grey and white matter, while FDG is physiologically picked up by normal brain, possibly masking areas of disease relapse.

MR

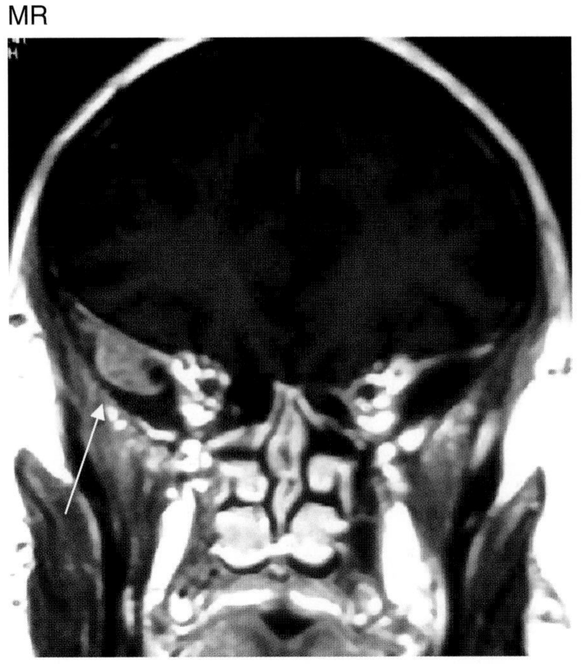

^{11}C-METH PET

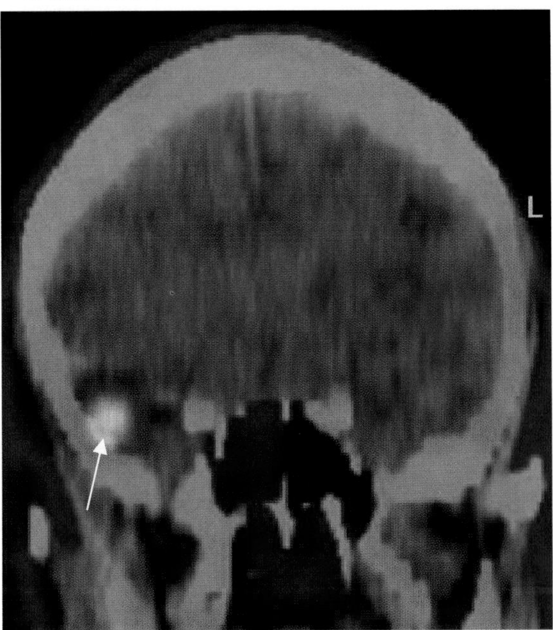

^{11}C-Methionine finding

PET is positive, confirming the diagnosis.

Teaching point

In this case a positivity of ^{11}C-METH PET leads to a prosecution of diagnostic follow-up, despite the very difficult site to biopsy, since the probability of malignancy is very high.

MR

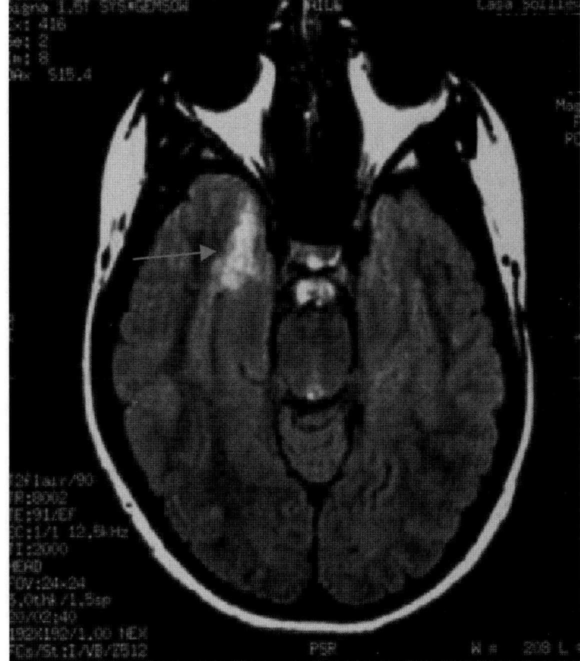

^{11}C-METH PET

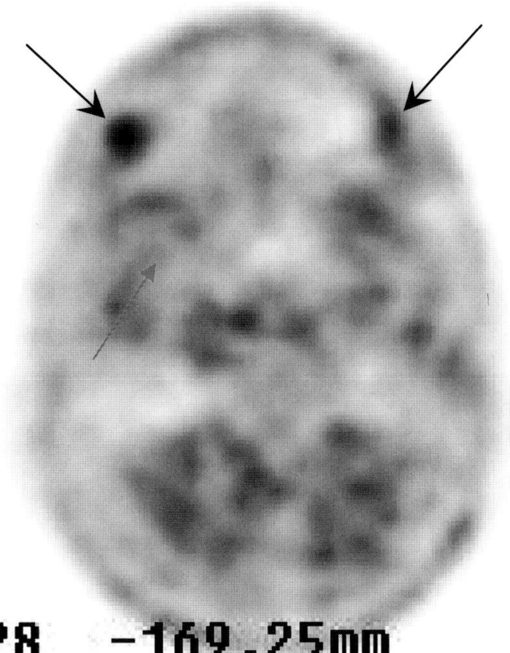

^{11}C-Methionine finding

PET is negative, confirming a subsequent diagnosis of displasia. *Black arrows* indicate normal uptake of lacrimal glands.

Teaching point

In this case, a negative ^{11}C-METH PET excludes with high probability the presence of a malignant disease, leading to a conventional imaging follow up and making an invasive diagnostic procedure not required.

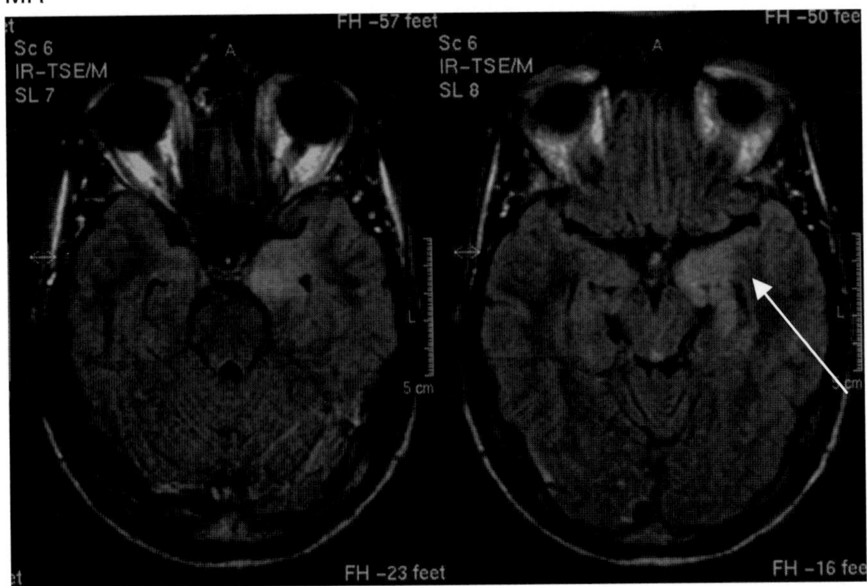

^{11}C-METH PET

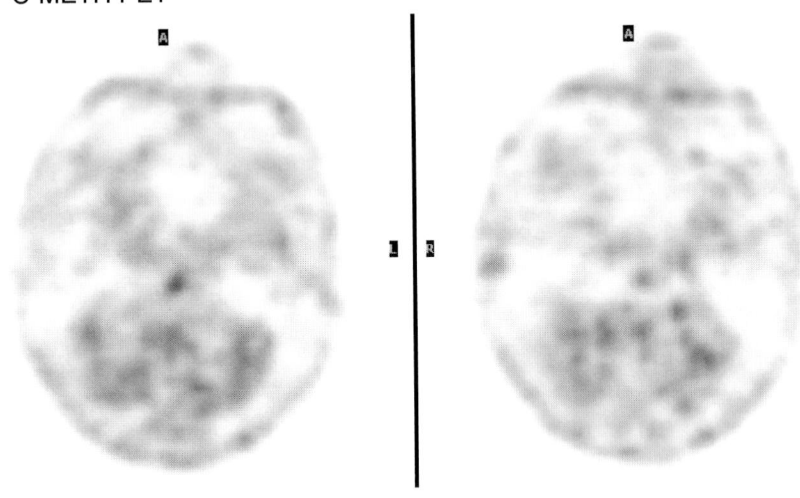

^{11}C-Methionine finding

PET is negative; follow-up data confirmed the diagnosis of nonmalignant disease.

^{18}F-FDG PET

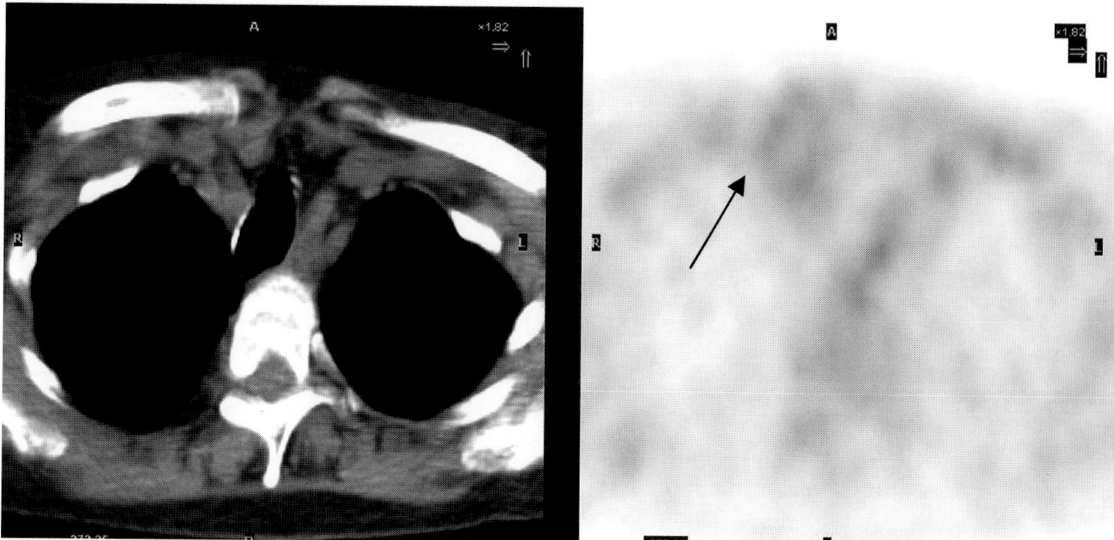

^{11}C-METH PET

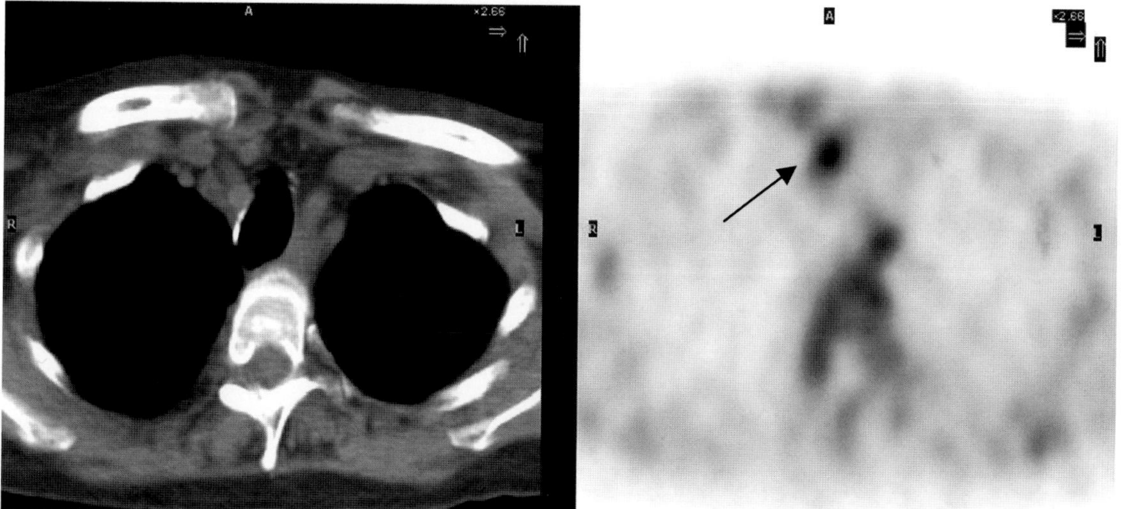

PET finding

^{18}F-FDG PET fails in identifying the hyperfunctioning gland.
^{11}C-METH PET identifies an increased tracer uptake in the hyperfunctionig parathyroid gland.

Teaching point

In this case, ^{11}C-METH PET identified an ectopic adenoma, which is very difficult to detect with standard scintigraphy due to its very small size. The support of corresponding CT can be used to guide the surgeon in finding the adenoma during intervention.

Chapter 5 Fluoride PET-CT

Roland Hustinx and Catherine Beckers

$[^{18}F]$fluoride was first introduced in 1962, and rapidly proposed as a radiotracer for bone exploration. The complex $[^{18}F]$NaF is injected intravenously, and it dissociates in the blood into Na^+ and $[^{18}F]$fluoride ion. The uptake of $[^{18}F]$fluoride results from ionic exchanges between hydroxyl groups of hydroxylapatite to form fluoroapatite and is thus directly related to bone metabolism. Both the blood flow and the osteoblastic activity influence the $[^{18}F]$fluoride accumulation, in proportions that are still discussed. $[^{18}F]$NaF-PET imaging, using appropriate modeling, can thus noninvasively assess bone metabolism. The advantage of $[^{18}F]$fluoride compared to other PET tracers is the synthesis, which is extremely simple and relatively inexpensive: $[^{18}F]$fluoride is rendered isotonic with a NaCl solution to form $[^{18}F]$NaF. Since the early sixties, the mechanism of uptake of $[^{18}F]$fluoride has been extensively studied. The accumulation of $[^{18}F]$fluoride in osteoforming areas of bone metastases was demonstrated in autopsy series and in rabbit experimental models. In mice, $[^{18}F]$NaF-PET clearly identified fractures as increased uptake foci up to 7 weeks after the initial trauma, human bone grafts 2 months after the implantation, and osteoblastic lesions induced by human prostate cancer cells. Lytic lesions from human prostate cancer cells (CL-1 et PC-3) were visualized either as foci of globally increased activity or, most frequently, as rim-like foci, surrounding the edge of the lesions. Quantitative uptake, measured as cps/pixel/min, was fairly reproducible in femoral and humeral ROIs drawn on four studies over a period of 4 weeks. The relationship between $[^{18}F]$NaF uptake and bone formation was clearly established using quantitative modeling in mini pigs, showing correlations of bone blood flow and metabolic activity, with histomorphometric indices of bone formation in the normal bone tissue. Furthermore, in patients with secondary hyperparathyroidism, the $[^{18}F]$NaF incorporation rate was correlated with the plasma parathormone level and with the bone formation rate.

Bone scintigraphy (BS) with ^{99m}Tc methylate diphosphonate (^{99m}Tc-MDP) remains the most widely used imaging method for detecting bone metastases. The reported sensitivity and specificity figures range from 62 to 100% and from 78 to 100%, respectively. Although bone scanning has proven highly valuable, the pharmacokinetic properties of $[^{18}F]$NaF appear more favorable than those shown by ^{99m}Tc-labeled compounds. In particular, the bone tissue first-pass retention is significantly higher and the blood clearance faster with $[^{18}F]$NaF than with ^{99m}Tc-MDP. As a result, the image acquisition can be started earlier after tracer injection, with higher bone to background activity ratio. The uptake time ranges from 30 to 60 min, and the injected activity is usually around 185–200 MBq. With the advent of faster and more sensitive PET devices coupled with high-end CT scanners, there has been renewed interest in $[^{18}F]$NaF imaging, especially in the oncology setting.

Schirrmeister et al. reported remarkably impressive results with $[^{18}F]$NaF PET in a series of prospective studies. They first showed that $[^{18}F]$NaF PET was significantly more sensitive than planar BS for detecting bone metastases from various cancers, mainly prostate and thyroid, and that it remained highly sensitive regardless of the location of the lesions, in contrast with BS. $[^{18}F]$NaF PET correctly evaluated the skeletal status in 27/28 breast cancer patients, without known bone metastases, as compared to 16/28 with BS. Although in this study, SPECT did not improve the detection rate, further evaluation in lung cancer patients showed similar diagnostic performances for $[^{18}F]$NaF PET and SPECT, both being more accurate than planar BS. Recent studies performed using PET-CT yielded further improved results. The group in Tel Aviv reported 85% sensitivity (99% when inconclusive foci were considered as positive) and 97% specificity in a series of 44 patients with various cancers, compared with 72% (90%) and 72% for PET alone, respectively. In another series of patients with prostate cancer and high risk of bone spread, PET-CT showed 100% sensitivity and 100% specificity, as compared with 61 and 87%, respectively, for BS with SPECT. These Authors considered suspicious foci on the $[^{18}F]$NaF PET images as positive, when there was no CT anomaly that could explain the PET lesions. Such perfect results are unlikely to be reproduced in the routine clinical setting and may be explained by the absence of a gold standard in these studies. Nevertheless, it clearly appears that low-dose CT improves the diagnostic accuracy, in particular by evidencing benign conditions that are responsible for nonspecific foci of increased $[^{18}F]$NaF uptake. Furthermore, all data conclude to a significantly higher sensitivity of $[^{18}F]$NaF PET for detecting lytic metastases as compared to bone scintigraphy. The combination of anatomical and structural information with better tracer properties and improved spatial resolution of PET appears extremely potent, enhancing both the sensitivity and the specificity of the test. Although PET-CT with $[^{18}F]$NaF appears to be intrinsically superior toBS, several drawbacks need to be overcome before reaching acceptable clinical performance. There is a steep learning curve for nuclear medicine physicians switching from BS to PET-CT. In addition, the collaboration of radiologists with a large experience in bone imaging enhances both the diagnostic accuracy and the confidence with which the report is released.

Several question marks remain considering a widespread use of [^{18}F]NaF PET-CT in oncology. The cost-effectiveness is yet to be appropriately evaluated, even though a report published in 2003 concluded to better ratios for BS compared to PET in lung cancer patients. PET imaging in general cannot be considered as inexpensive, but [^{18}F]NaF is much cheaper than other tracers such as FDG, and the increased availability of both PET-CT and cyclotrons also influences the cost-effectiveness of the analysis. Such analysis should also take into account the recurrent shortage in molybdenum-99 supply in both Europe and USA. Also, up to date PET-CT technology should be compared with the most recent monophotonic technology, i.e., SPECT/CT. Such studies are currently inexistent. Finally, radiation dose to the patient is not really an issue, as the effective doses (for an adult) of the commonly injected activities of [^{18}F]NaF and ^{99m}Tc-MDP are very similar. The low-dose CT procedure of PET-CT increases the dose but similarly, it will probably be increasingly performed with new SPECT/CT systems.

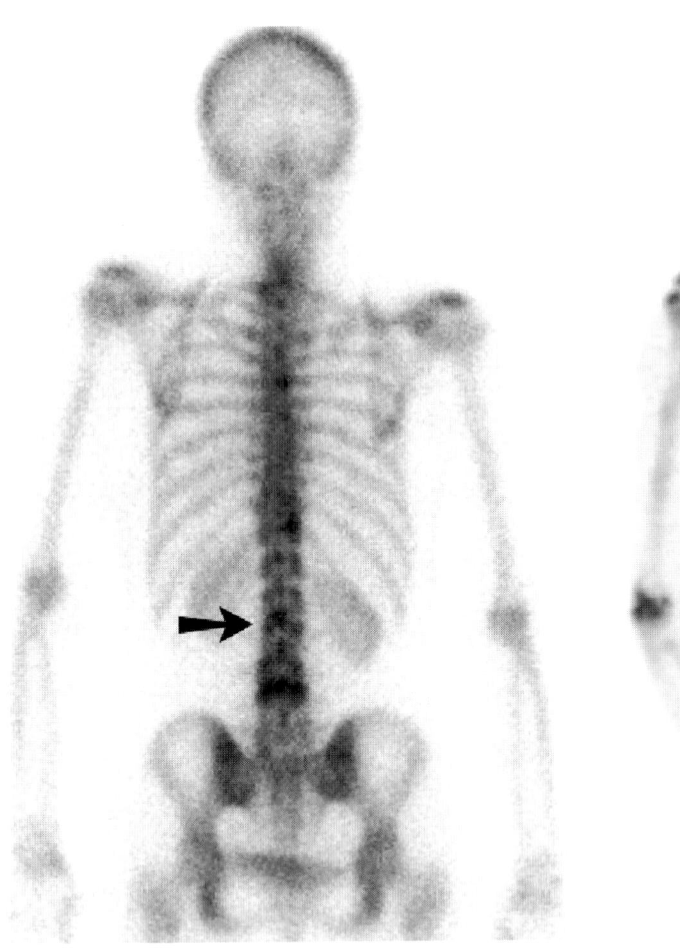

^{99m}Tc-MDP

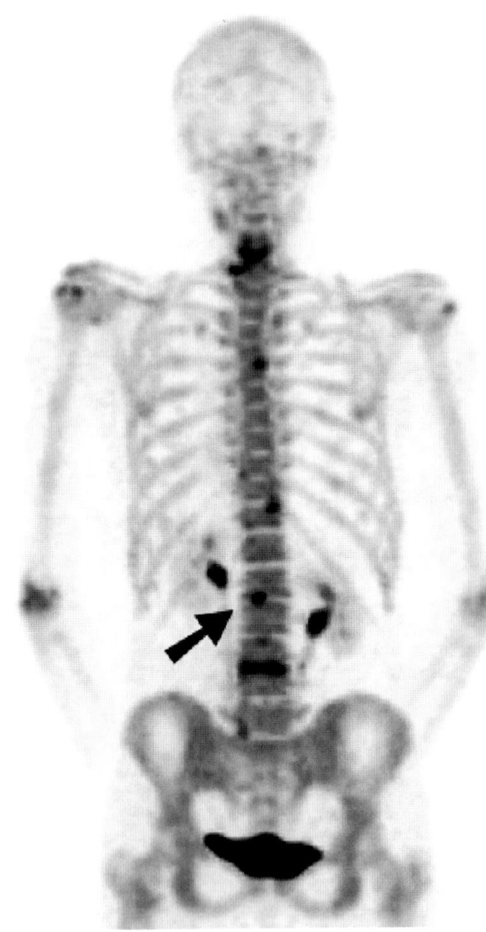

^{18}F-NaF

^{99m}Tc-MDP finding

Bone scan performed as part of the systematic follow-up demonstrates a new hot spot in the superior lumbar spine.

^{18}F-NaF finding

The hot spot is precisely located near the L1/L2 disk.

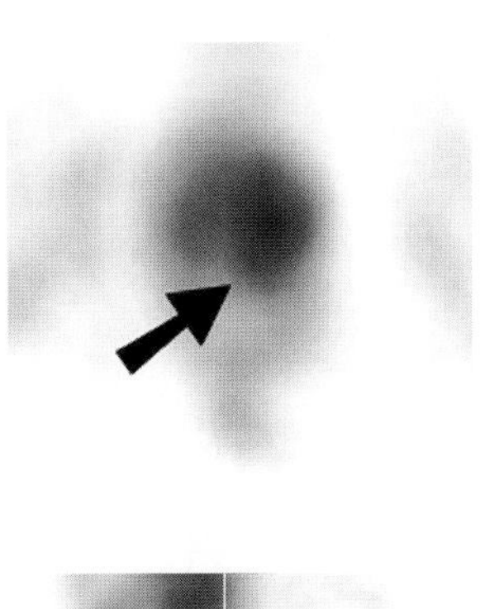

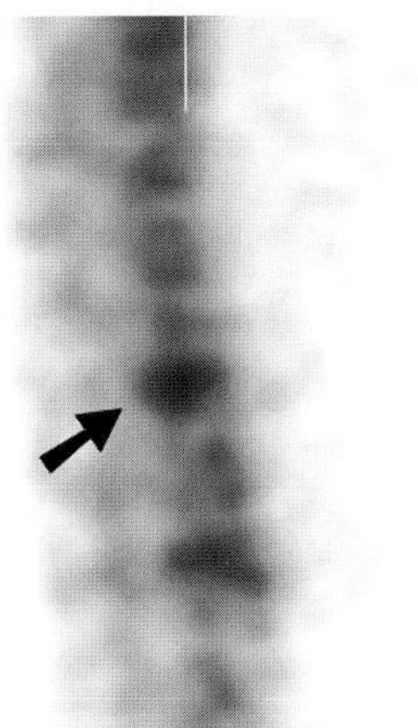

^{99m}Tc-MDP

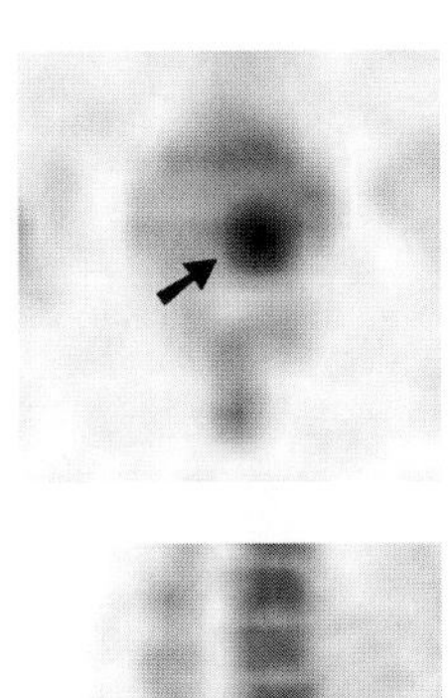

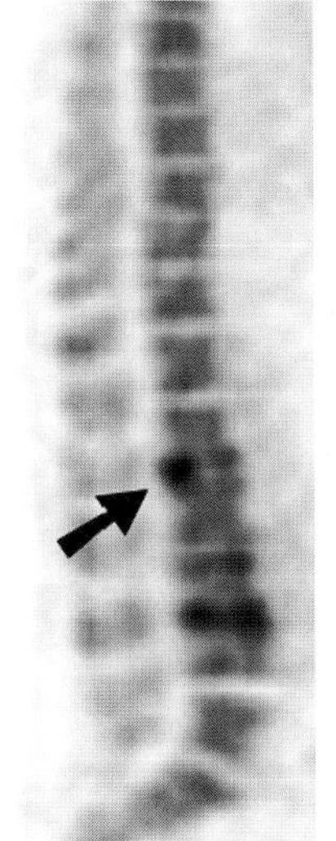

^{18}F-NAF

T1 TSE FS

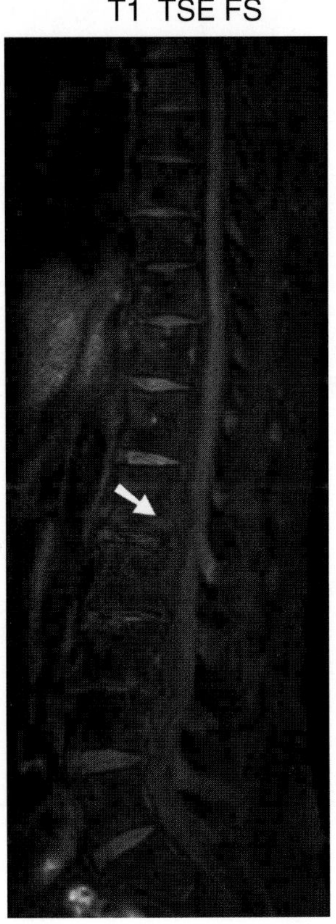

T1 TSE FS+Gd

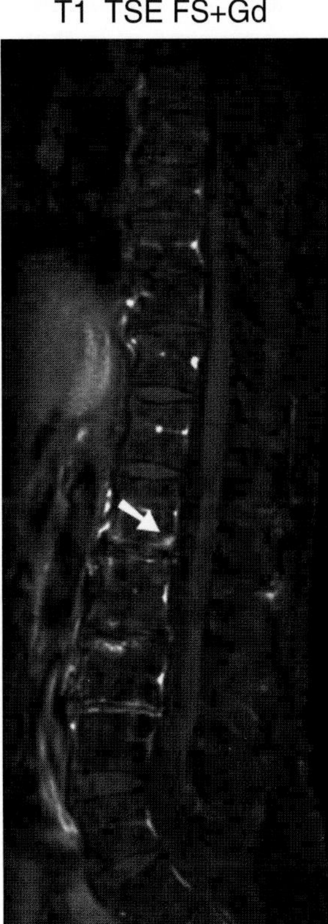

T1 TSE

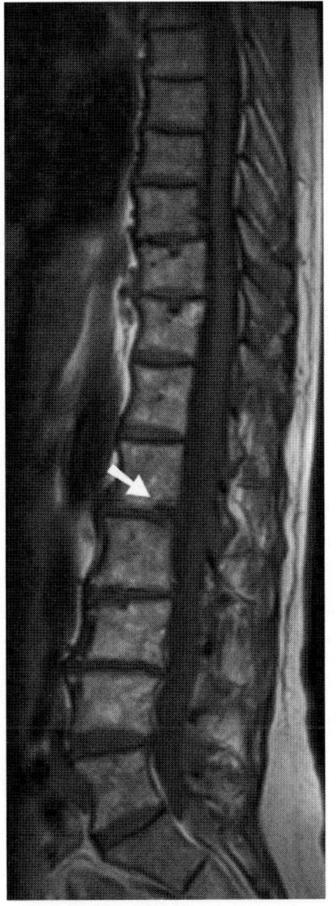

T2 TSE

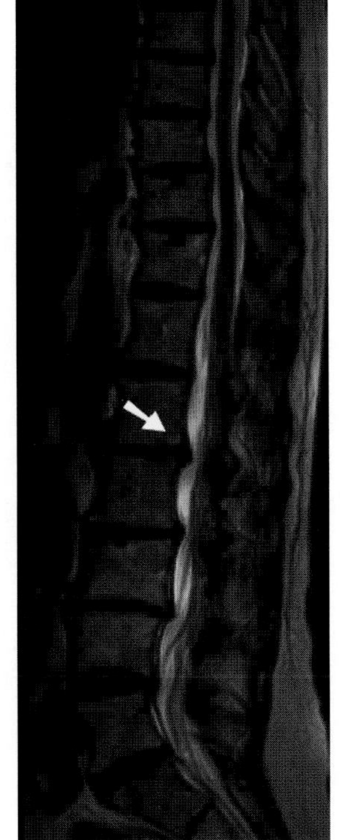

Teaching point

^{18}F-NaF PET has a better bone to background ratio and a higher spatial resolution than bone scan. It thus allows a better delineation and location of the lesion. In this case, the peridiscal location of the hot spot with the narrowing of the disk space excludes with a high probability a bone metastasis, as confirmed by MRI demonstrating L1/L2 degenerative disk disease with corporeal posterior edema. As a result, 5 years after the onset of the disease, the patient is considered in clinical remission and the follow-up will be performed annually by the GP (CA 15.3 and mammography).

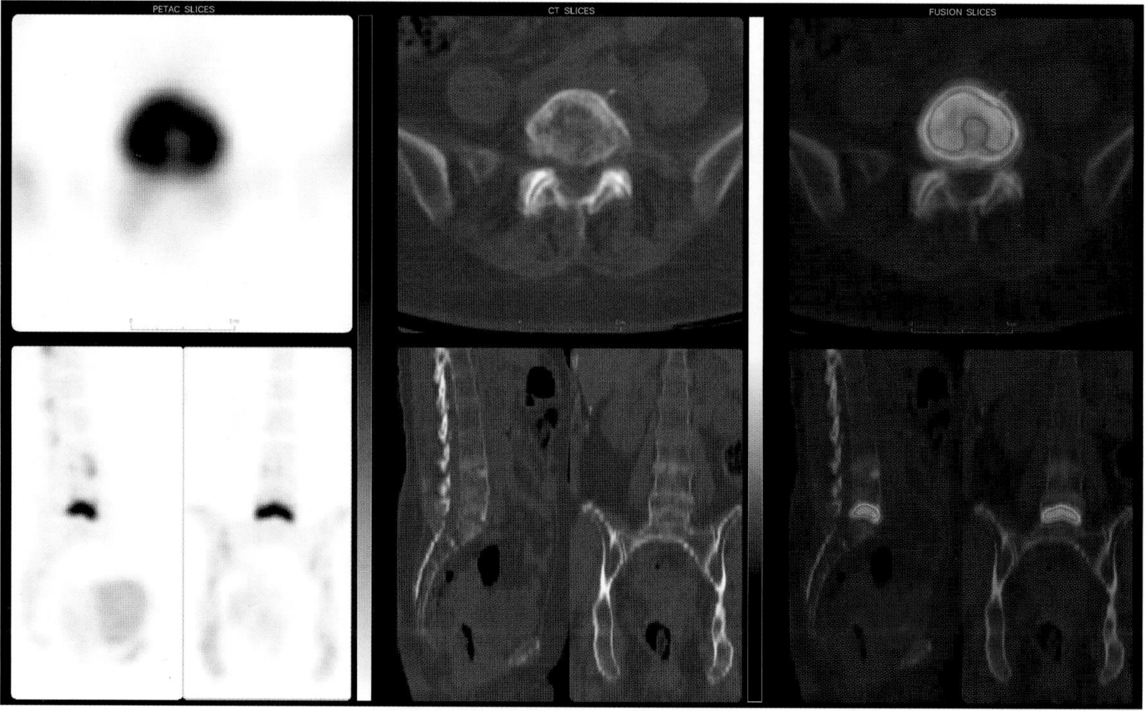

■ ^{18}F-NaF finding

Highly increased uptake in the body of L5. Low-dose CT shows heterogeneous density and compression fracture of its inferior endplate.

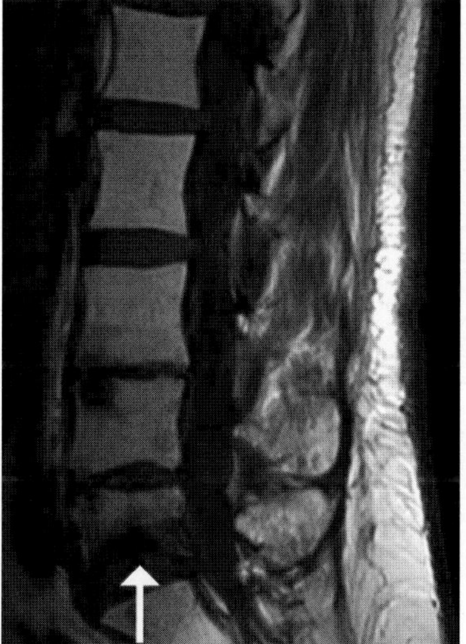

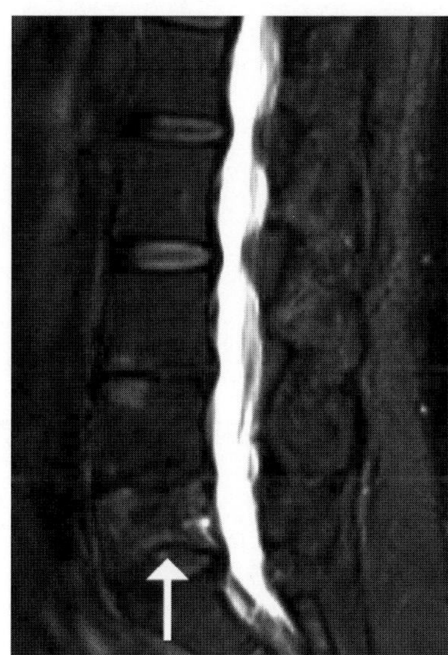

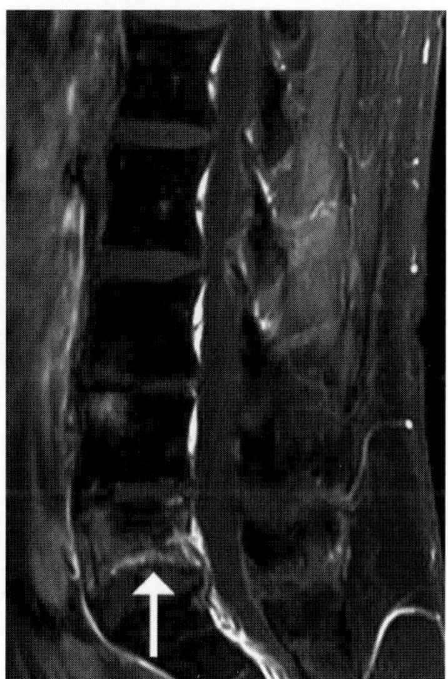

Teaching point

The combination of ^{18}F-NaF PET and low-dose CT is very powerful for characterizing the lesions. In this case, CT was highly suggestive of a pathological fracture. As a whole-body survey PET is also able to determine whether the metastatic spread is monostototic or polyostotic, thus helping centering complementary imaging if necessary. In this case, MRI confirms the malignant etiology of this fracture (*arrows*). MRI also shows degenerative changes on L3–L4. Radiotherapy is programmed and zoledronic acid introduced.

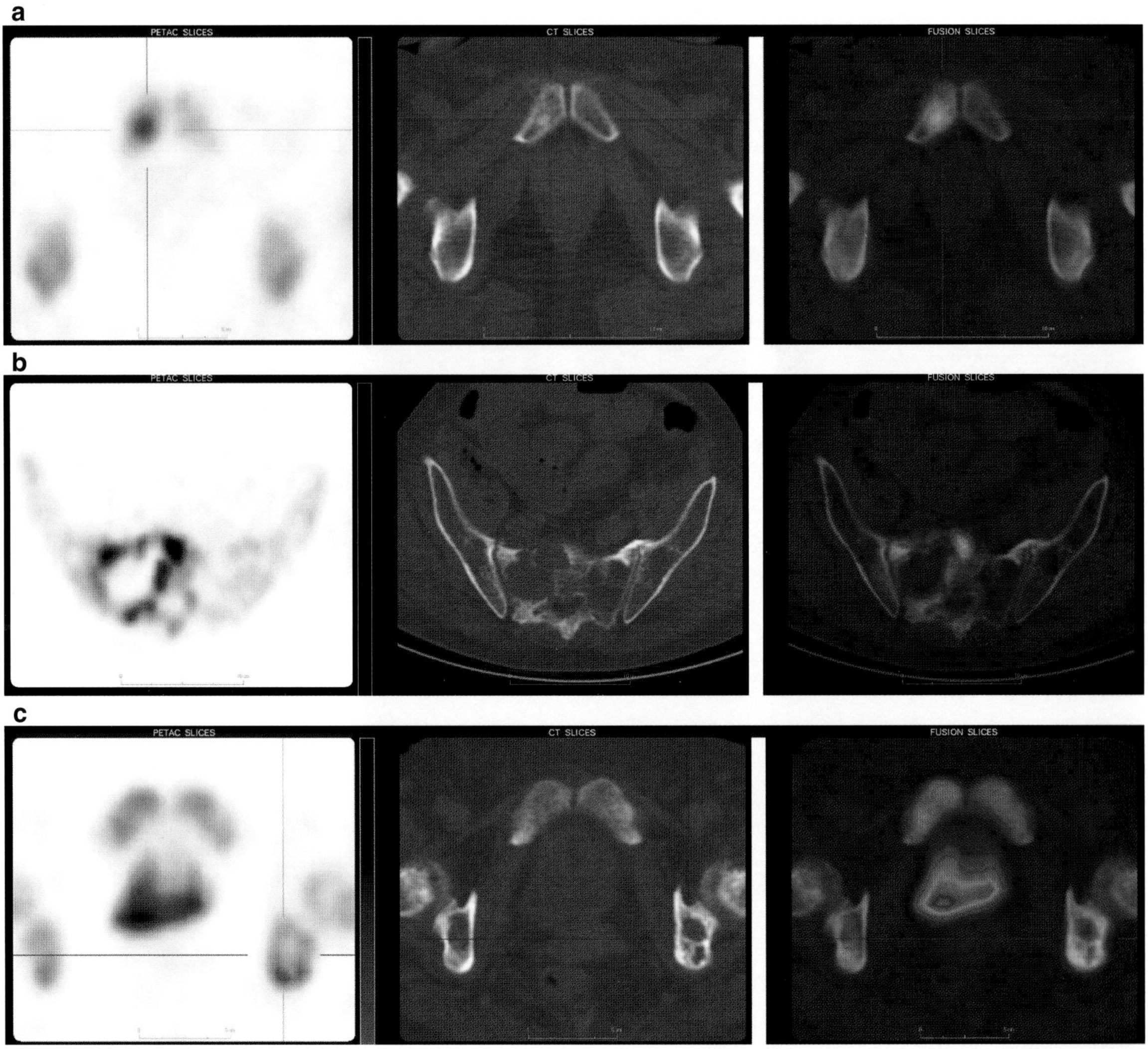

a

PETAC SLICES CT SLICES FUSION SLICES

b

PETAC SLICES CT SLICES FUSION SLICES

c

PETAC SLICES CT SLICES FUSION SLICES

^{18}F-NaF finding

Hot spot in (a) a very small pubic osteoblastic metastasis of a SCLC, (b) a large sacral osteolytic metastasis of a renal cell carcinoma, and (c) an ischiatic mixed metastasis of a breast cancer.

Teaching point

^{18}F-NaF is preferentially deposited at sites of high bone turnover and remodeling, and bone metastases are seen indirectly because uptake depends on surrounding bone reaction to the tumor. Metastases may be predominantly lytic, blastic, or mixed. Most are associated with increased ^{18}F-NaF uptake. Changes may be very subtle though and careful examination of all data sets is required, as shown in this case (c).

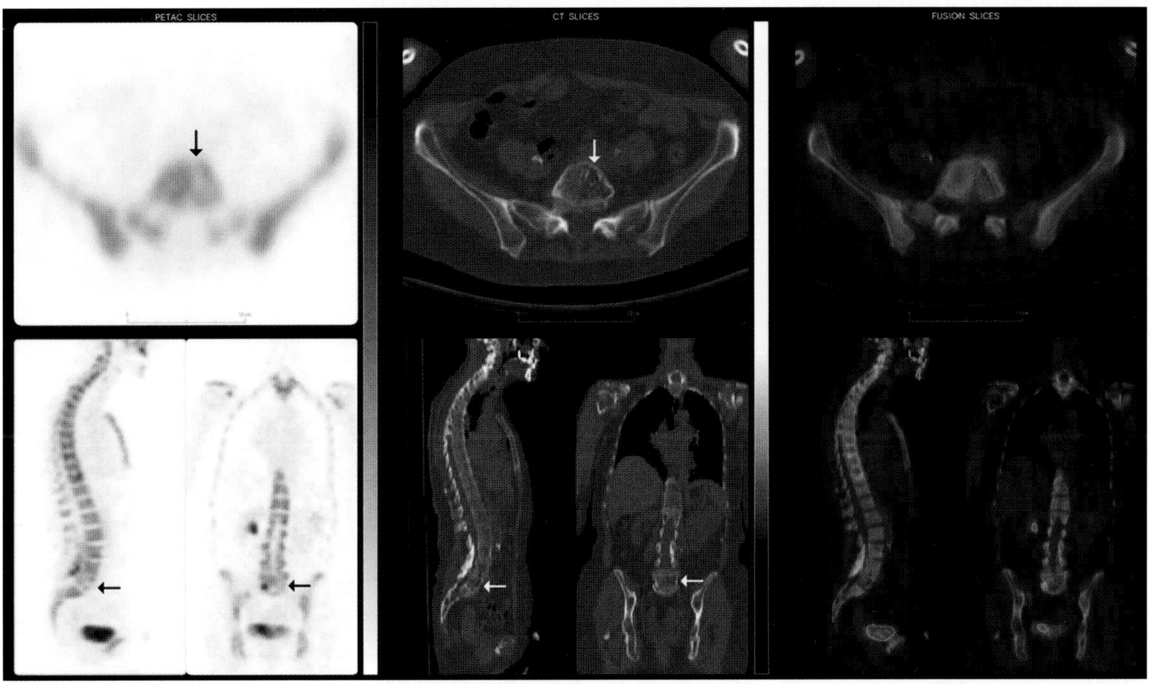

^{18}F-NaF finding

Cold spot in the left part of the body of L5.

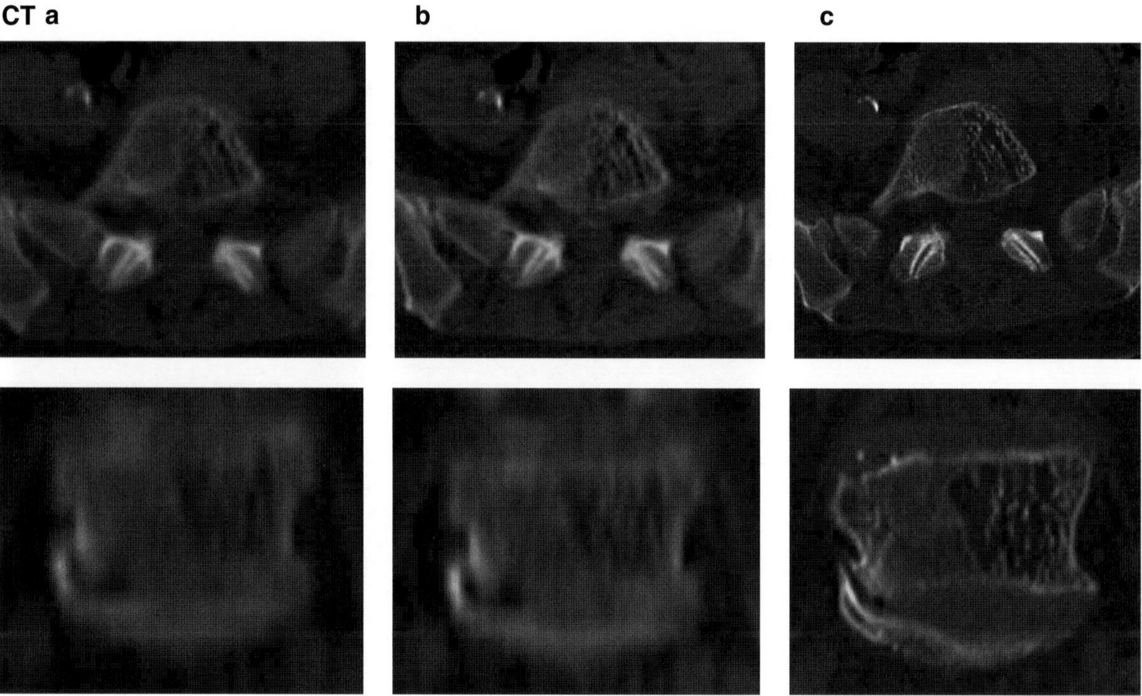

CT finding

Low-dose CT with (a) 5 mm-thick reconstructed slices; (b) 3 mm-thick reconstructed slices, and (c) diagnostic CT with isotropic 0.6 mm-thick slices (transaxial and coronal slices in all three cases). There is a low-density lesion with coarsened vertical trabeculae surrounded by fat with normal cortex and surrounding soft tissues, which is a characteristic pattern of hemangioma.

Teaching point

In renal cell carcinoma as in squamous cell lung carcinoma, breast and thyroid cancers, bone metastases are usually lytic and may appear as a cold spot on the ^{18}F NaF PET images. In many cases, the low-dose CT provides useful information as regards to the nature of the lesion although it must be kept in mind that a 5 or 3 mm-thick CT does not provide the spatial resolution and wealth of structural details provided by a dedicated CT study, as shown by the various CT sections in this case. Here, the cold spot corresponds to an hemangioma, which is the more frequent benign lesion with decreased uptake.

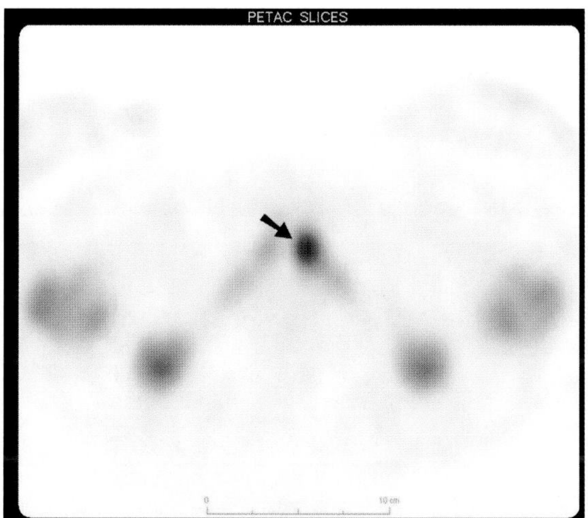

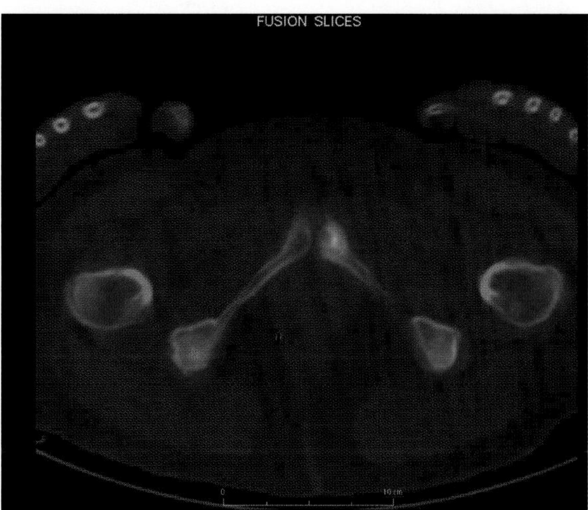

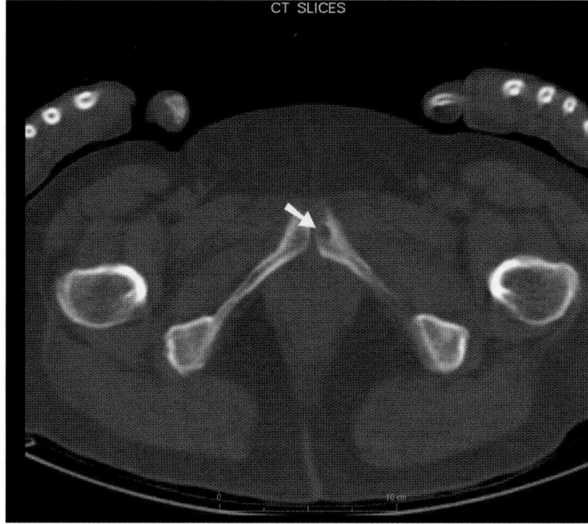

^{18}F-NaF finding

Seven millimeter gap in the left part of the pubis with increased ^{18}F-NaF uptake (SUV_{max} 12).

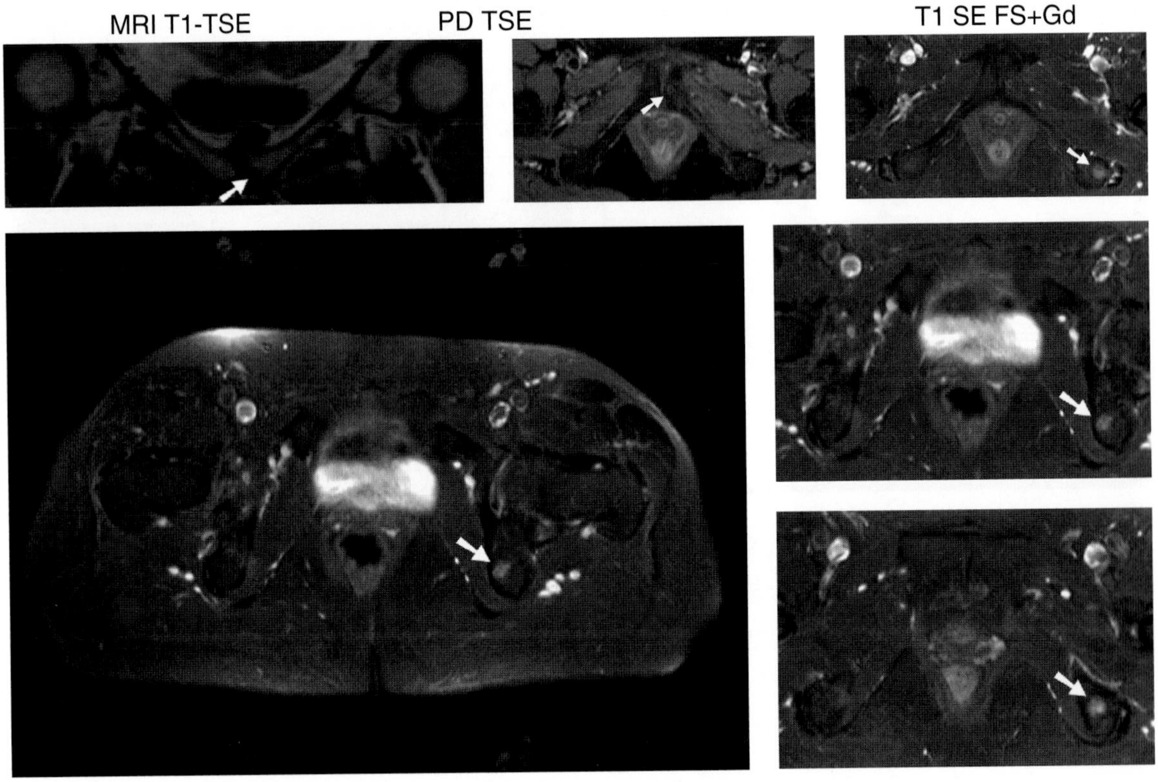

MRI T1-TSE

PD TSE

T1 SE FS+Gd

Teaching point

The high intensity of the ^{18}F-NaF uptake does not sign malignant etiology. MRI is often considered as the noninvasive gold standard for bone metastases. In this case, although it clarifies the pubic lesion as degenerative, it shows additional ischiatic enhanced abnormalities that may be mistaken for bone metastases. This case illustrates the difficulty of reliably assessing all bone lesions, and that MRI is an imaging technology that requires a large expertise. Image artifacts may mimic pathologies as in this case where pulsatility artifacts mimic enhancing lesions if superimposed over the bone.

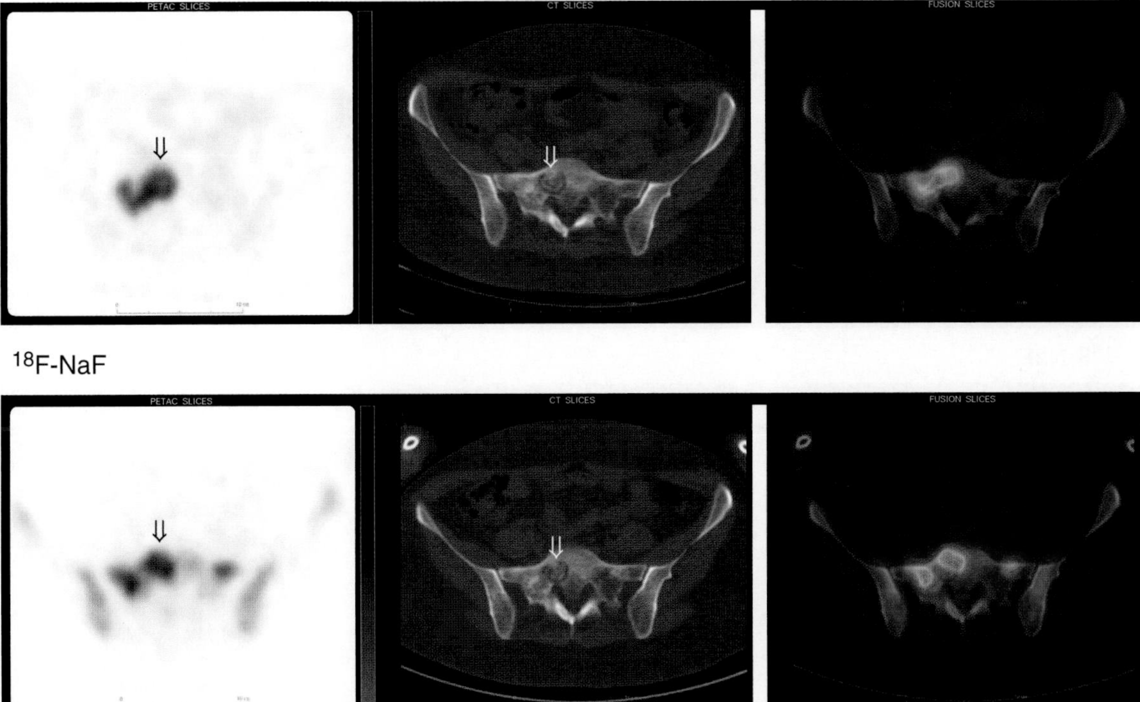

PET finding

There is a mixed lesion of the right sacral ala showing increased uptake of both ^{18}F-NaF (*first row, open arrow*) and FDG (*second row, open arrow*).

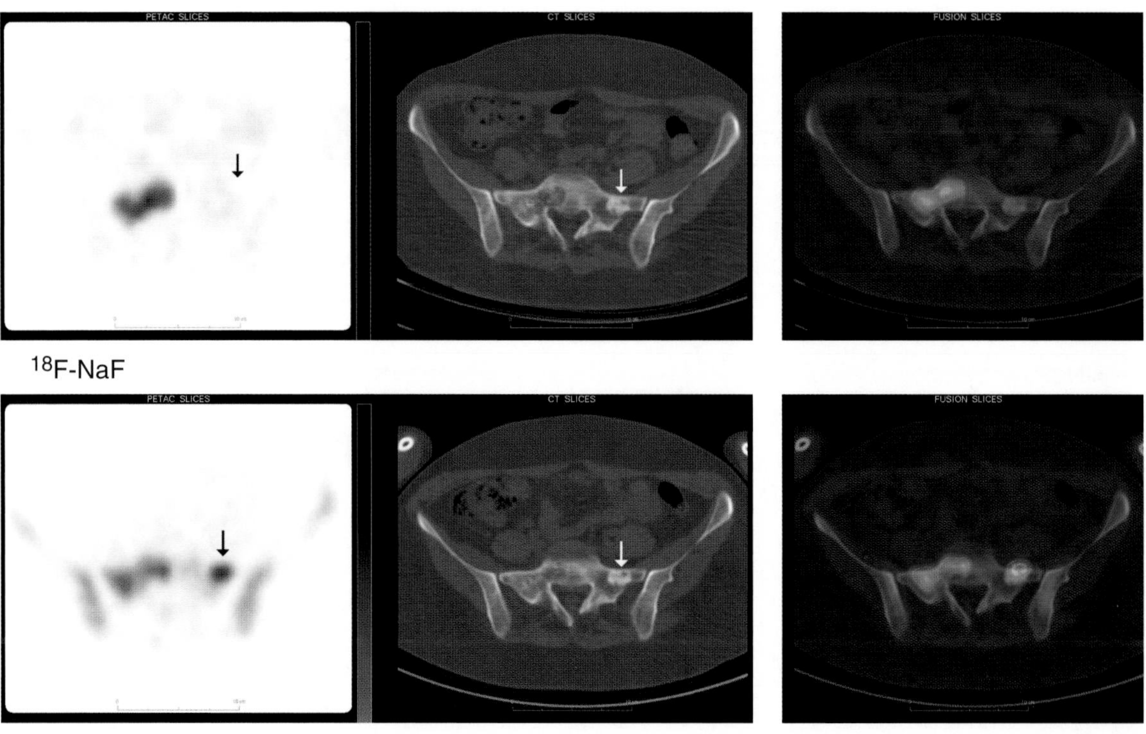

PET finding

In addition, there is a sclerotic lesion of the left side of the sacrum with increased ^{18}F-NaF uptake (*first row*, *arrow*) but negative on the FDG scan. These findings are consistent with bone metastases.

Teaching point

The osteoblastic lesions are sometimes earlier detected by the ^{18}F-NaF PET scan than with the FDG PET as shown on the left sacral ala. The progressive metastatic disease led to therapeutic changes (first line chemotherapy).

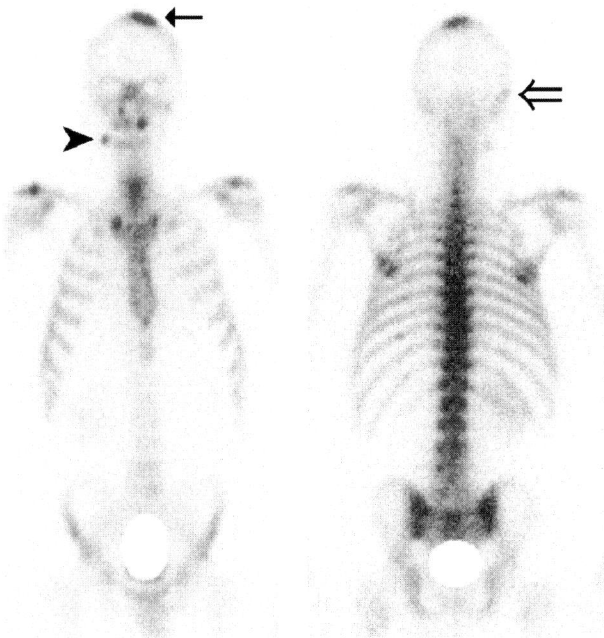

^{99m}Tc-MDP

^{99m}Tc-MDP finding

There are several hot spots over the facial bones and skull, but only one at the top of the skull seems consistent with a metastasis (*arrow*).

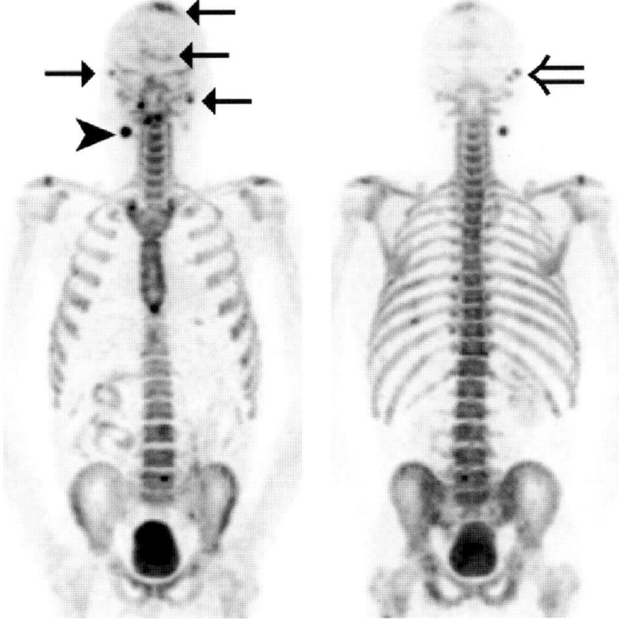

^{18}F-NaF

^{18}F-NaF finding

Several additional hot spots are visualized (*arrows*). The lesion at the top of the skull takes the typical "rosette-like" uptake pattern of a lytic metastasis, which was confirmed by the low-dose CT.

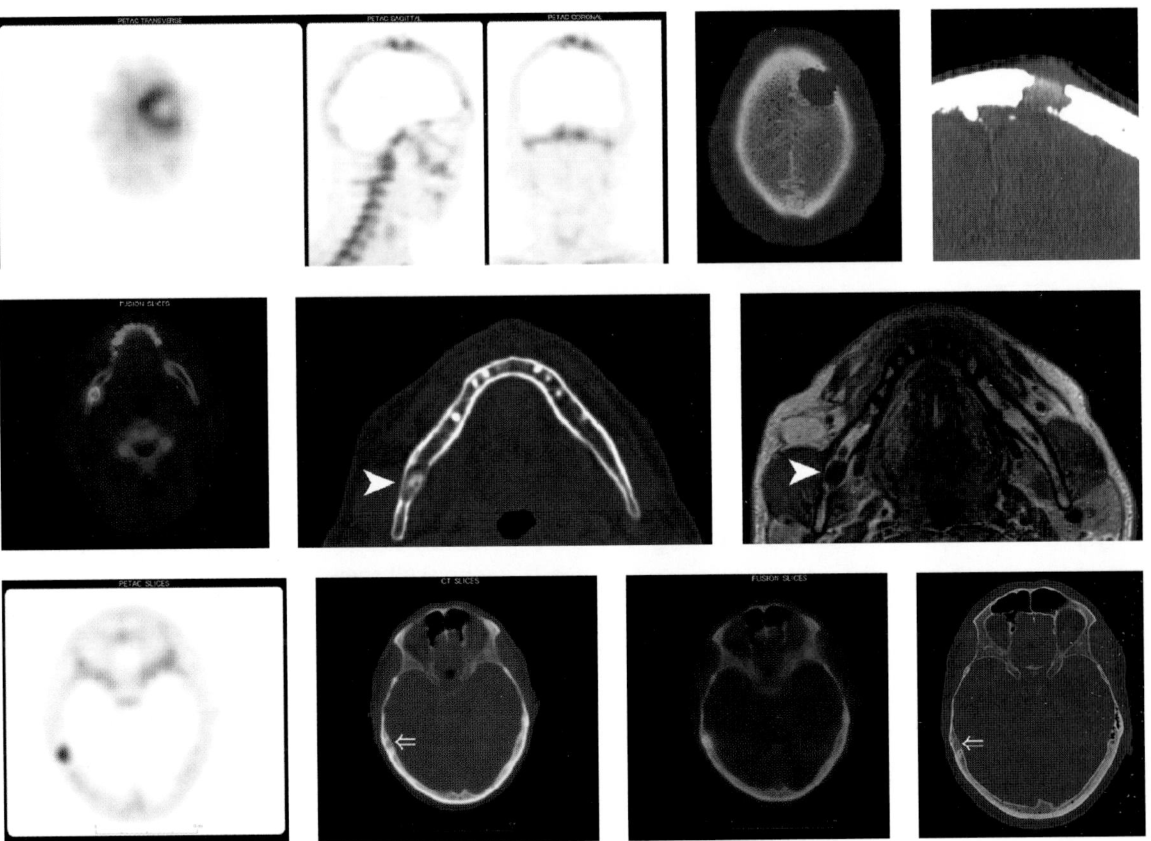

Teaching point

This case illustrates the higher sensitivity of ^{18}F-NaF PET as compared to bone scan, and the added value of low-dose CT. Only the parietal lesion was clearly identified as metastatic with both modalities. The other lesions were missed on the bone scan, although in retrospect some showed a very faint uptake, as the lytic lesions seen in the right occipital bone (*open arrows*). Both the low-dose Ct and the diagnostic Ct studies are shown. Additionally, thanks to the low-dose CT, the right mandibular lesion (*arrow head*) is located behind the last tooth and identified as a sclerotic lesion consistent with fibrous dyslasia, which was confirmed by MRI. Therefore this lesion was depicted as benign, although it was the one showing the highest ^{18}F-NaF uptake. This is a reminder that uptake intensity is not a valid criterion for characterizing abnormal foci.

Chapter 6 Tyrosine PET-CT

Mohsen Farsad and Gabriele Pöpperl

Radiolabeled amino acids are attracting increasing interest in nuclear medicine over the past years mainly because amino acid tracers appear to be more specific than FDG for brain tumor imaging. The uptake of amino acids, especially of O-(2-[F-18]fluoroethyl)-L-tyrosine (FET) (less of MET) in macrophages and other inflammatory cells seems to be lower than FDG.

FET is used as a tumor imaging tracer since 1999. FET accumulates in malignant transformed cells probably, mainly due to increased expression of amino acid transporters and amino acid transport. There is no relevant participation of FET in protein synthesis or any other metabolic pathway. FET uptake is considered to be slightly higher in tumor tissues with than in those without a disrupted blood-brain barrier. Therefore, probably an additional passive influx of FET contributes to the higher FET uptake.

FET is one of the first F-18-labeled amino acids with high radiochemical yields which can be produced in large amounts. Therefore FET is not restricted, unlike the most commonly used amino acid PET tracer C-11-labeled methionine, to a few PET centers with a cyclotron on site and can be distributed in a satellite concept similar to the widely used FDG.

FET shows the highest activities in the urinary tract. All other organs with visible F-18 accumulation have only moderate FET uptake with low standardized uptake values (SUVs). Noticeable is a faint accumulation in the pancreas, skeletal muscles, and the heart which is in the range of the liver uptake. No increased radioactivity uptake is seen in the bones, the bone marrow, the lung parenchyma and the biliary tract. Similar distribution of the tracer can be seen in all organs in late acquisitions (after 3 h post injection). Following tracer injection, normal brain tissue shows a very faint FET uptake which steadily increases up to 1 h. In contrast, high-grade gliomas show an early peak of FET uptake between 5 and 15 min after tracer injection followed by slightly decreasing values up to 40 min after injection. Less aggressive low-grade tumors as well as radiation induced changes behave more like normal brain tissue with increasing FET uptake over time. Therefore, it can be recommended to acquire a series of static limited field tomographic images of 10 min duration each in a time period between 10 and 40 min after injection of FET (180–370 MBq). For the evaluation of time-activity curves, the single time frames may be evaluated, or alternatively dynamic acquisition (list mode) may be performed after injection of the tracer for a time period of 40 min. For semiquantitative evaluation, the most common method is to calculate a tumor to background ratio in a static image (about 20–40 min p.i.).

The main application field of FET PET is brain tumor imaging. In the absence of data from a large series of patients, FET PET seems to have a few emerging useful clinical applications for patients with brain tumors. The most common clinical indication for FET PET brain imaging is the identification of tumor recurrence and differentiation from delayed radiation-induced lesions in patients with unclear findings on morphological imaging. An earliest possible and reliable differentiation is necessary to determine the most appropriate further treatment. While radiation necrosis may be treated by steroids, or in extensive cases, by debulking surgery, recurrent tumor requires continuation of therapy, change of ineffective treatment or palliative care only. Conventional structural imaging methods are of limited value in this setting, since recurrent tumor and posttherapeutic lesions may both appear as mass lesion coming along with edema and contrast enhancement due to a breakdown of the blood brain barrier. FET PET shows a high diagnostic accuracy in this setting (due to a higher specificity compared to conventional MRI) and helps to shorten the time of diagnosis in these patients. Therefore, inclusion of FET PET in the diagnostic workup improves patient management and avoids undertreatment and overtreatment.

An important role has also been suggested for biopsy target definition. Implementation of FET PET in biopsy planning reduces the number of required trajectories in patients with brain tumors, especially in those patients with widespread abnormalities in MRI or lesions located in high risk or functional areas. Metabolic FET PET imaging with fusion techniques enhances the diagnostic yield to assess the metabolically most active and most representative area within the tumor.

Concerning brain tumor delineation which is especially relevant for treatment planning, amino acid tracers are also very helpful and are clearly superior over FDG. Amino acid PET helps to define the optimal volume for percutaneous or stereotactic radiation therapy. Early studies have shown significantly longer survival times following a combined treatment planning concept including functional and morphological information, compared to treatment planning based on morphological data alone.

FET PET seems also to be sensitive enough to assess therapeutic effects early on and to distinguish between harmless reactive lesions induced by different treatment modalities (intralesional radioimmunotherapy, radiation therapy and systemic chemotherapy) and tumor regrowth. Furthermore, decreasing metabolic activity of brain tumors during chemotherapy rather points to a success of therapy while increasing uptake values suggest tumor progression. However, because of few and small-sized studies, the diagnostic reliability of FET PET remains unknown in this setting and deserves further prospective evaluation.

The differential diagnosis of solitary intracerebral lesions with FET PET seems to be less reliable. Some benign lesions such as brain abscesses and demyelinating lesions may show pathological FET accumulation. Moreover, one third of patients with low-grade gliomas do not show increased FET uptake. Therefore, a negative FET PET scan does not exclude a tumor. However, FET PET may depict some high-grade gliomas in unclear lesions with widespread T2 abnormalities in MRI, which based on MRI are classified as low-grade gliomas with the differential diagnosis of an encephalitis/encephalomyelitis.

To avoid potential pitfalls, some uptake characteristics of FET-PET brain imaging should be mentioned. FET concentration in the blood compartment, especially in the early phase but also in the later phase, may be relatively high. Therefore, the visualization of large vessels in the brain, for example, the large venous sinus should not be misinterpreted as pathologic uptake.

Slightly increased and homogeneous FET uptake surrounding the tumor cavity following treatment (surgery and/or radiation therapy) should be attributed to a passive influx of FET. This uptake is usually less intense and more homogeneous compared with the FET uptake in tumor tissue and it is probably caused by benign posttherapeutic changes. This has been attributed mainly to the disruption of the blood-brain barrier induced by benign changes which corresponds, in most cases, to more or less intense contrast enhancement on MRI or CT scans.

FET PET has been also used in other cancers than brain tumors. However, the available preliminary data indicate that the diagnostic performance of FET PET in peripheral tumors is not high enough. In contrast to most cerebral lymphoma or metastases, surprisingly, peripheral lymphoma and also most peripheral adenocarcinomas do not show any FET PET uptake. This might be caused by expression of different subtypes of the amino acid transporter in the brain compared to peripheral organs. Only some head and neck cancers show increased FET accumulation with a somewhat higher specificity, compared to FDG which showed some false-positive results in patients with inflammation. However, the diagnostic sensitivity of FET PET in these patients is lower compared to FDG PET, and therefore, FET PET is not useful for the management of these patients.

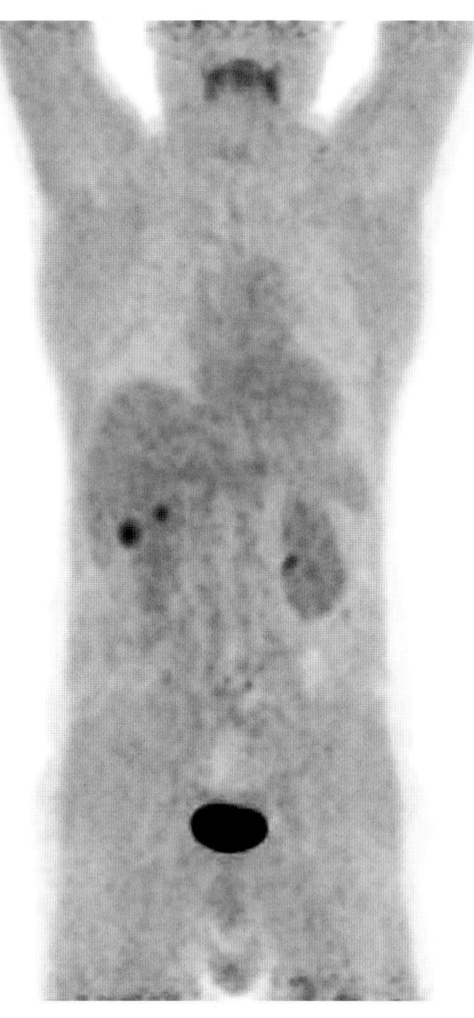

Liver, spleen and stomach uptake

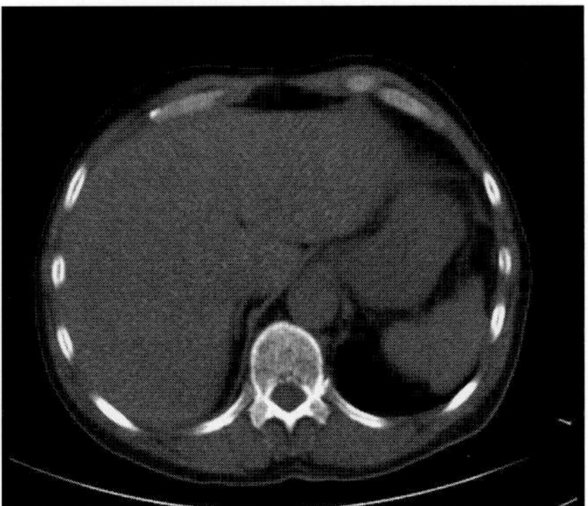

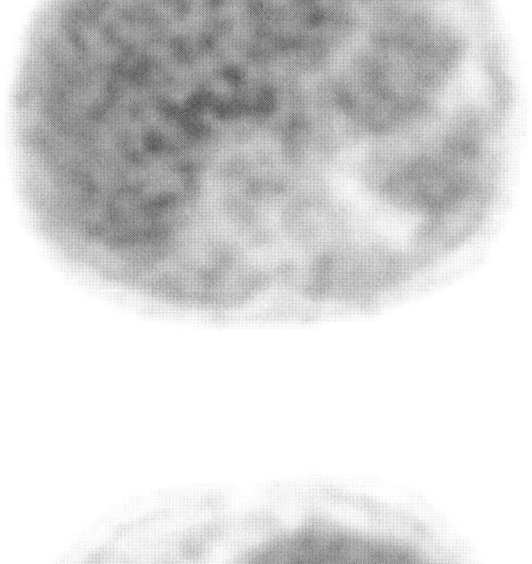

Heart uptake

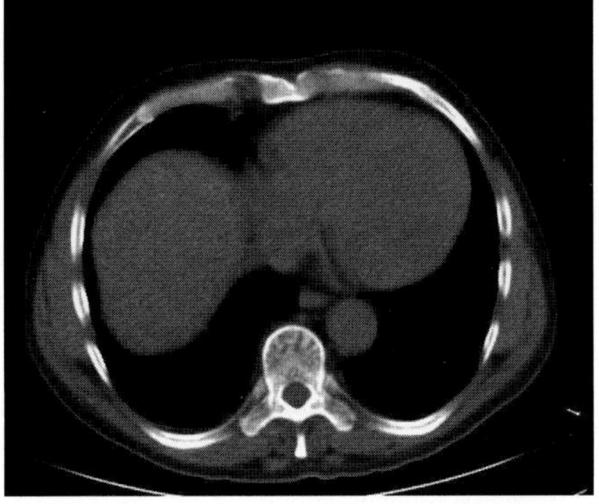

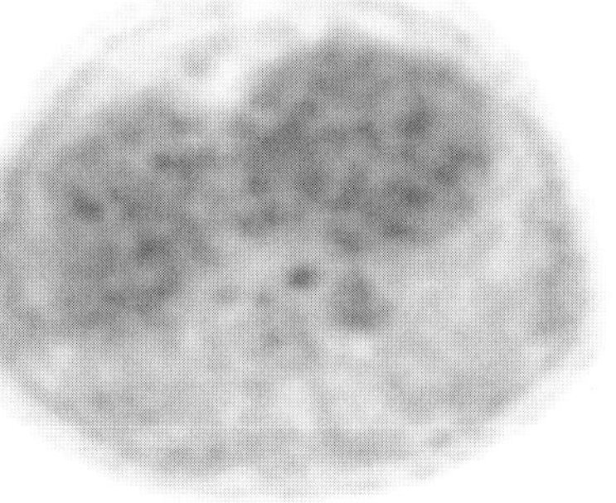

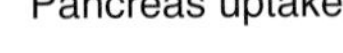

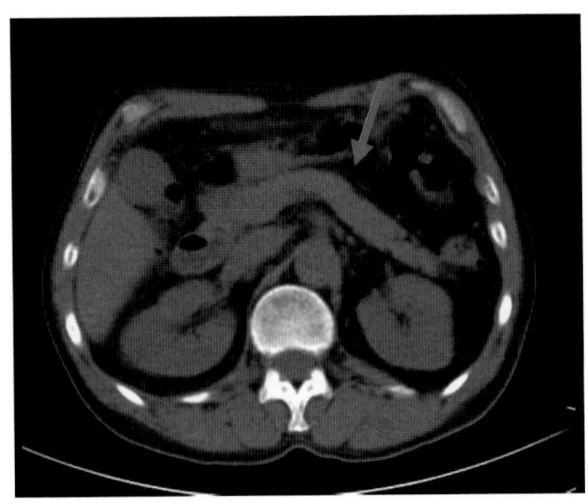

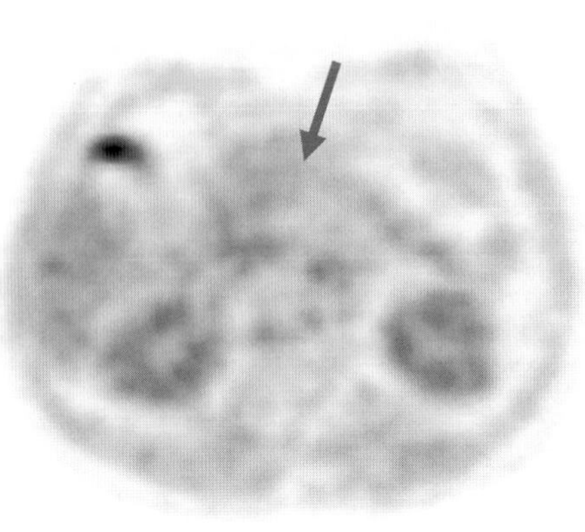

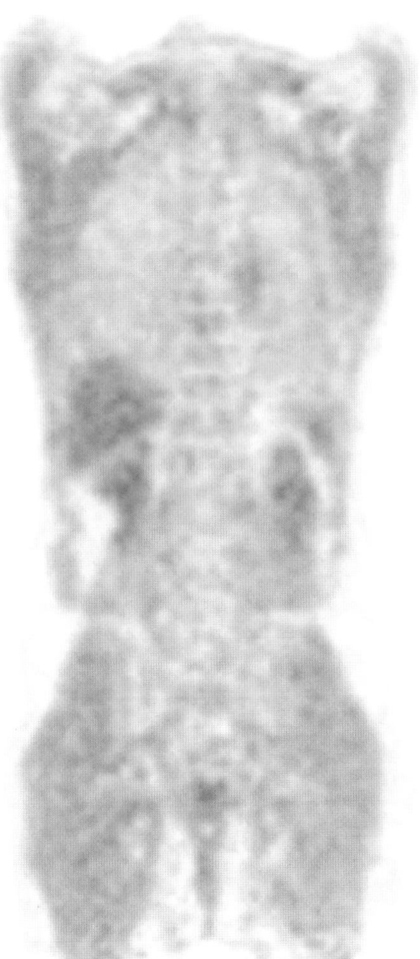

Skeletal muscle uptake

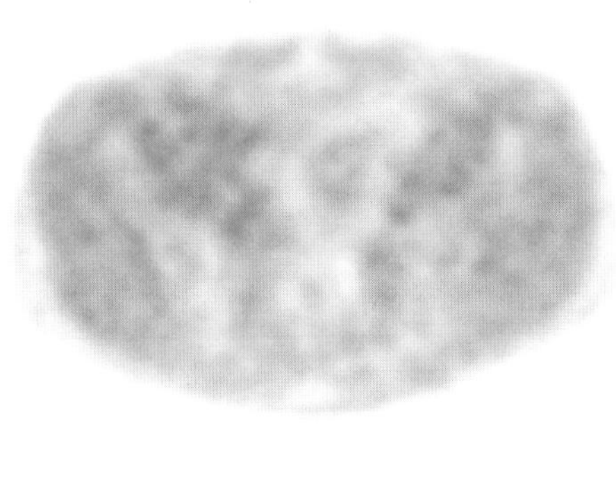

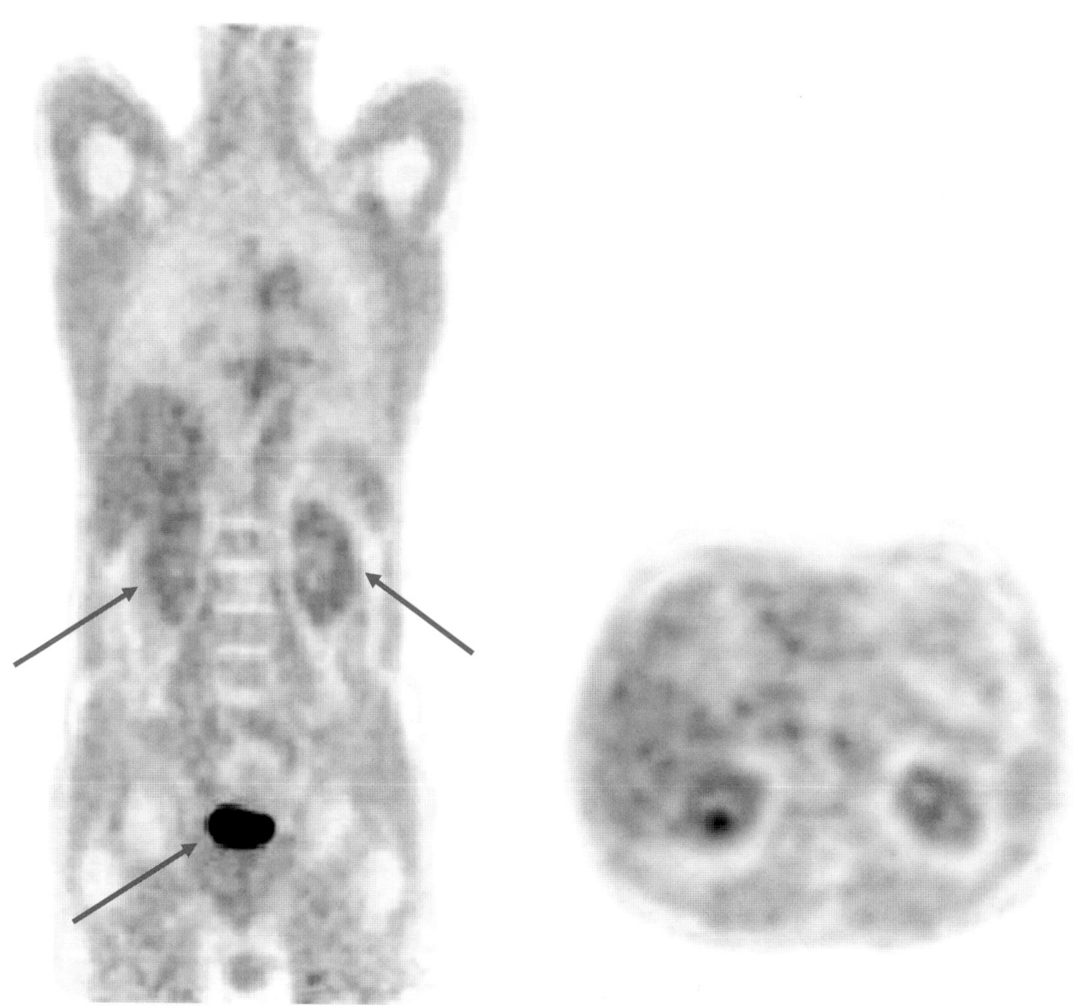

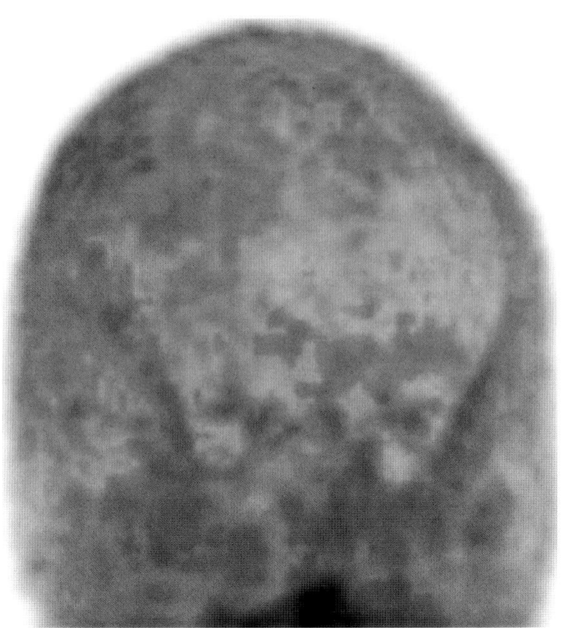

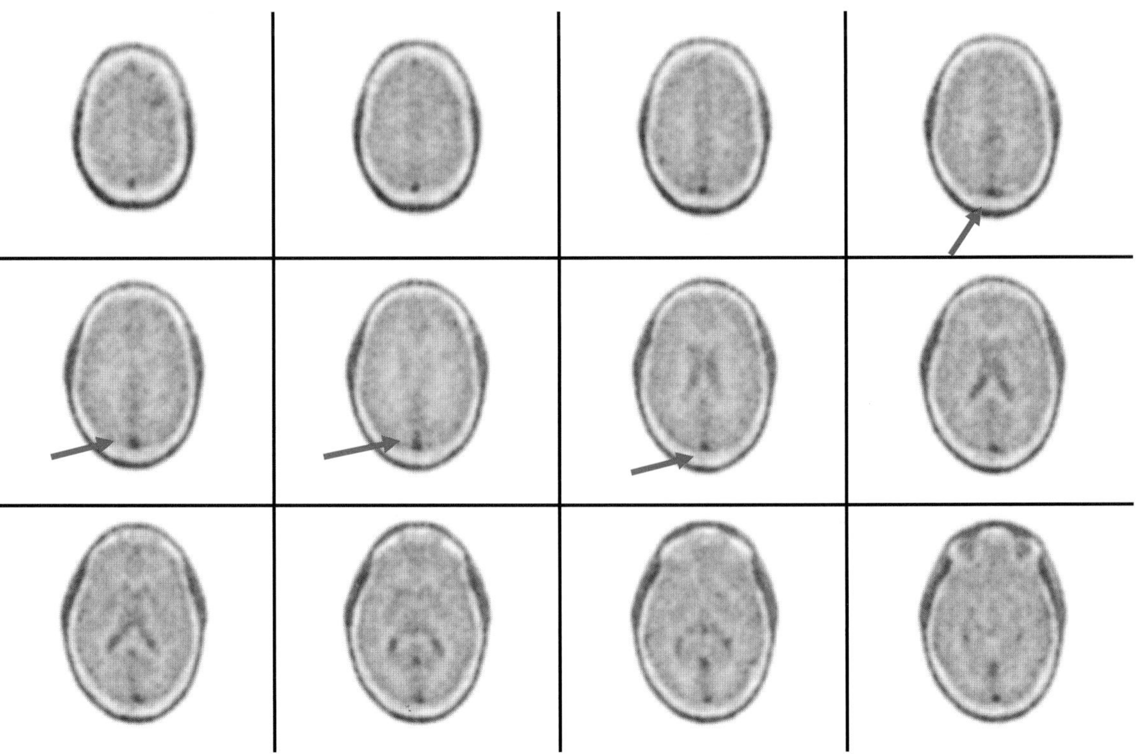
Sinus sagittalis superior

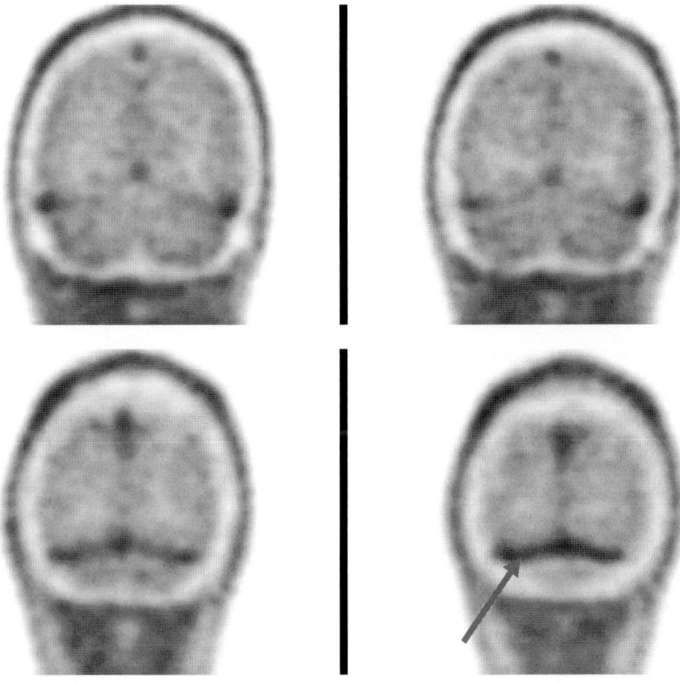

Sinus transversus

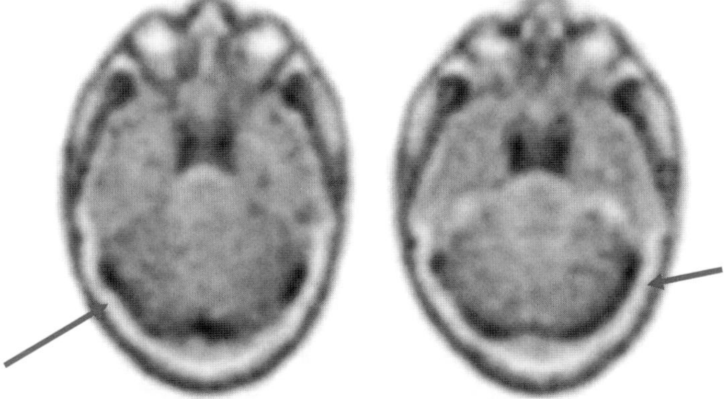

Teaching point

F-ET concentration in the blood compartment is relatively high in the first hour after injection, which could cause visualization of large vessels in the brain, for example, the large venous sinus. This should not lead to misinterpretation in brain tumors especially in the early images.

Female 61 years

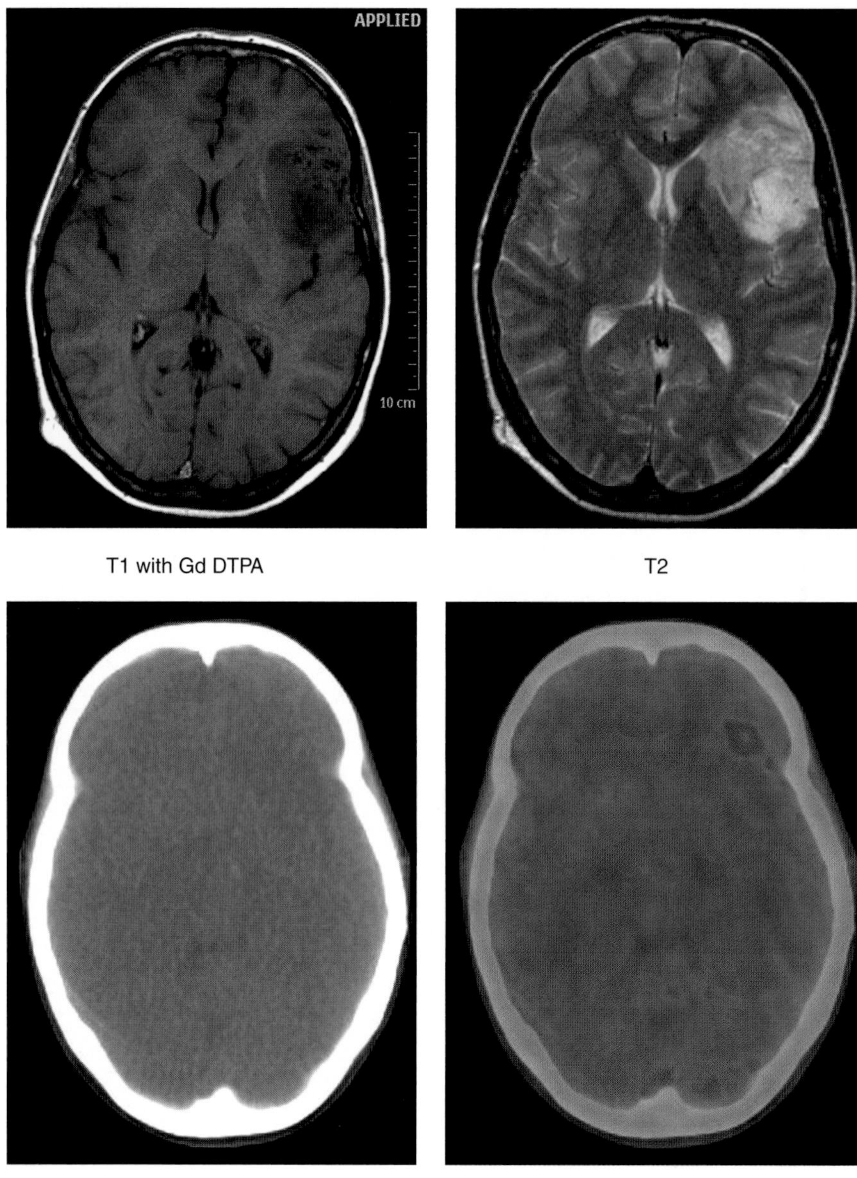

T1 with Gd DTPA

T2

Low dose-CT

Fused PET-CT

MRI finding

MRI confirms low-grade glioma but do not allow to identify any focus transformed to high-grade tumor.

^{18}F-ET finding

^{18}F-ET PET shows a focal area of hypermetabolism (SUV_{max}/BG = 4). This area was confirmed as anaplastic transformation with a relatively higher proliferative index (Ki-67 index = 20%) at stereotactic biopsy.

Female 61 years

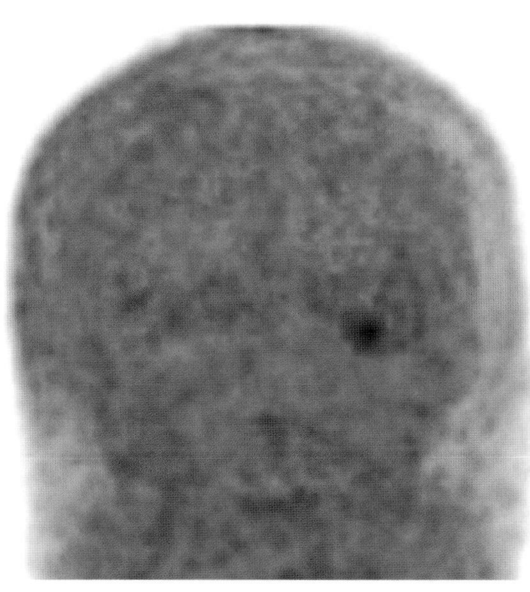

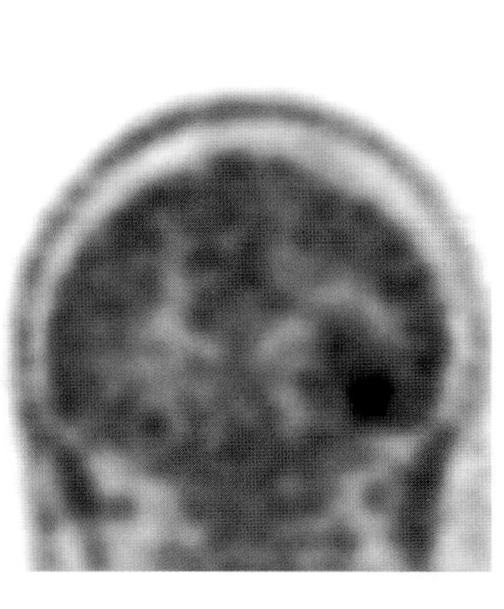

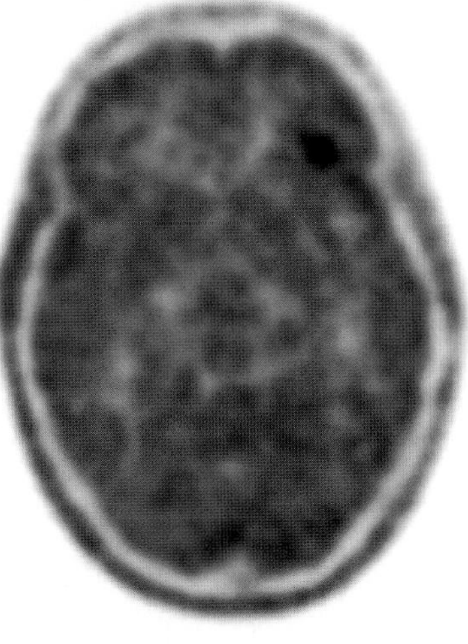

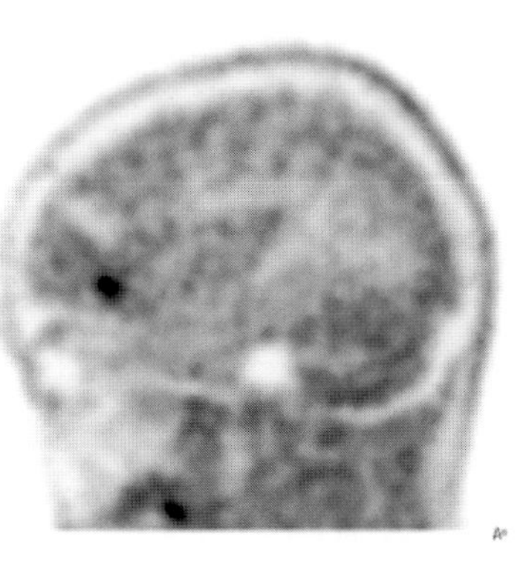

Coronal PET Axial PET sagital PET

Teaching point

Prognosis evaluation of patients with low-grade glioma is clinically very important. In some patients the tumor remains stable for many years while the majority develop tumor growth and progress to high-grade gliomas. ^{18}F-FET PET showed promising results for tumor behavior evaluation of low-grade gliomas.

Male 44 years

T2 T1 with Gd DTPA

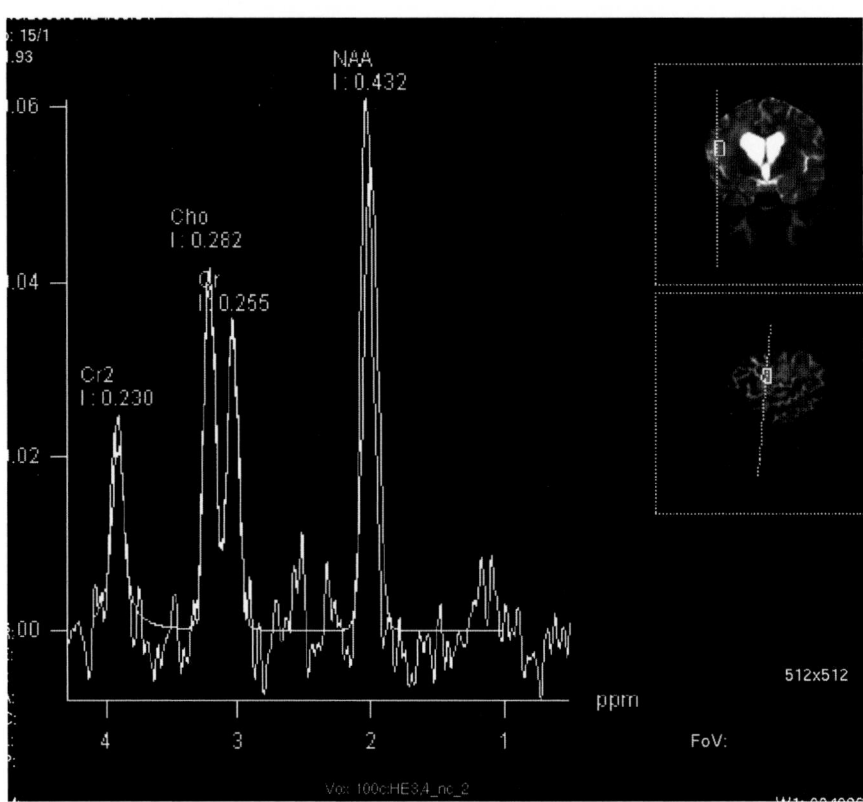

MR finding

MR suspected tumor recurrence.
MR spectroscopy could not confirm tumor recurrence (choline peak not high enough).

Male 44 years

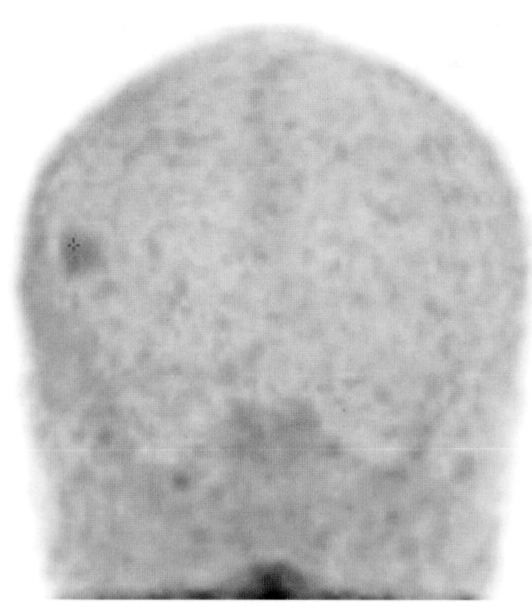

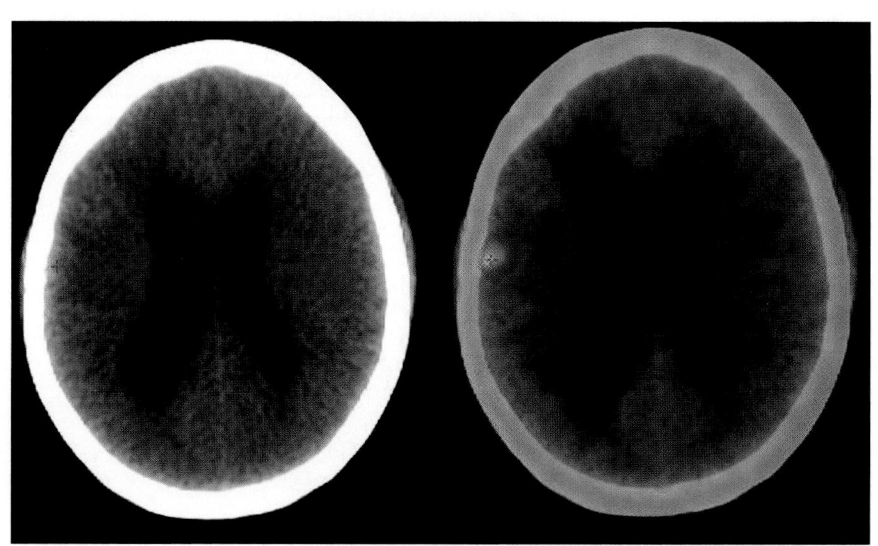

Low dose - CT Fused PET - CT

^{18}F-ET finding

^{18}F-ET PET shows a focal area of hypermetabolism (SUV_{max}/BG = 3.2). This area was confirmed as tumor recurrence at surgery.

Teaching point

^{18}F-ET PET is applied for the identification of tumor recurrence in patients with unclear findings on morphological imaging. ^{18}F-ET PET imaging allows to shorten the time to diagnosis in these patients.

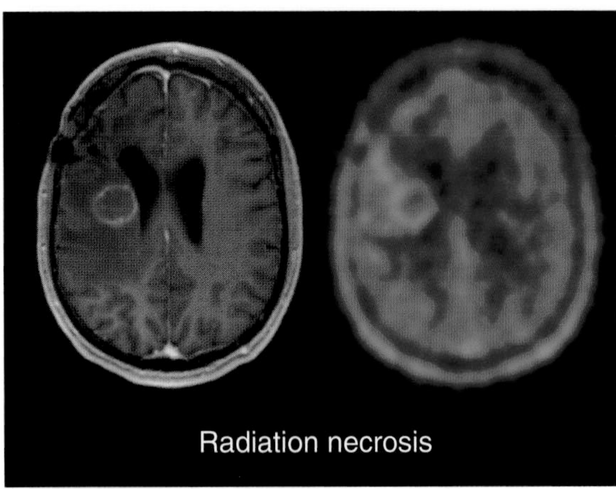

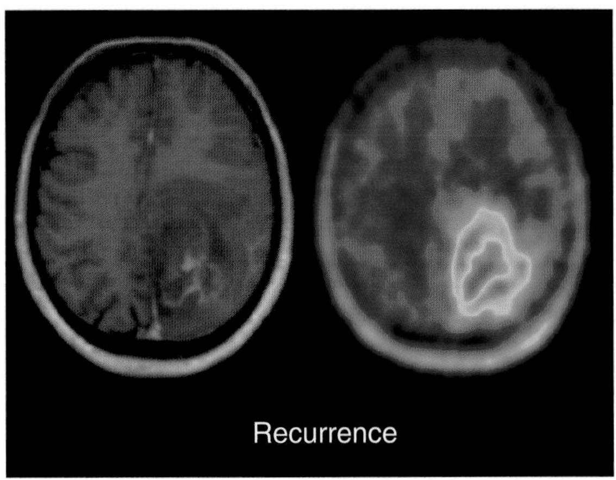

MR finding

MR shows an irregular contrast enhancement with perifocal edema in both cases of glioblastoma following percutaneous radiation therapy.

^{18}F-ET finding

^{18}F-ET PET shows only a slight and homogeneous uptake surrounding the necrotic area caused by a passive influx of F-ET via the disrupted blood brain barrier in case of radiation necrosis (SUV_{max}/BG_{mean}: 1.7). In contrast the histologically confirmed recurrent glioblastoma on the right side shows an intense F-ET uptake (SUV_{max}/BG_{mean}: 3.8).

Teaching point

^{18}F-ET PET is applied for the identification of tumor recurrence and differentiation from radiation induced benign changes in patients with unclear contrast enhancement in MRI following radiation therapy. ^{18}F-ET PET Imaging allows to determine the most appropriate treatment in these patients.

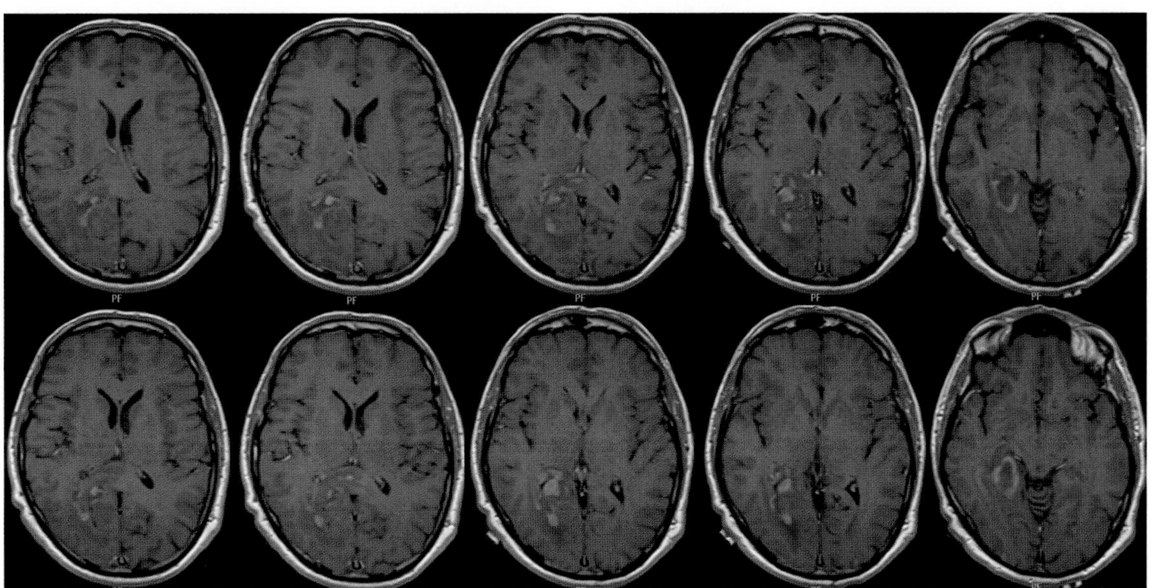

T1 with Gd DTPA

MR finding

MR shows widespread abnormalities on the right occipito-temporal and meso-temporal regions.

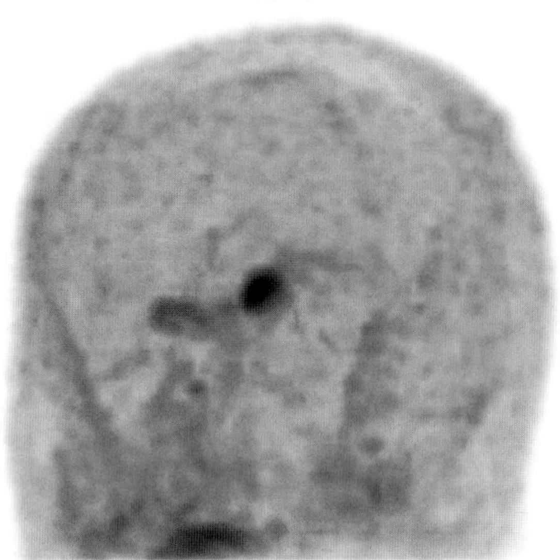

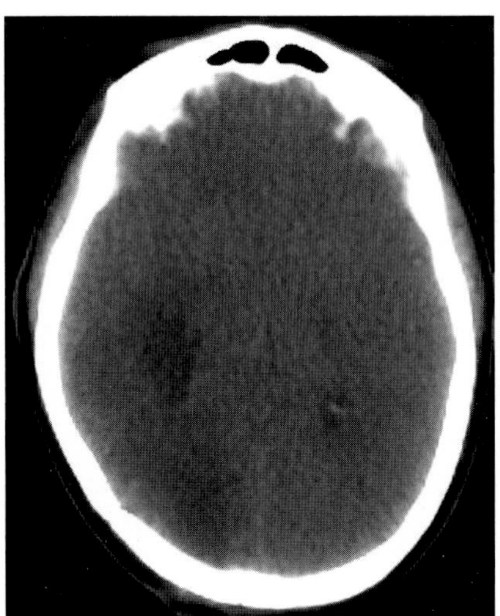

Low dose - CT

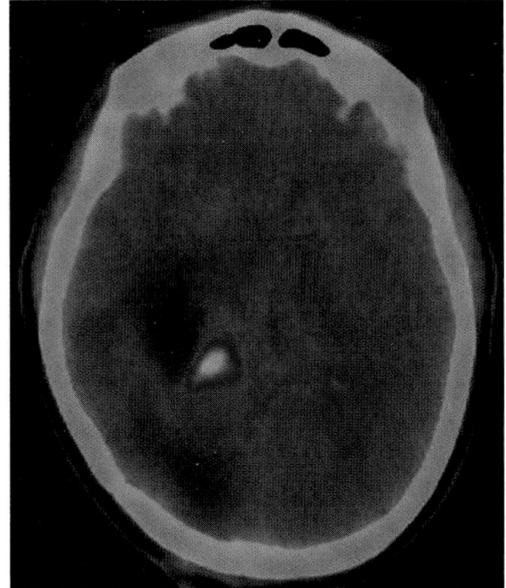

Fused PET - CT

^{18}F-ET finding

^{18}F-ET PET shows a focal area of pathologic uptake. Metabolic guided biopsy revealed high grade glioma.

Teaching point

^{18}F-ET PET is very helpful to identify the tumor tissue in diffuse gliomas with widespread abnormalities in MR. To enhance the diagnostic yield, metabolic imaging with fusion techniques may be useful for biopsy target definition.

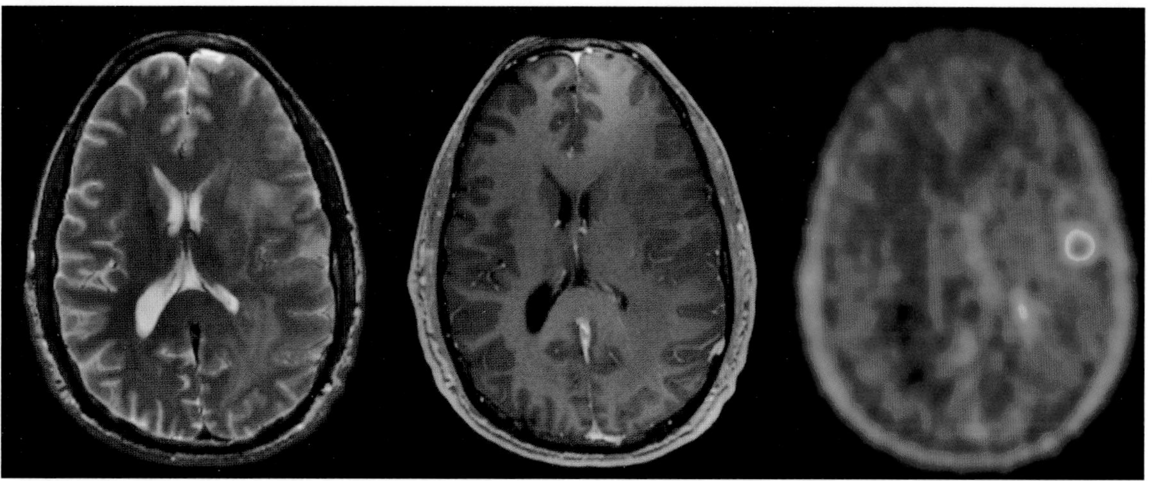

MR finding

MR shows widespread and diffuse T2 abnormalities in the left hemisphere without showing a solid lesion or any contrast enhancement pointing to a malignant tumor. Findings were rated unclear with differential diagnosis of encephalomyelitis (ADEM) vs. diffuse low grade astrocytoma.

^{18}F-ET finding

^{18}F-ET PET shows slightly increased uptake within the widespread lesion with a clear metabolic focus. PET guided biopsy taken from this area revealed an anaplastic astrocytoma in this area.

Teaching point

^{18}F-ET PET is very helpful to identify tumor tissue within widespread diffuse lesions showing only T2 hyperintensites in MRI. In this case F-ET PET was clearly superior to conventional MRI to establish the diagnosis of a brain tumor and to define the most reliable target volume.

Female 54 years

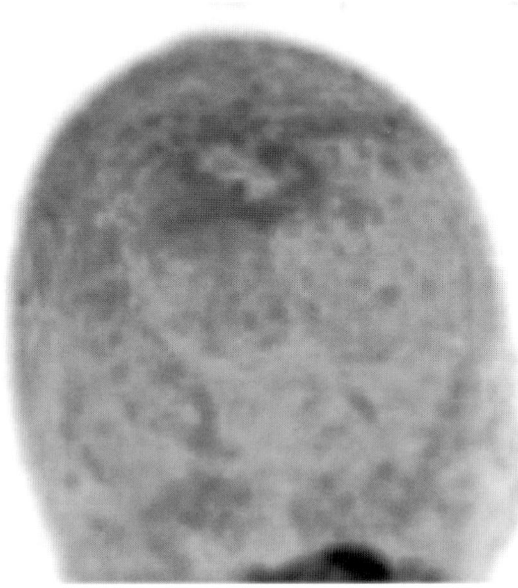

^{18}F-ET finding

Mild ^{18}F-ET uptake surrounding the surgical cavity.

Teaching point

Pretreated patients may demonstrate slightly increased F-ET uptake surrounding the tumor cavity. The uptake is less intense and shows a more homogeneous pattern compared with the F-ET uptake in tumor tissue. Quantitative evaluation (tumor/background ratio), in addition to visual assessment, may be helpful to reliably distinguish between uptake, indicating tumor recurrence and uptake representing therapy-induced alterations.

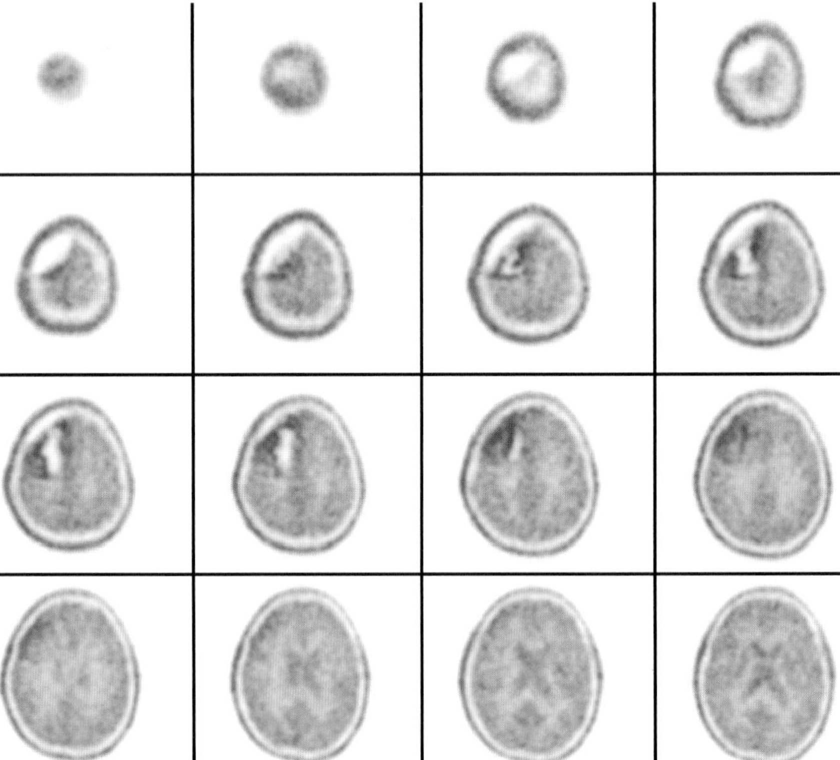

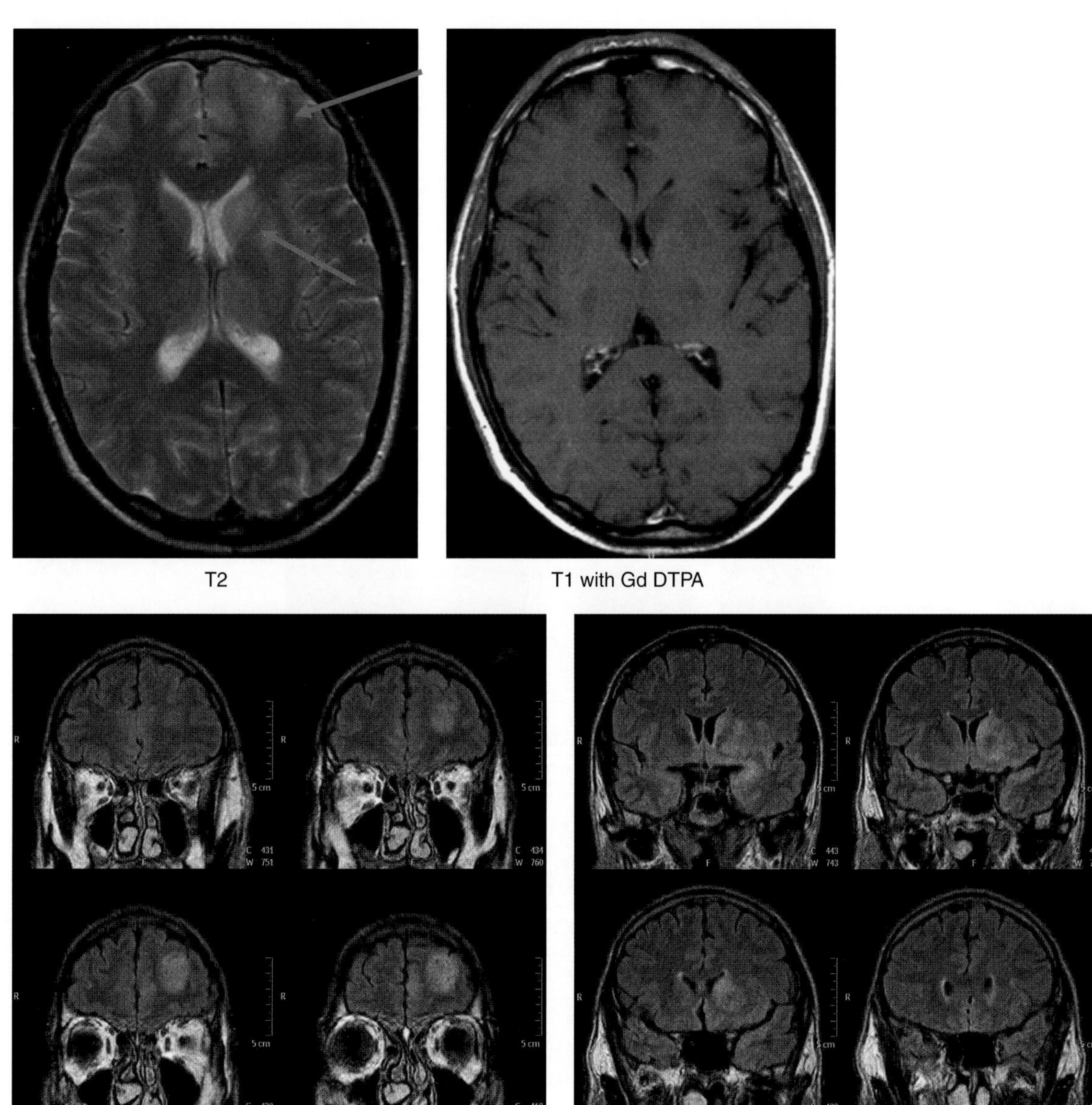

T2

T1 with Gd DTPA

TIRM

TIRM

MR finding

MR shows multifocal areas of abnormal signal in the left frontal region, left basal ganglia, and temporal cortex without contrast enhancement on T1 with Gd DTPA. (Tumor? Postencephalitic disorders?)

Male 47 years

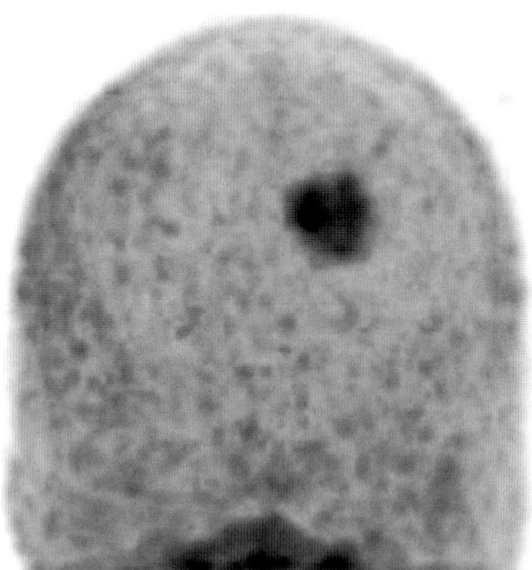

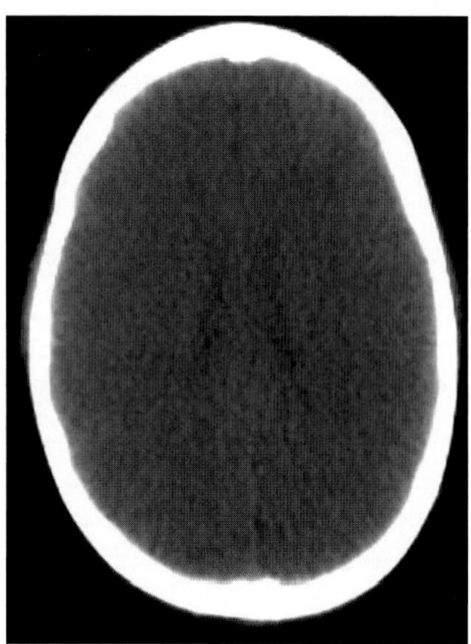

Low dose - CT

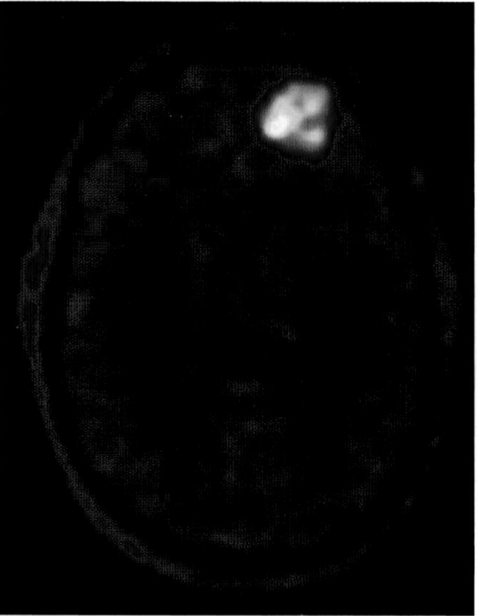

Fused PET - CT

^{18}F-ET finding

^{18}F-ET PET shows only one focal area of hypermetabolism in the left frontal region confirmed at surgery as glioblastoma. The other regions turned out to be postencephalitic alterations.

Teaching point

^{18}F-ET PET may be helpful to clarify doubtful findings at conventional Imaging. Areas with intense ^{18}F-ET uptake result to be highly suspicious for malignant lesions and need to be further investigated.

Chapter 7 Somatostatin Receptor PET-CT

Valentina Ambrosini, Paolo Castellucci, GianCarlo Montini, and Stefano Fanti

Somatostatin receptor PET-CT employs positron emitting tracers (68Ga-DOTA-peptides) that specifically bind to somatostatin receptors (ssr) expressed on tumor cell surface and has been used mainly for the assessment of neuroendocrine tumors (NETs). NETs derive from neuroendocrine cells widely dispersed in the human body and present an increased expression of ssr, particularly of ssr2. 68Ga-DOTA-peptides are very accurate for the assessment of well-differentiated NETs, since being slow-growing tumors, they are not clearly visualized on 18F-FDG PET-CT scans.

Several different somatostatin analogues derived from octreotide, lanreotide, or vapreotide (DOTA-TOC, DOTA-TATE, DOTA-NOC) have been employed in the clinic. The most relevant difference among the various compounds is the variable binding affinity to ssr-subtypes. Although DOTA-TOC, DOTA-TATE, and DOTA-NOC can bind to ssr2, the predominant receptor-type in NET, and to ssr5, only 68Ga-DOTA-NOC presents also a good affinity for ssr3.

At present, there are no published studies directly comparing 68Ga-DOTA-peptides for the assessment of NET or papers investigating if ssr-subtypes expression differences on tumor cells are related to any specific clinical setting. However, considering the more favorable dosimetry and the wider ssr-subtypes spectrum affinity, 68Ga-DOTA-NOC seems to be the most promising tracer for NET imaging.

68Ga-peptides present several technical and biological advantages for NET PET imaging, compared to other commonly used tracers (such as 18F-FDG and 18F-DOPA) and to SRS (somatostatin receptor scintigraphy).

First of all, the synthesis and labeling process is quite easy and economic. Gallium can be easily eluted from a commercially available Ge-68/Ga-68 generator, therefore not requiring an on-site cyclotron. 68Gallium ($t1/2 = 68$ min) presents an 89% positron emission and negligible gamma emission (1,077 keV) of 3.2%. The long half life of the mother radionuclide 68Ge (270.8 days) makes it possible to use the generator for approximately 9–12 months depending upon the requirement, rendering the whole procedure relatively economic. In particular, for 68Ga-DOTA-NOC, a radio-labeling yields of >95% can usually be achieved within 15 min and 300–700 MBq of 68Ga DOTA-NOC can be obtained within 20 min.

68Ga-DOTA-peptides PET-CT technical procedure consists of the intravenous administration of approximately 100 MBq (75–250 MBq) of the radiolabeled peptide (such as 68Ga-DOTA-NOC, DOTA-TOC, etc). Image acquisition usually starts after an uptake time of 60 min (30–180 min). DOTA-peptides are primarily excreted through the kidneys. 68Ga-DOTA-NOC physiologic uptake areas include the pituitary gland, the spleen, the liver, the adrenal glands, the head of the pancreas, the thyroid (very mild uptake), and the urinary tract (kidneys and urinary bladder). Some centers require somatostatin analogue treatments to be interrupted before PET. A better visualization of gastro-entero-pancreatic tumors can be achieved by oral pre-medication with gastrografin.

A 68Ga-DOTA-peptides PET-CT scan is a single-day examination that can be performed in a couple of hours, being more patient friendly than SRS.

Another advantage of 68Ga-peptides is that they directly bind to ssr and provide an indirect measure of tumor cell differentiation (ssr are expressed in well-differentiated forms), offering data not only on disease extension but also on tumor cell receptor expression status, particularly relevant before starting targeted nuclide therapy.

Indications to perform 68Ga-DOTA-peptides PET-CT in NET cases include disease staging/re-staging, detection of unknown primary tumor sites, selection of patients candidated to nuclide therapy and evaluation of treatment response.

NET Staging and Re-Staging

68Ga-DOTA-TOC was the first compound to be used to assess NET patients: in 2001 Hofmann reported a higher detection rate for DOTA-TOC as compared to 111In-octreotide-scinitgraphy.

The largest patient population studied by 68Ga-DOTA-TOC PET was reported by Gabriel et al. in 2006: 84 patients with NET were studied with PET, SRS, and CT. Sensitivity and specificity for the different imaging modalities were compared with each other and clinical follow up and histology were used as standard of reference. PET sensitivity was significantly higher than SRS and CT (97 vs. 52 vs. 61% respectively) with an overall accuracy of 96% for PET, 58% for SRS, and 63% for CT. In particular, PET with 68Ga-DOTA-TOC was superior to the other imaging modalities for the detection of NET lesions at bone and node level.

In the same year, in a limited population of 15 cases, PET with 68Ga-DOTA-TOC was used to select patients with tumors expressing ssr that were therefore initiated to nuclide therapy.

Although the experience with 68Ga-DOTA-NOC PET-CT is less extensive, recent studies on limited populations report its higher sensitivity compared to CT and its relevant impact on patient management. In a series of 11 patients with bronchial carcinoid, studied for staging and re-staging, PET-CT findings were concordant with c.e. CT in only 3/11 cases; of the remaining 8 cases, PET-CT detected a higher number of lesions in 5/8, and excluded malignancy at sites reported as positive on c.e. CT in 3 patients. In the majority of cases, 68Ga-DOTA-NOC PET allowed the detection of a higher number (37 vs. 21) of tumor lesions, in particular at lymph nodes, liver, and bone level. The authors concluded that PET contributed to a better evaluation of disease extent, and to a change in the clinical management of 3 patients.

In the literature, there is only one paper directly comparing 68Ga-DOTA-NOC and 18F-DOPA findings in NET patients: although the studied population was small, 68Ga-DOTA-NOC identified more lesions than 18F-DOPA (71 vs. 45), especially at liver, lung, and lymph node level. 68Ga-DOTA-NOC was also more sensitive for the detection of lesions at pancreatic/peripancreatic level, known sites of increased 18F-DOPA uptake.

A more recent paper, published online ahead of print, compared 68Ga-DOTA-TATE PET with 18F-DOPA PET. Also using 68Ga-DOTA-TATE, PET detected a higher number of metastatic lesions (54 of 55 positive metastatic tumor regions) than 18F-DOPA (29 of 55).

Overall, 68Ga-DOTA-peptides are accurate for staging and restaging of well-differentiated NETs or forms presenting a high ssr-expression. In this clinical setting, 68Ga-DOTA-NOC seems to be the most interesting tracer for the wider ssr affinity range, the favorable dosimetry, and the easy and economic synthesis process.

Detection of the Site of the Unknown Primary Tumor

The identification of the unknown primary tumor site (CUP) is another indication to perform 68Ga-DOTA-peptide PET-CT. In fact, conventional imaging procedures fail to detect the primary tumor site in almost one third of cases (20–27%). Therefore patients with biopsy-proven secondary NET lesions and negative physical examination, laboratory tests and conventional imaging procedures (including chest X-ray, abdominal and pelvic CT, mammography in women, etc.) should be addressed to 68Ga-DOTA-peptides PET-CT. From a clinical point of view, the identification of the primary tumor site is crucial to choose the most appropriate line of therapy intervention.

Until today, no studies addressing this issue have been published, due to the very recent introduction of PET-CT for the detection of NET.

Considering the very good results obtained using PET-CT for NET staging/restaging with 68Ga-DOTA-peptides and the good accuracy documented for PET with FDG for the detection of primary tumors of other histologies, PET-CT with 68Ga-peptides seems to be a potentially useful tool for the detection of the primary site in patients bearing NE metastasis.

Evaluation of the Response to Therapy

18F-FDG PET is routinely used for the assessment of patients during and after therapy for the early detection of therapy response.

Regarding NET, although good results have been obtained using cold or targeted somatostatin analogues for treatment, the studies published until now used clinical parameters as standard of reference to assess therapy response. To our knowledge, there are no studies evaluating the role of PET in this particular clinical setting.

However, considering the high accuracy of PET for the detection of NET and for the selection of patients' candidate for targeted therapy, PET will be more and more used with this indication.

Patients Selection to Targeted Therapies

Surgical resection and cold somatostatin analogues represent the main stain treatment for NET, while targeted radionuclide therapies have been increasingly used as a third-line treatment option.

As stated before, 68Ga-DOTA-peptides PET-CT scan provides not only information on the disease extension but also indicates patients who present a high ssr expression on tumor cells; therefore, PET is crucial to identify patients who will more likely respond to targeted therapy (either with cold somatostatin analogues or with peptide radionuclide targeted therapy).

Moreover, the semi-quantitative and visual interpretation of the uptake of 68Ga-DOTA-NOC measured by PET-CT is used to guide the quantity of radiation and the timing for targeted radionuclide therapy (using 177Lu or 90YDOTA-TOC). In this setting, 68Ga-DOTA-NOC represents an indispensable procedure before planning-targeted treatment.

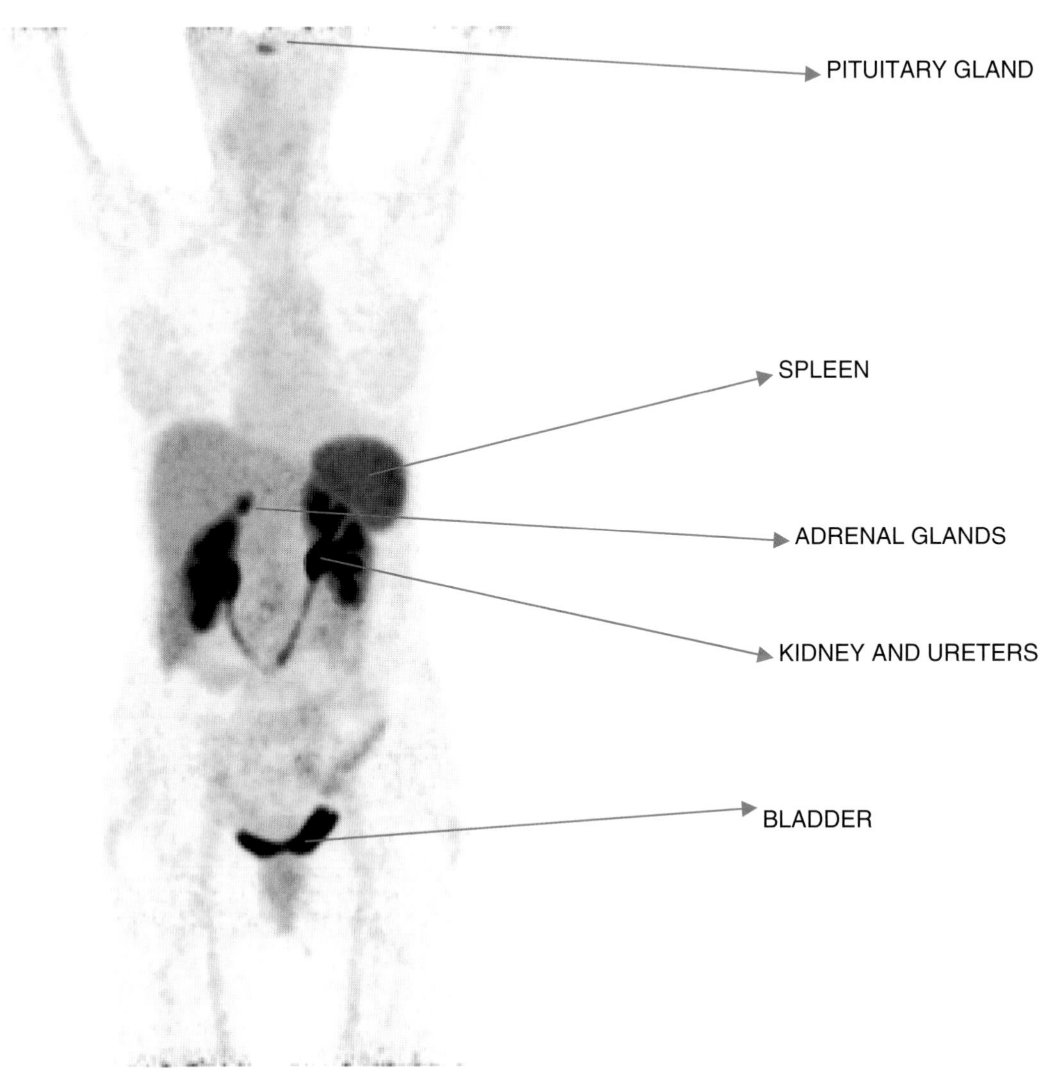

Teaching point

The uptake within the spleen is diffuse and more intense than in the liver.

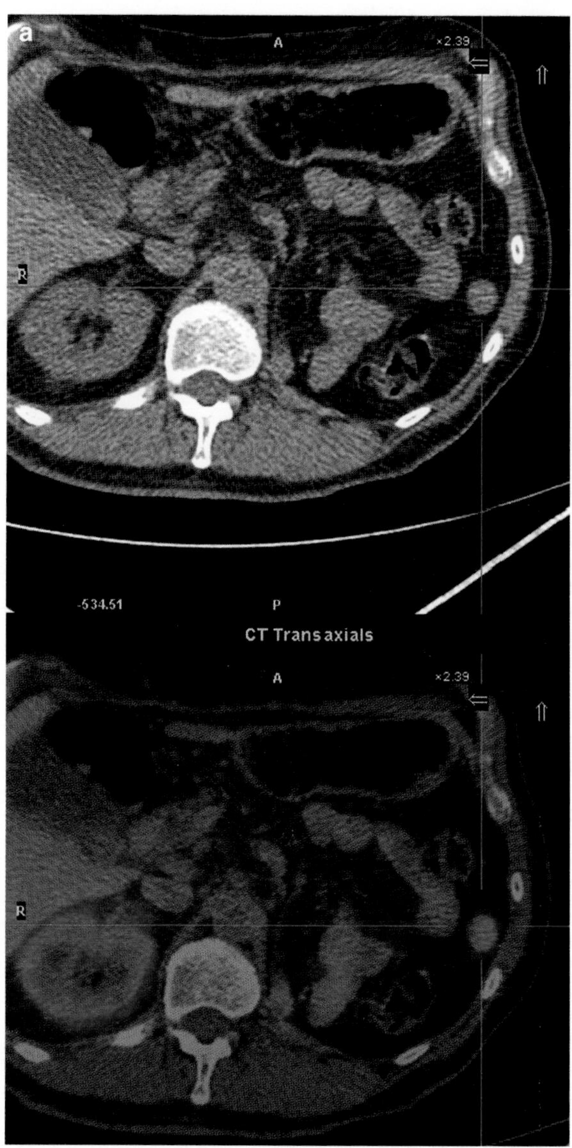

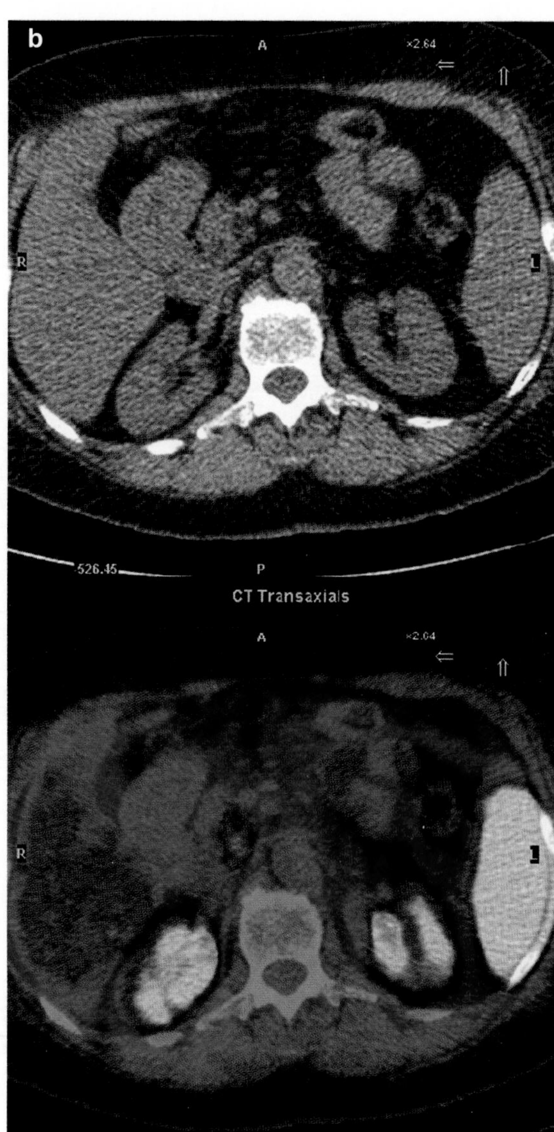

^{68}Ga-DOTA-NOC finding

Mild ^{68}Ga-DOTA-NOC uptake can occur in accessory spleen (a) and pancreatic head and should not be interpreted falsely as secondary uptake.

Teaching point

Some evident uptake in the pancreatic head can be observed in 20–50% of cases, it has to be considered when a mass is known or suspected at this level. The physiologic uptake is less intense and not focal.

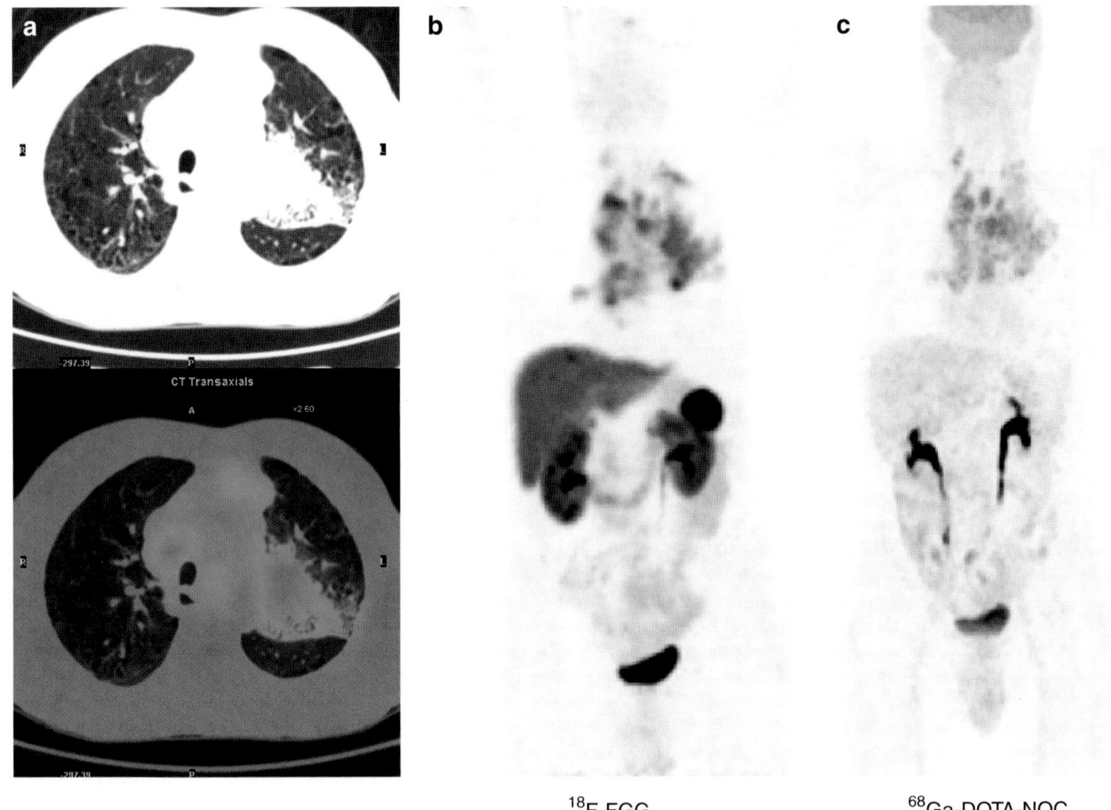

PET findings

Patient with sarcoidosis studied with ^{68}Ga-DOTA-NOC PET (a: transaxial, b: MIP) and with ^{18}F-FDG PET/CT (c). Increased tracer uptake is present in both scans.

Teaching point

Teaching point: activated lymphocytes present an increased ^{68}Ga-DOTA-NOC uptake due to ssr expression. Therefore, chronic inflammation may interfere with correct ^{68}Ga-DOTA-NOC image interpretation.

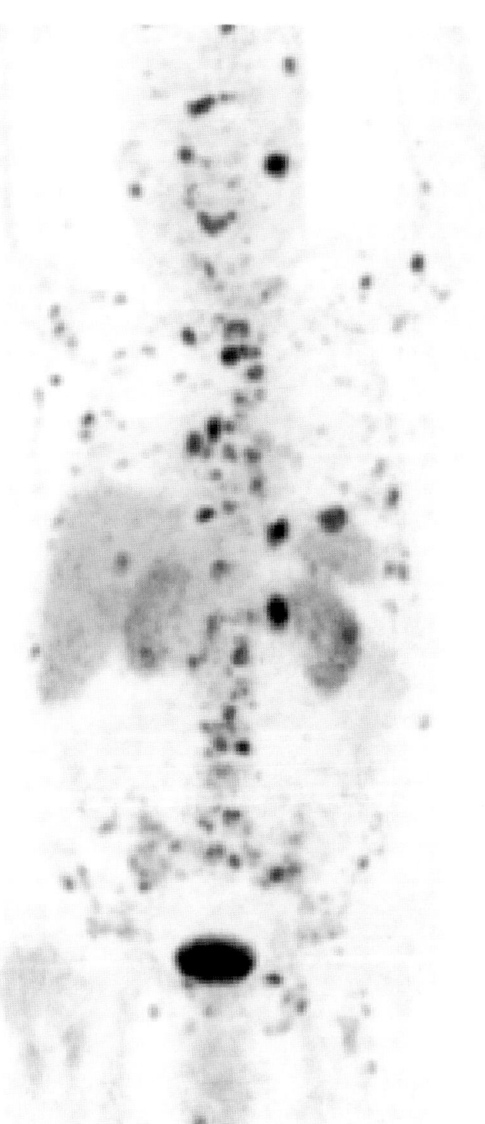

^{68}Ga-DOTA-NOC finding

Patient with bronchial carcinoid and diffuse secondary lesions; lesions at bones (a, b, d), liver (c), brain, optic nerves, bone marrow (f), nodes (b), right testicule.

Teaching point

PET-CT allows the detection of very small-sized lesions.

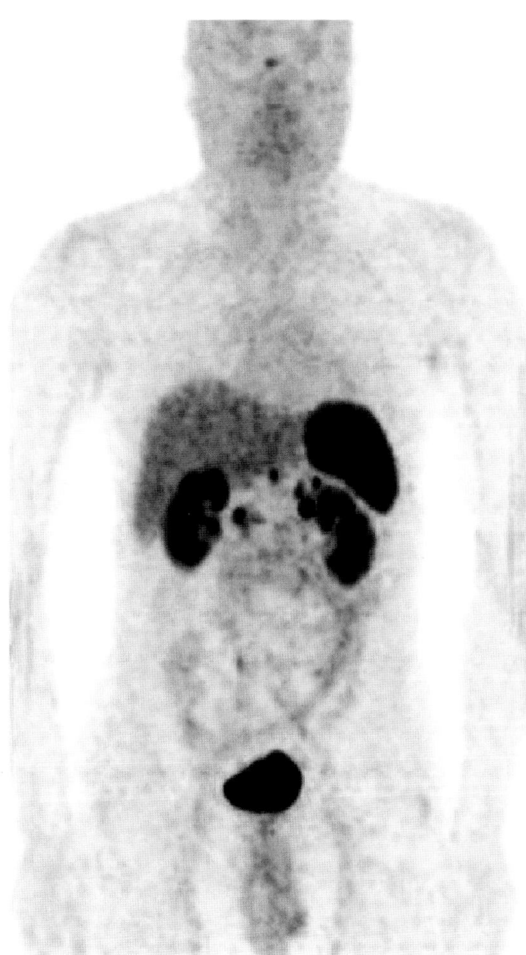

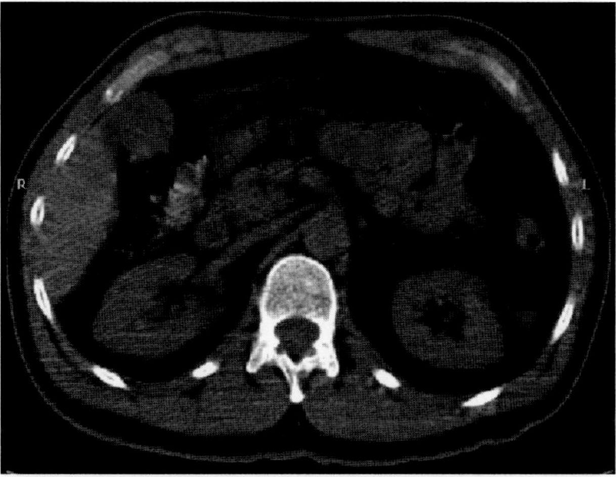

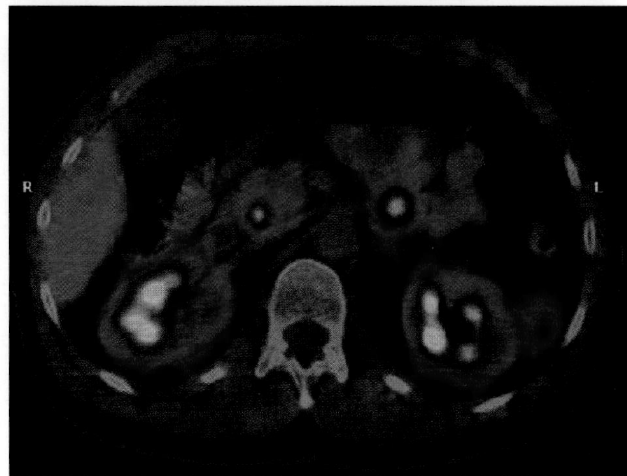

^{68}Ga-DOTA-NOC finding

PET-CT shows the primary NET and some secondary peripancreatic lymph nodes.

Teaching point

Somatostatin receptor PET has a high sensitivity also for small primary lesions.

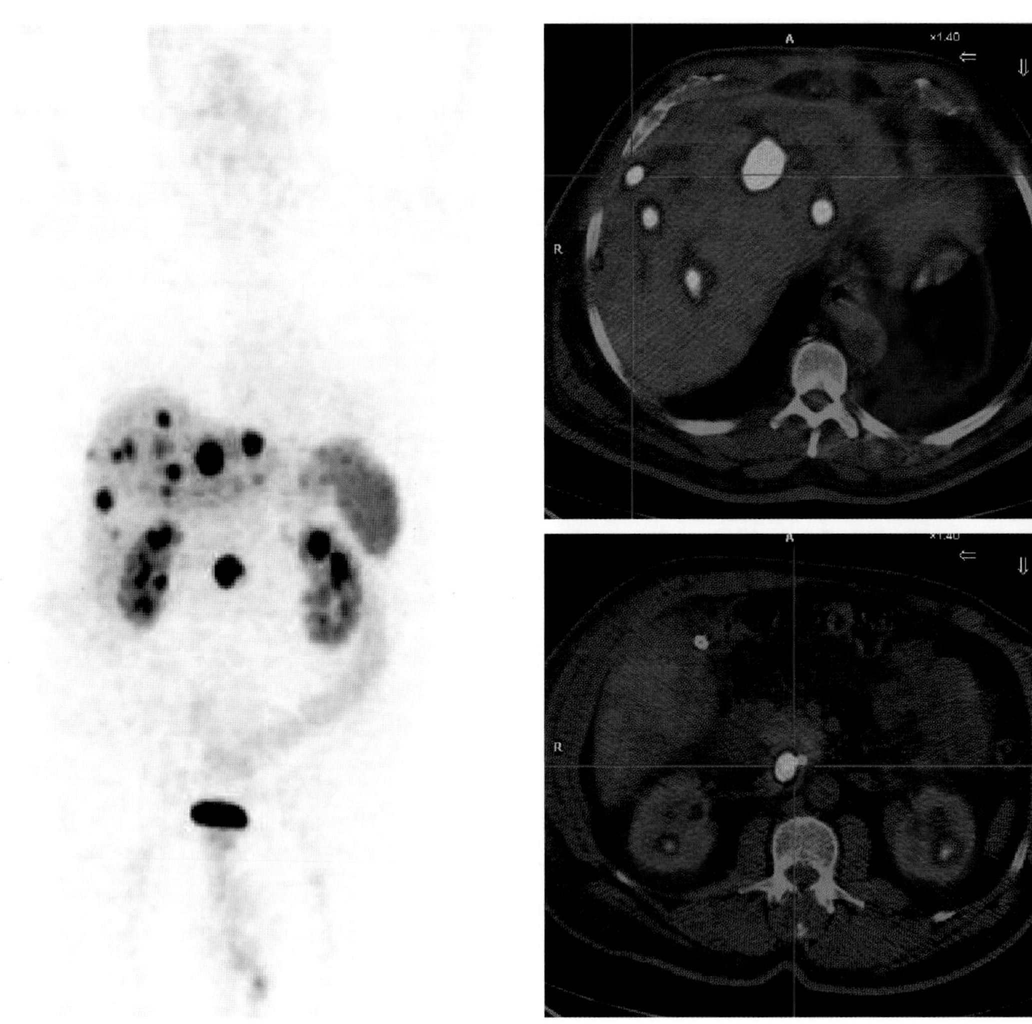

^{68}Ga-DOTA-NOC finding

PET-CT allows to identify pancreatic tumor as well as lymph nodes and multiple liver lesions.

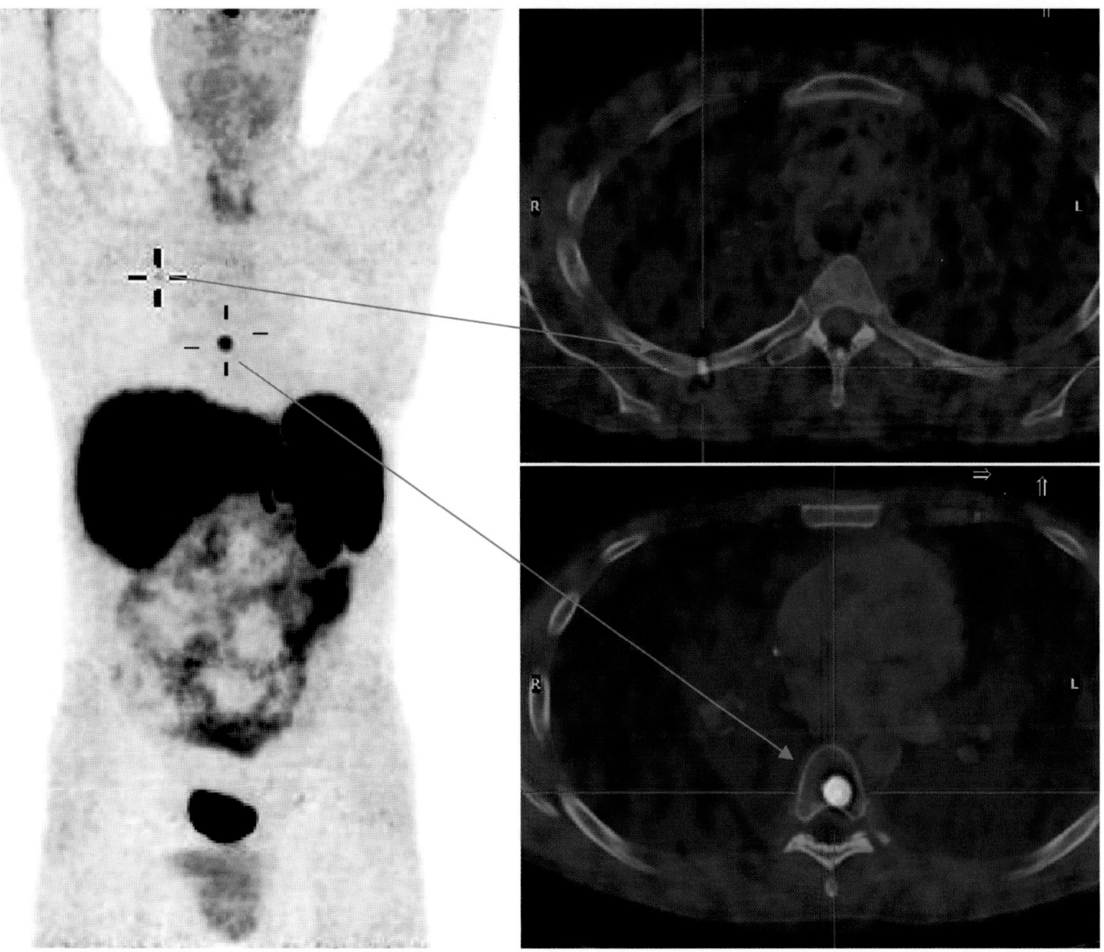

^{68}Ga-DOTA-NOC finding

PET scan performed one year after the last radioimmunotherapy cycle shows a pathologic uptake at D7 and smaller lesions at the fifth right rib and at the fourth liver segment.

Teaching point

Somatostatin receptor PET has a high sensitivity for demonstrating disease relapse.

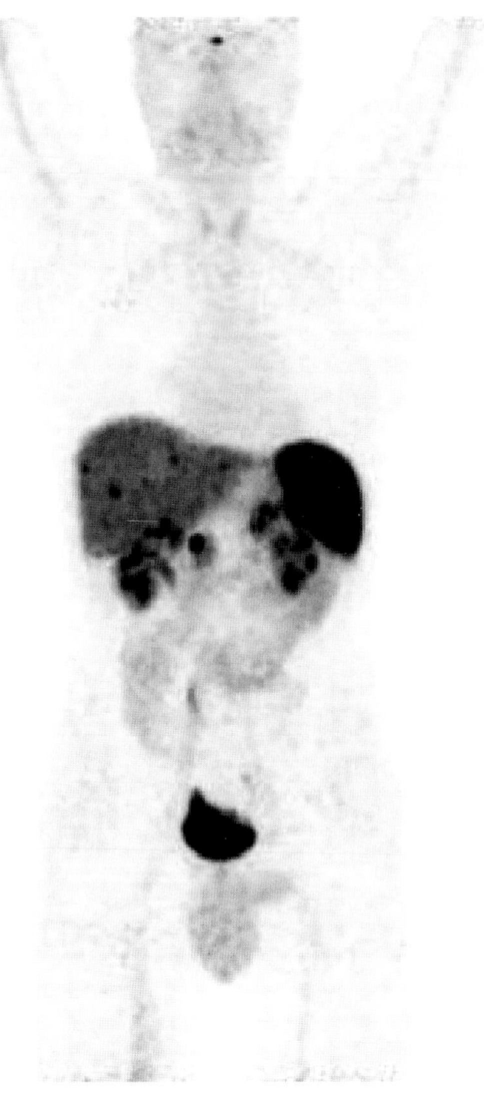

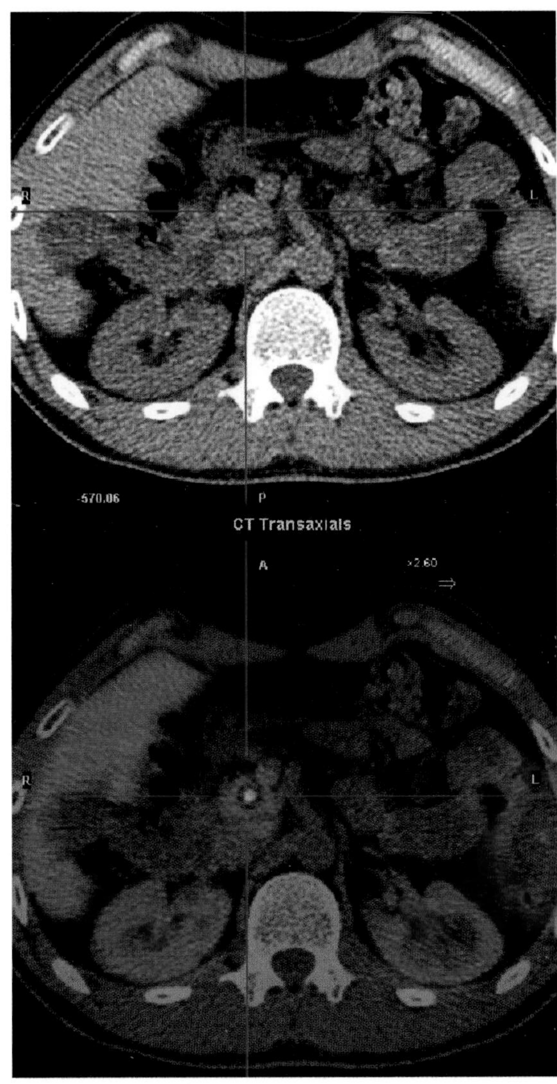

CT and other finding

CT demonstrates liver lesions (4th and 5th/8th segment), while somatostatin receptor scintigraphy was negative.

^{68}Ga-DOTA-NOC finding

PET-CT confirmed liver involvement and showed a mesogastric lesion that could be referred to peripancreatic nodes or the pancreatic head.

Teaching point

PET-CT was determinant to up-stage the disease and to candidate the patient to radioimmunotherapy.

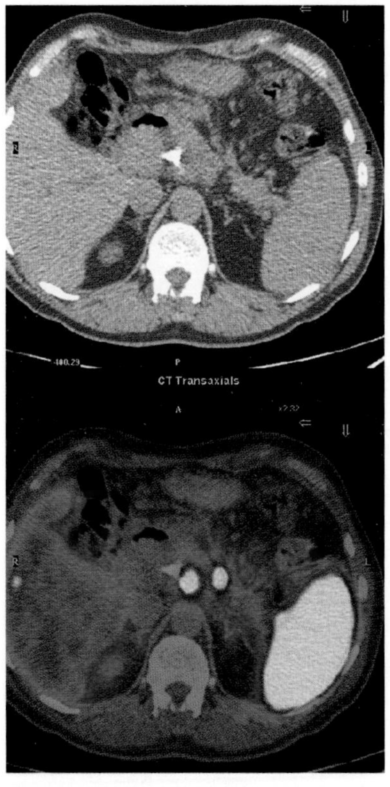

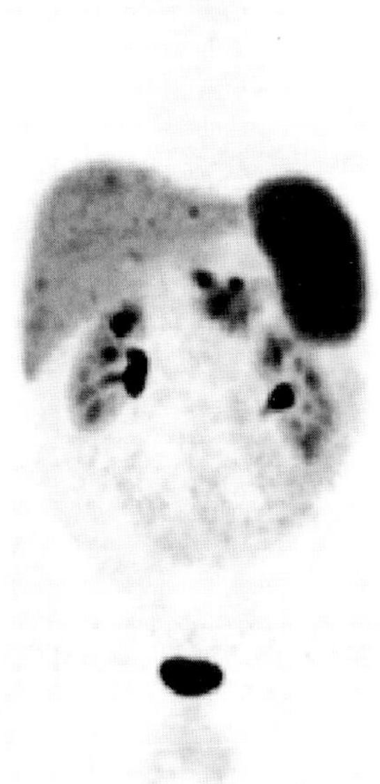

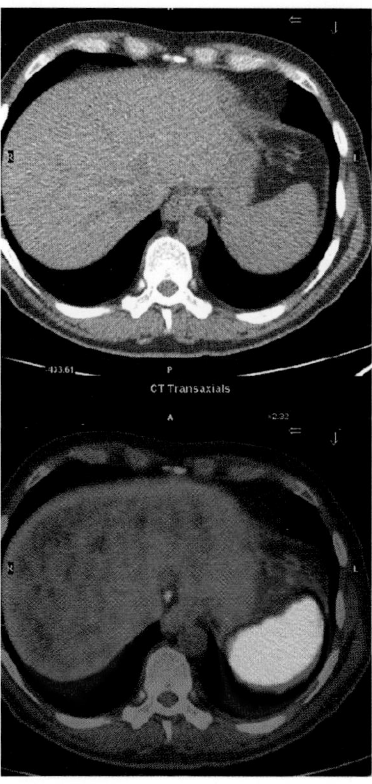

MR and other finding

MR showed a suspicious liver lesion while ^{18}F-FDG PET identified only a suspicious uptake at pancreas level.

^{68}Ga-DOTA-NOC finding

PET-CT confirmed the presence of relapse at pancreatic level (head and body) and five small liver lesions.

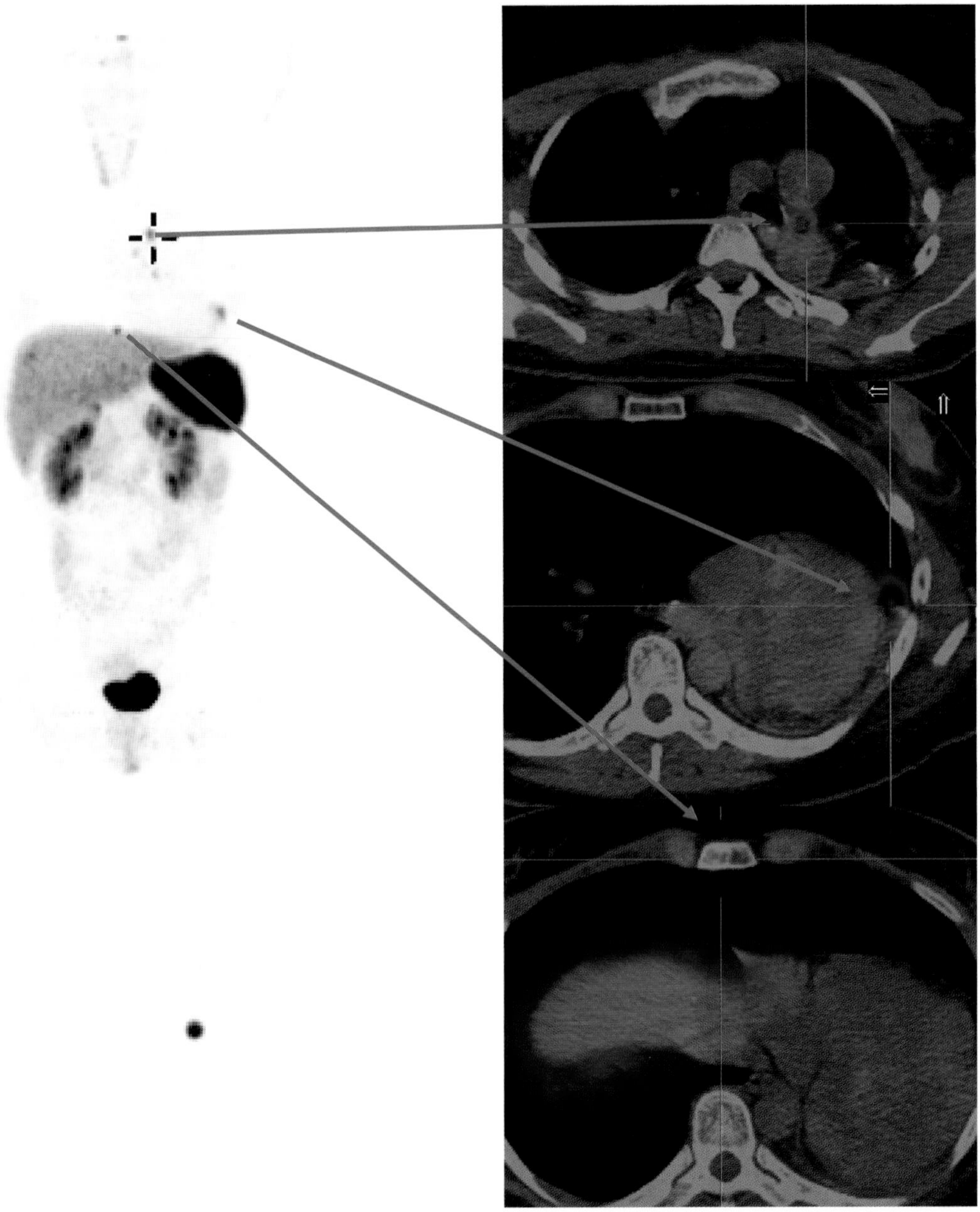

CT and other finding

Patient with metastatic atypical lung carcinoid already treated; at follow-up CT shows liver lesions and suspect lung nodules.

^{68}Ga-DOTA-NOC finding

PET-CT scan confirms liver lesions and identifies one adenopathy at the pulmonary-aortic window, one at the heart apex and bone involvement (left femur and sternum).

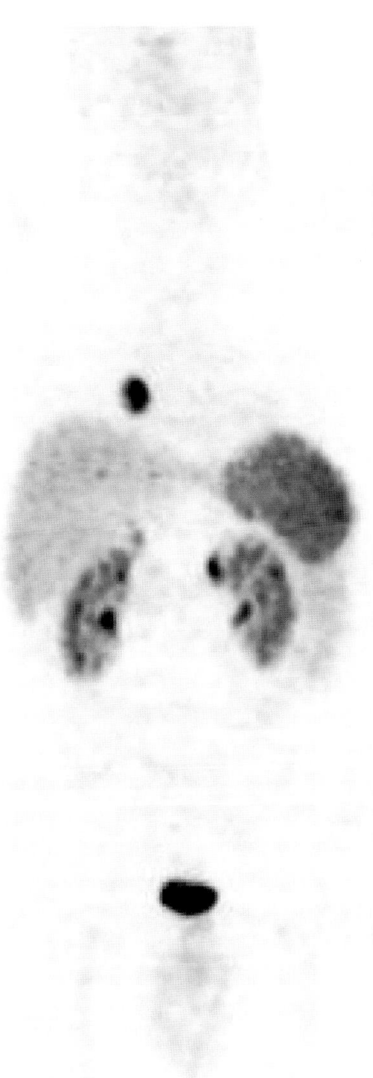

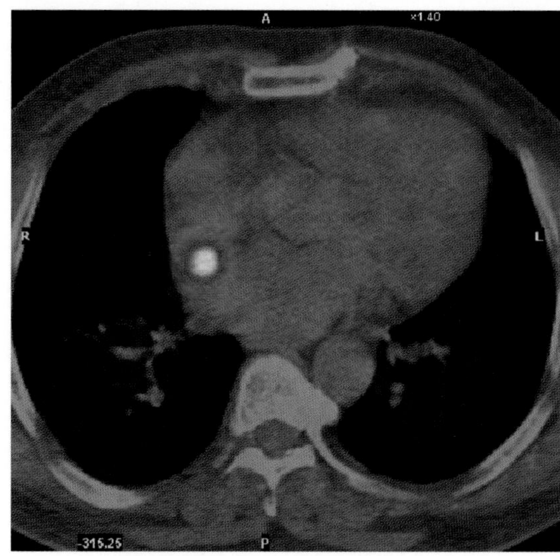

^{68}Ga-DOTA-NOC finding

PET-CT shows a lesion close to the cava superior. Surgery confirmed the PET finding to be recurrent paraganglioma.

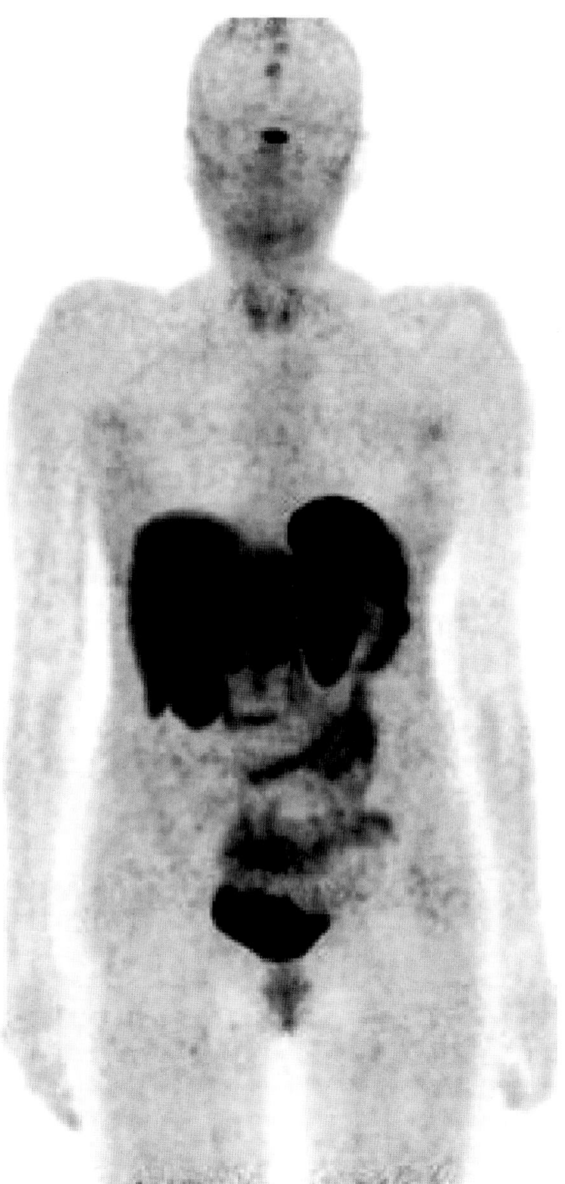

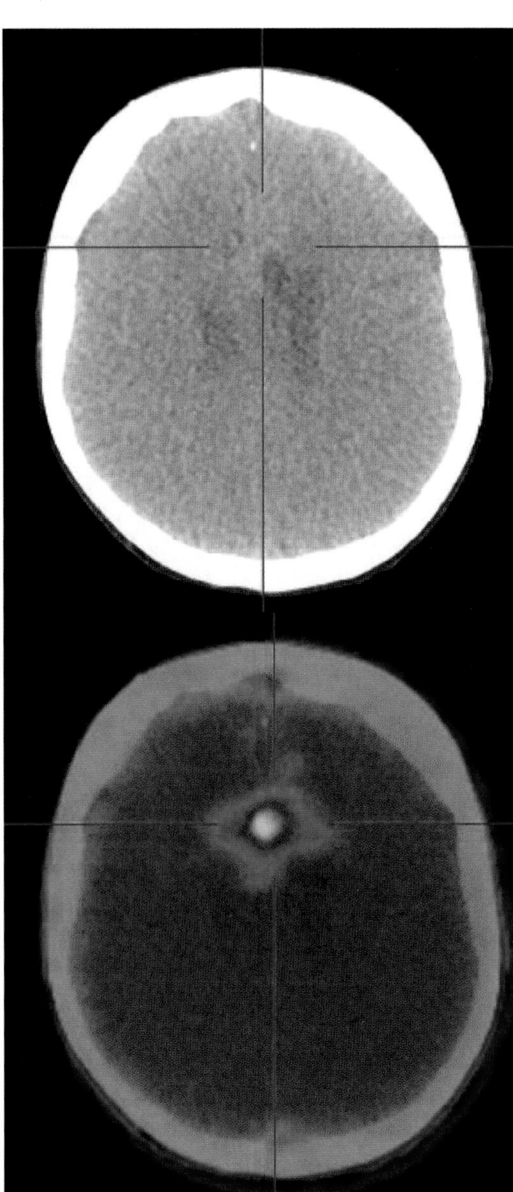

^{68}Ga-DOTA-NOC finding

PET-CT identifies the presence of a focal area of residual disease.

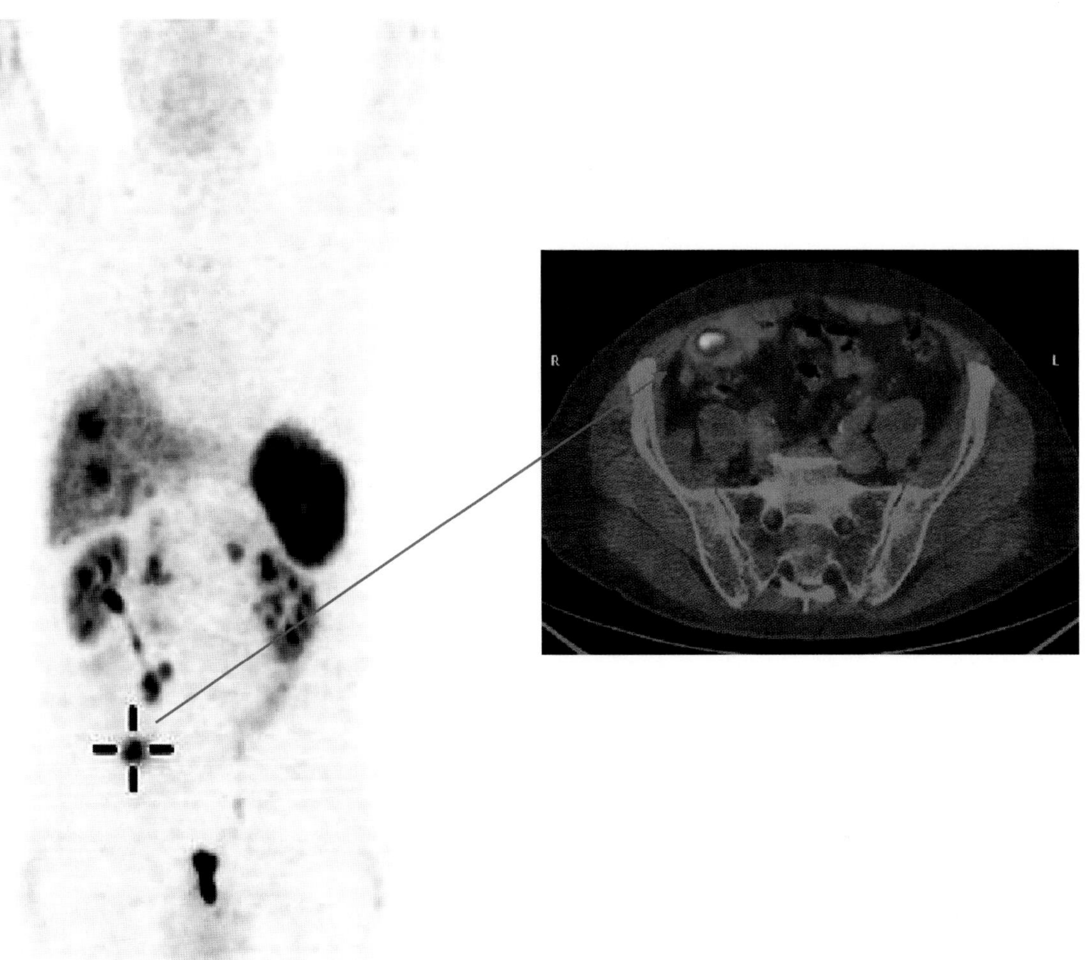

CT and other finding

Patient with biopsy-proven NET liver lesions and unknown primary tumor. CT positive at liver; negative other imaging methods.

^{68}Ga-DOTA-NOC finding

PET-CT confirmed liver involvement and demonstrated a pathologic uptake at ileum, then confirmed to be the primary tumor.

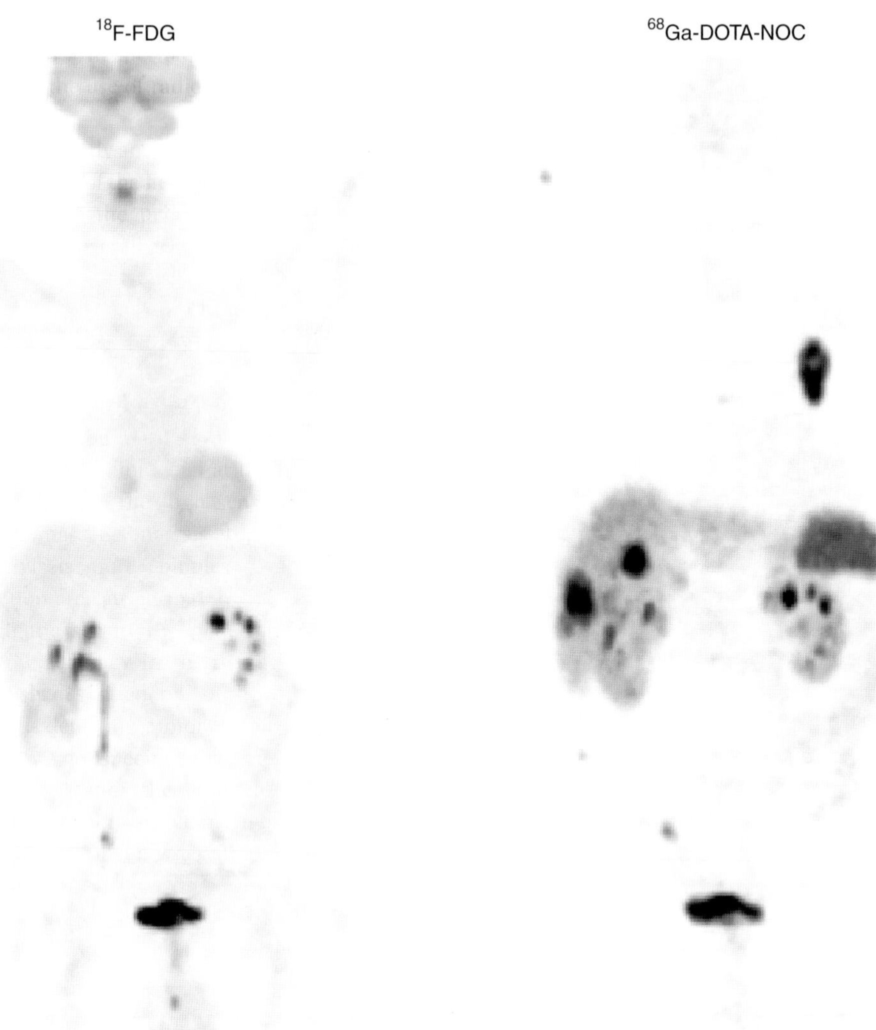

PET finding

^{18}F-FDG PET/CT was negative, while ^{68}Ga-DOTA-NOC PET/CT confirmed liver involvement and demonstrated a pathologic uptake at left lung level (primary tumor), as well as secondary lesions at bone level (vertebrae, right iliac, homerus) and one abdominal adenopathy.

^{18}F-FDG

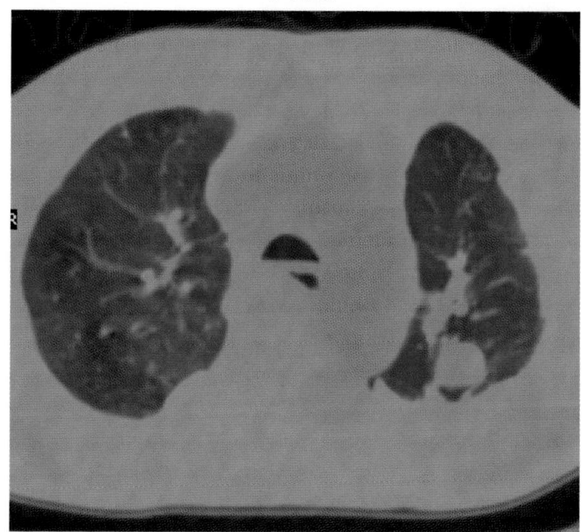

^{68}Ga-DOTA-NOC

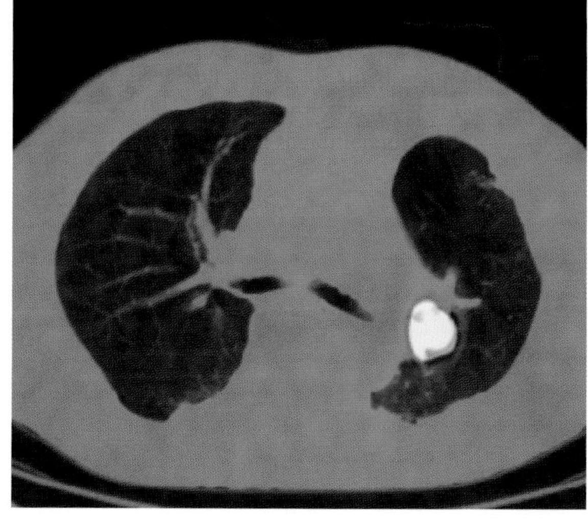

Teaching point

PET-CT with ^{68}Ga-DOTA-NOC performs better than ^{18}F-FDG for the assessment of well-differentiated NET.

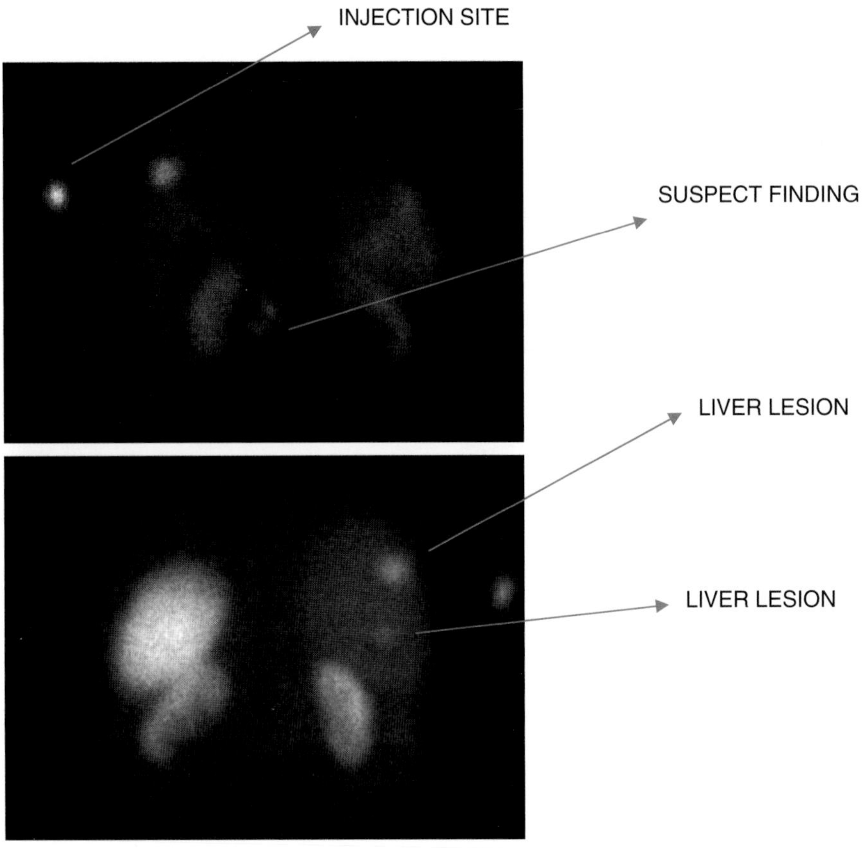

SPECT finding

Patient with pathology-proven NET. At somatostatin receptor scintigraphy two liver lesions and suspect mesogastric uptake.

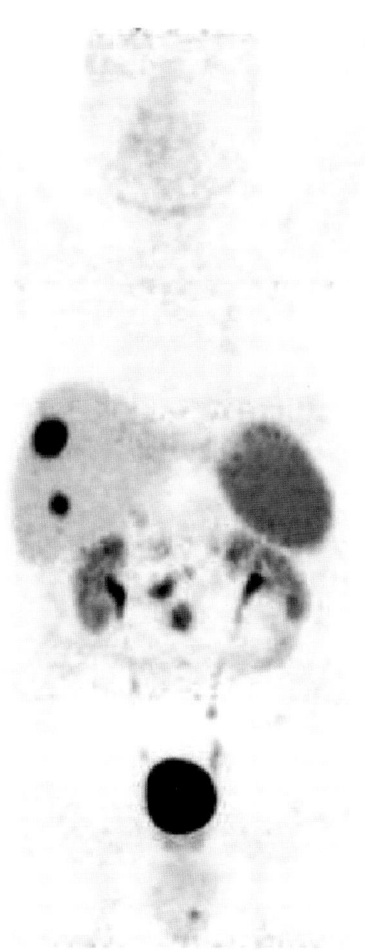

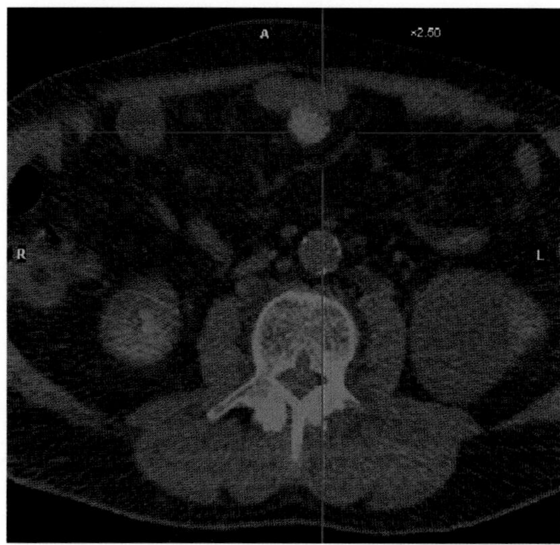

^{68}Ga-DOTA-NOC finding

PET-CT confirmed liver metastasis and showed two additional abdominal areas of pathologic tracer uptake at mesogastric level: one lesion in close proximity to small bowel and the other just below the kidney vessels.

Teaching point

Better spatial resolution of PET over SPECT allows better lesion localization.

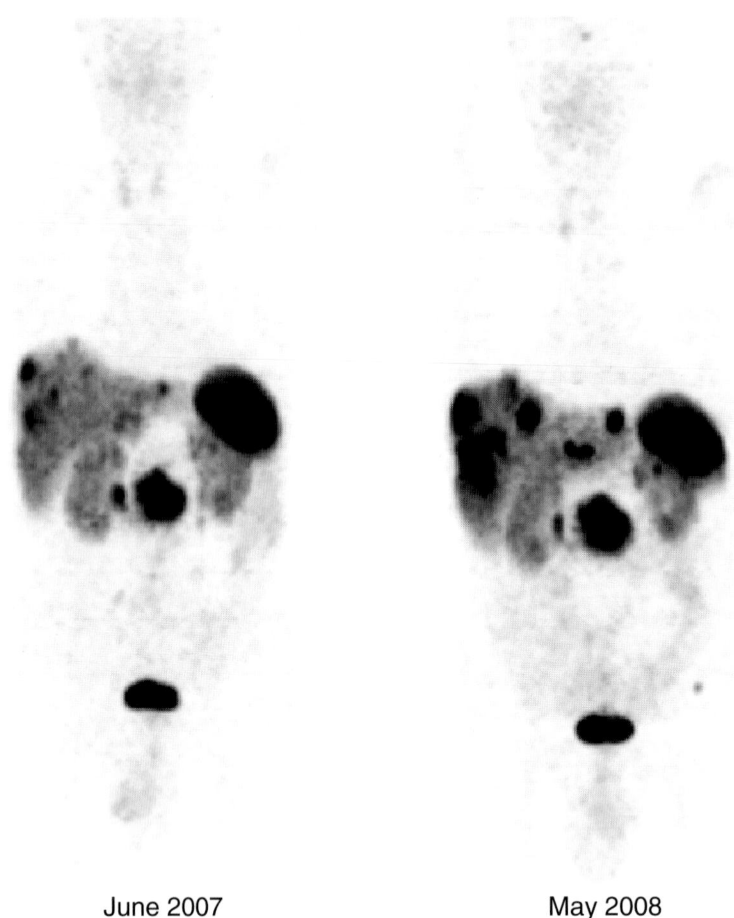

^{68}Ga-DOTA-NOC finding

PET-CT scan shows disease progression (increased number and SUV_{max} at liver and pancreatic level, additional bone lesion at left iliac level).

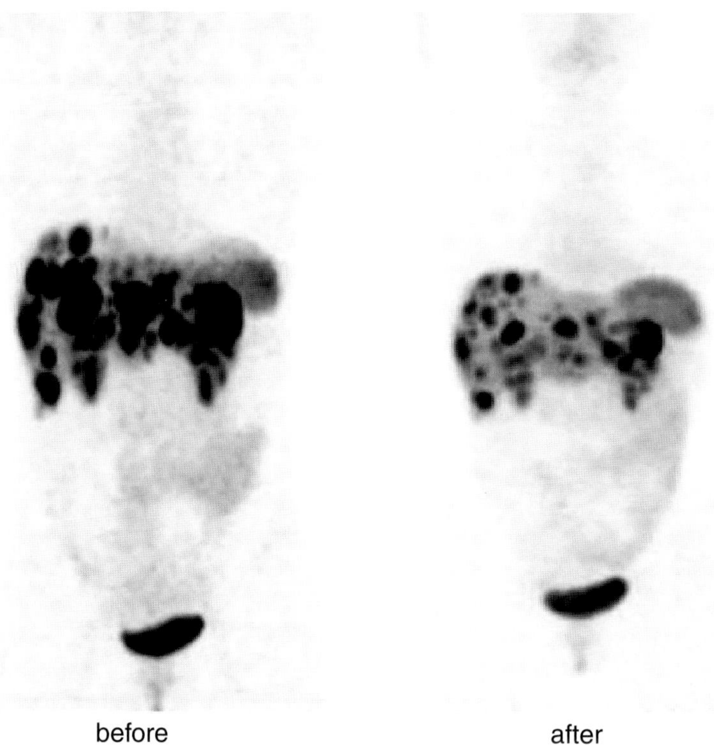

^{68}Ga-DOTA-NOC finding

PET-CT scan shows good partial response after treatment with radiometabolic treatment (decreased number of lesions and less intense uptake).

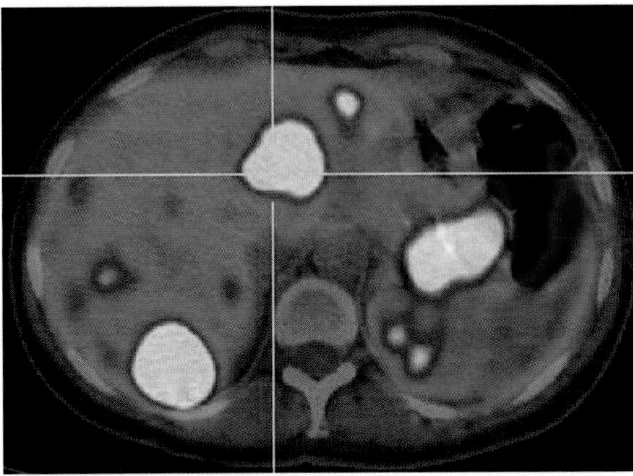

before

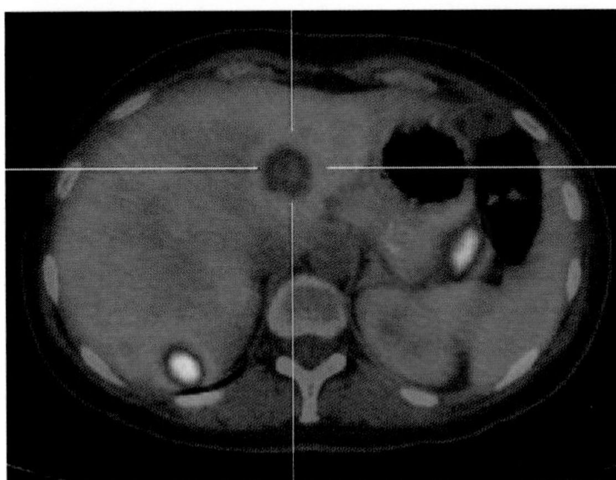

after

Teaching point

Somatostatin receptor PET is fundamental for identifying candidate to treatment with radiometabolic treatment (peptides labelled with ^{90}Yttrium or ^{177}Lutetium), and can be usefully employed to evaluate response to therapy.

Chapter 8 Acetate PET-CT

Mohsen Farsad, Franca Chierichetti, and Stefano Fanti

Acetate is a metabolic substrate of β-oxidation and precursor of amino acid and sterol. ^{11}Carbon labeled Acetate (ACE) was first used in the early 1980s for the evaluation of the myocardial oxidative metabolism. ^{11}C-Acetate is rapidly taken up in the myocardium and subsequently metabolized to CO_2 via the Krebs cycle. Therefore, kinetic analysis of accumulation and washout curves of radiolabeled acetate allows to analyze myocardial oxygen consumption and myocardial blood flow.

The use of ACE PET in tumor imaging has been suggested in various malignancies (brain, nasopharyngeal, ovarian, liver and prostate tumors). It should be pointed out that the mechanism of tumor uptake is different from that of myocardium, in which ^{11}C-Acetate is channeled mainly to the Krebs cycle. The participation in free fatty acid synthesis is believed to be the dominant method of incorporation in tumors. However, the metabolic pathways of Acetate are different in various tumor types.

^{11}C-Acetate like ^{11}C-Choline is the most studied PET tracer suitable for prostate cancer imaging. The value of these two appears nearly identical and none of them can be favored. It is hypothesized that the anabolic pathways in fatty acid and sterol synthesis may account for the retention of Acetate in prostate cancer. Like Choline, the Acetate uptake of normal prostate and benign hyperplasia overlap significantly with those for prostate cancer and therefore, ACE PET has a limited value for identification of primary prostate tumors. At present, the only clinical indication for ACE PET in prostate cancer imaging is the evaluation of suspected recurrence after first-line treatment. Available data indicate the successful use of ACE PET in identifying both local and distant metastasis in patients with prostate cancer relapse. Although not the "perfect" radiotracer for prostate cancer imaging, nevertheless, ACE PET generally shows more sites of disease compared to all conventional imaging methods together. In more than half of patients with rising PSA after surgery or radiation therapy, ACE PET detects the site of disease recurrence, even in the presence of low PSA values. Moreover, in our experience, it seems that PSA value is not sensitive to differentiate patients with local relapse or diffuse disease, while ACE PET seems useful to decide the proper treatment.

A minor role of ACE PET has been suggested for diagnosis of hepatocellular carcinoma. Some authors report the complementary role of ACE PET to FDG PET in the detection of hepatocellular carcinoma. The well-differentiated hepatocellular carcinomas demonstrate a high ACE and a low FDG uptake, while poorly differentiated ones have a low ACE and a high FDG uptake. In those tumors that are both ACE and FDG positive, authors suggest that these tracers are taken up by different parts of a moderately differentiated tumor. However, ACE PET is not a specific tracer for hepatocellular carcinoma. Benign liver lesions, like hepatic adenoma and focal nodular hyperplasia also show increased ^{11}C-Acetate uptake.

^{11}C-Acetate has also been used for detection and characterization of brain tumors. ACE PET shows, despite the low background activity of normal brain, low sensitivity for detection of high-grade gliomas. Furthermore, ACE PET seems not to be useful in differentiating high-grade from low-grade brain tumors. In order to establish the clinical role of ACE for brain tumor imaging and for differentiation of recurrent brain tumor from radiation necrosis, more studies are needed. An interesting application in brain lesions seems to be the power of ACE PET in identifying meningial tumors with respect to other lesions as neuromas. In our experience, ACE PET was positive in all meningial tumors and negative in a case of lymphoma and in patients with fibrillary neuromas.

Other oncological applications of ACE PET were explored with equivocal results. The diagnostic accuracy of ACE PET for detection of well-differentiated lung tumors and head and neck cancers is still to be addressed.

Like Choline, labeling of Acetate with a longerlived positron emitter such as ^{18}F has been investigated for prostate and brain cancer imaging. Methods for safe and efficient synthesis for a routine clinical use are still under investigation.

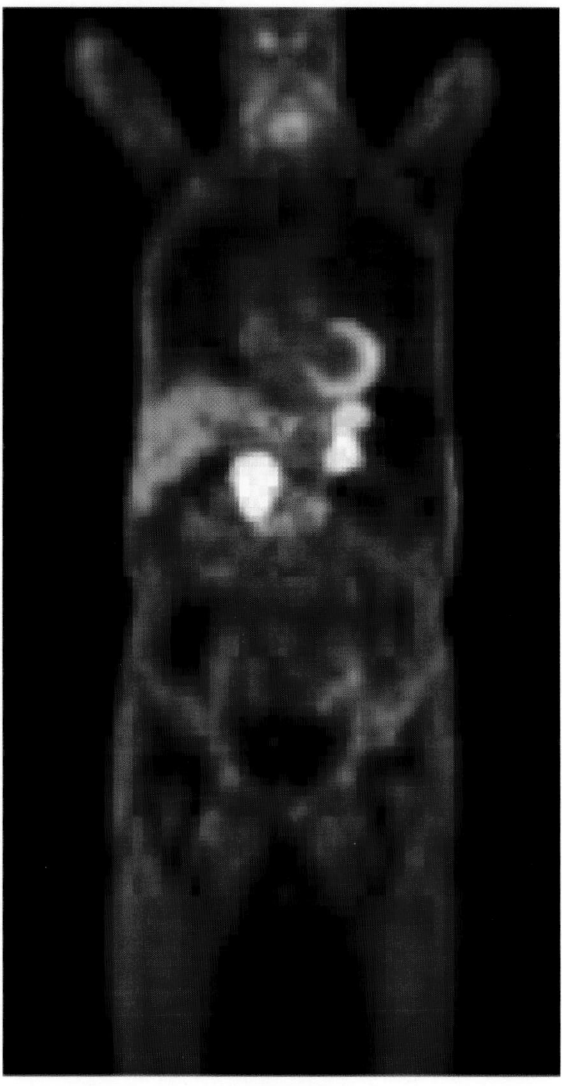

^{11}C-Acetate

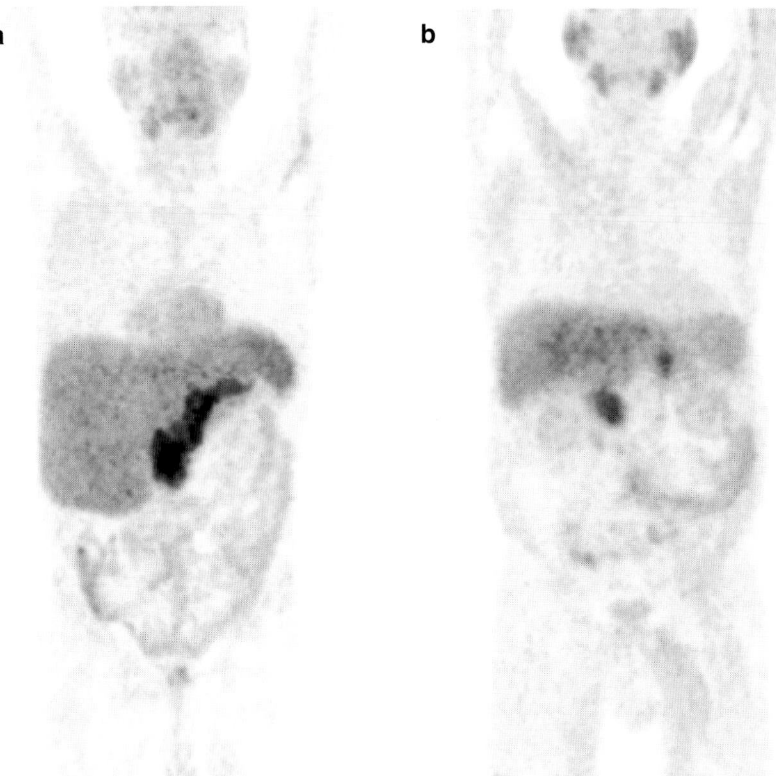

Teaching point

Pancreatic uptake of ^{11}C-acetate choline may vary, with cases showing intense diffuse uptake (a) and cases with only partial uptake (b). Notice the very low bladder excretion.

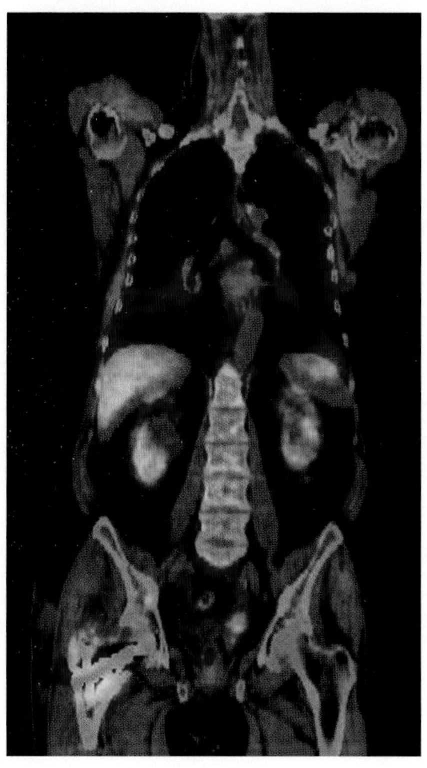

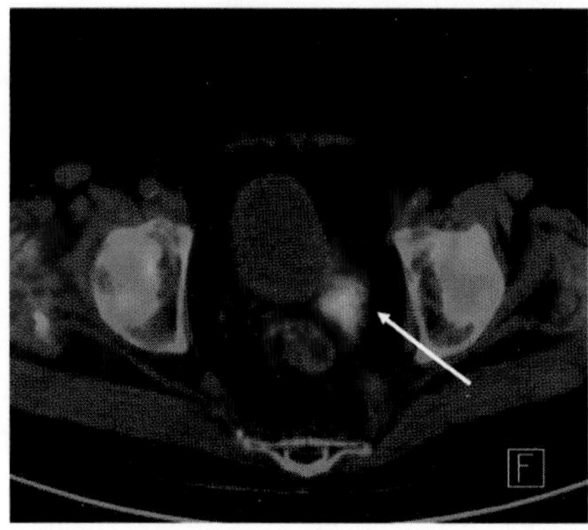

^{11}C-acetate finding

After partial prostatectomy, pathologic increased uptake in left seminal gland.

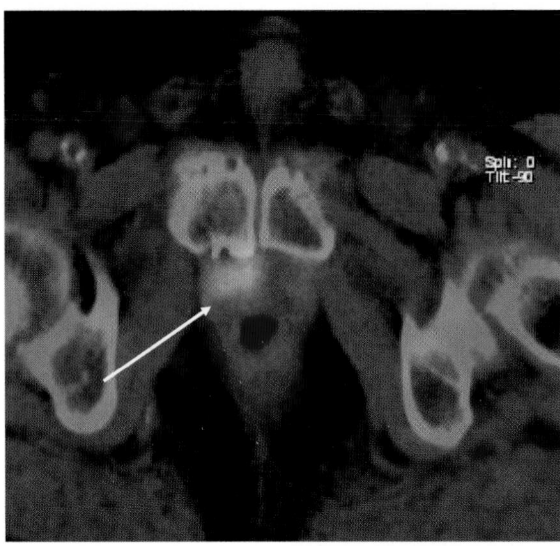

^{11}C-acetate finding

After prostatectomy, pathologic local relapse.

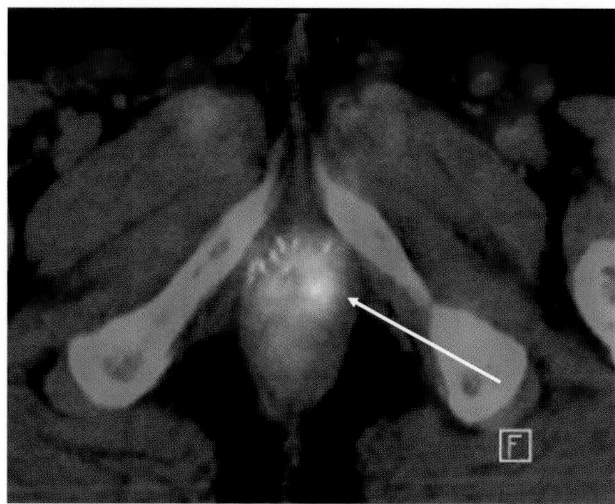

^{11}C-acetate finding

After brachitherapy, pathologic local relapse.

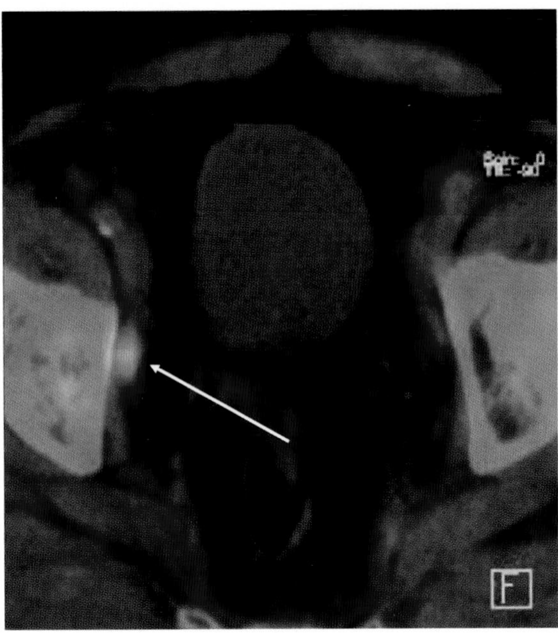

^{11}C-acetate finding

After prostatectomy, pathologic increased uptake in right obturatory lymph node.

Teaching point

^{11}C-acetate has a high sensitivity also for small nodal lesions.

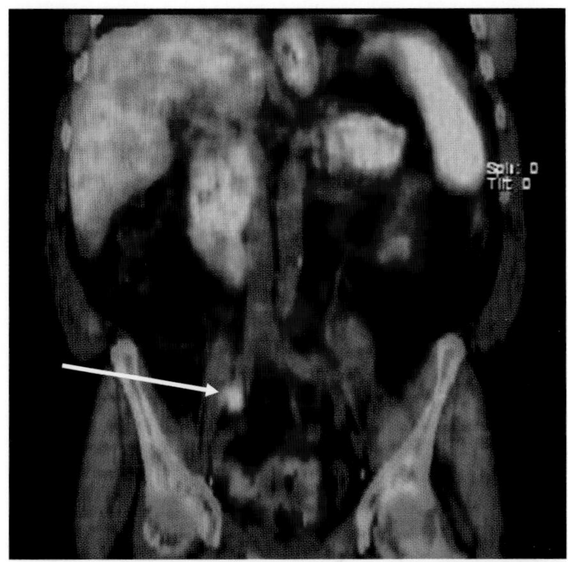

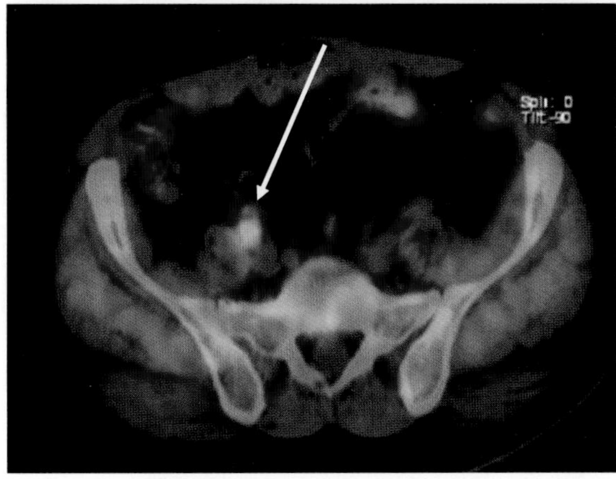

^{11}C-acetate finding

After prostatectomy, pathologic increased uptake in presacral lymph node.

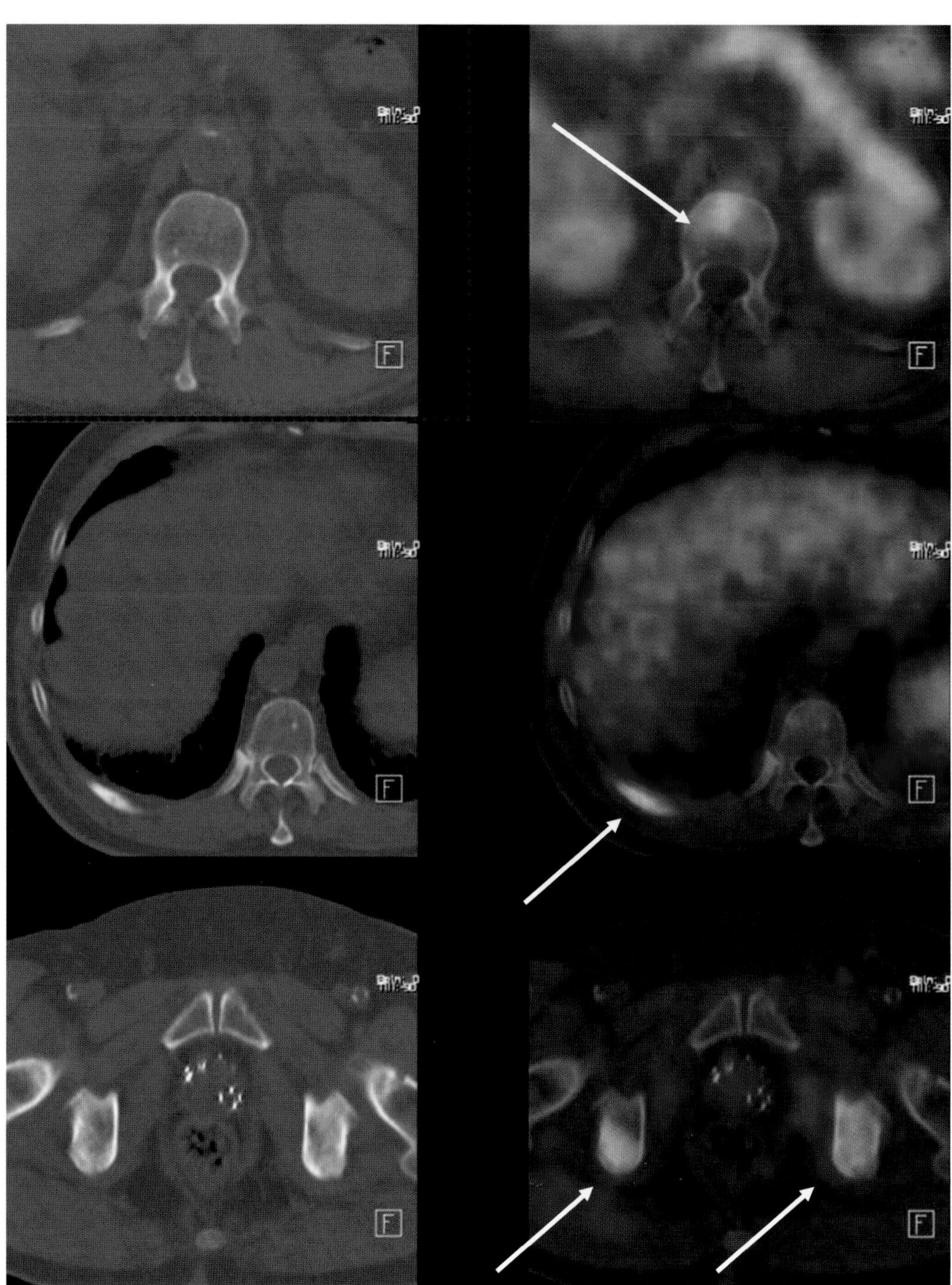

^{11}C-acetate finding

After brachytherapy, pathologic increased uptake in several bones.

Teaching point

^{11}C-acetate can frequently be positive before CT.

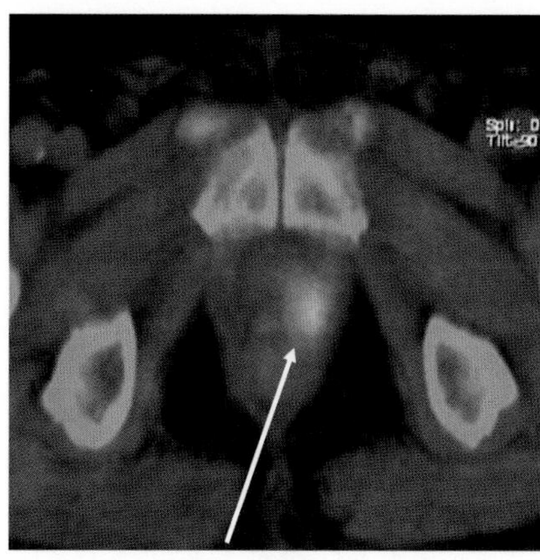

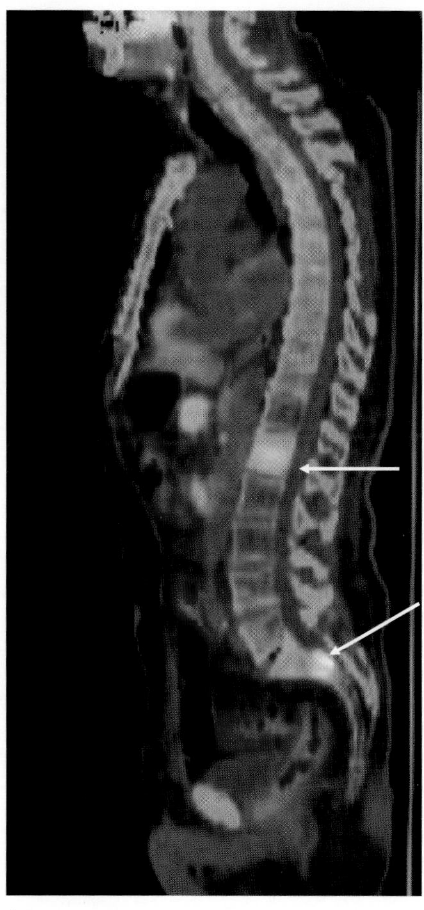

■ ^{11}C-acetate finding

Pathologic increased uptake in prostate bed and several bones.

Teaching point

PSA was 1.6; PSA values do not necessarily correlate with the number and the sites of relapse.

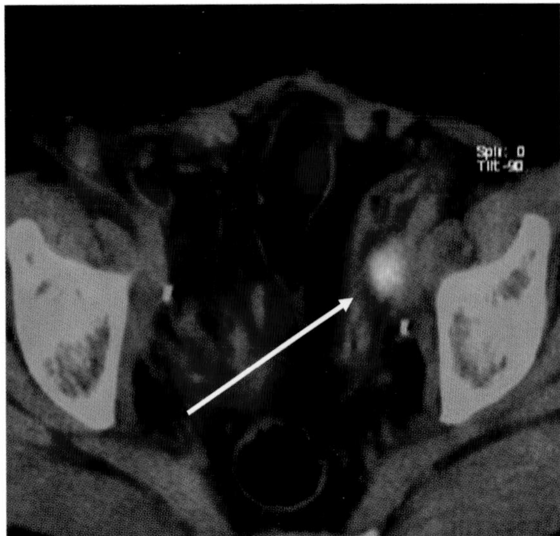

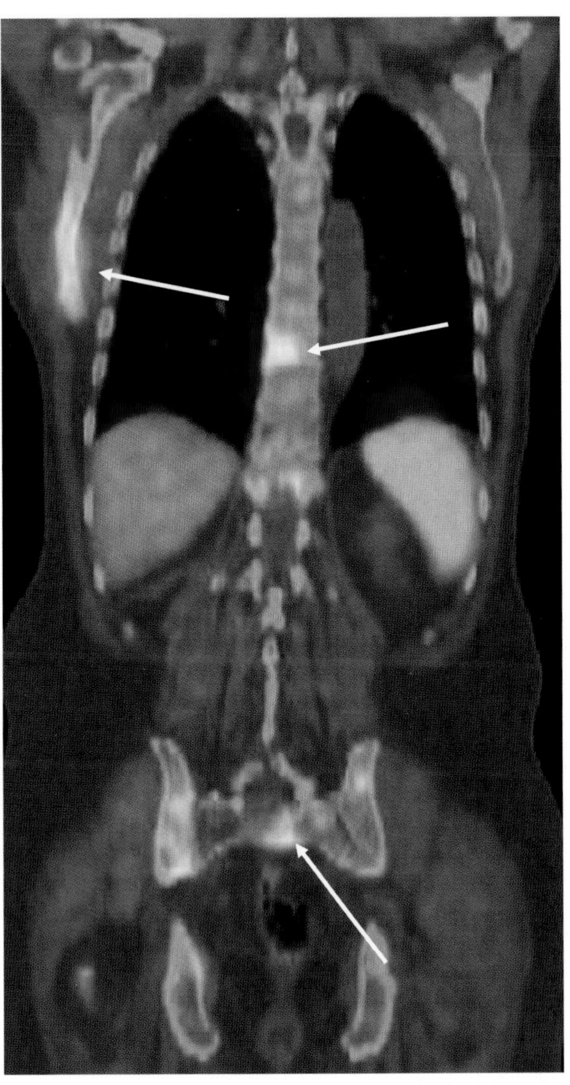

^{11}C-acetate finding

Pathologic increased uptake in a lymph node and several bones.

Teaching point

PSA was 19; PSA values do not necessarily correlate with the number and the sites of relapse.

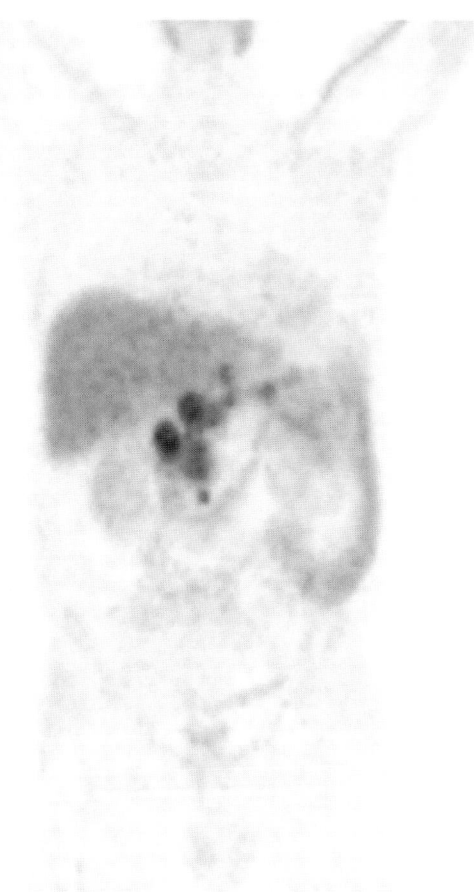

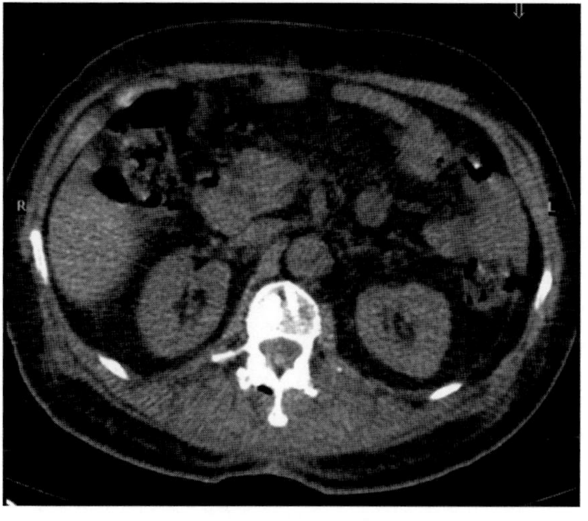

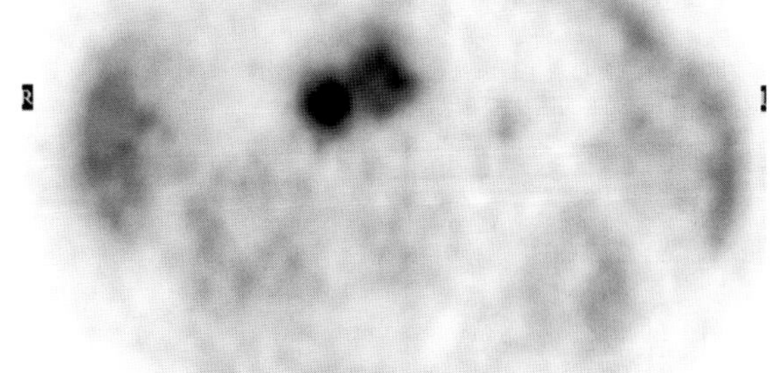

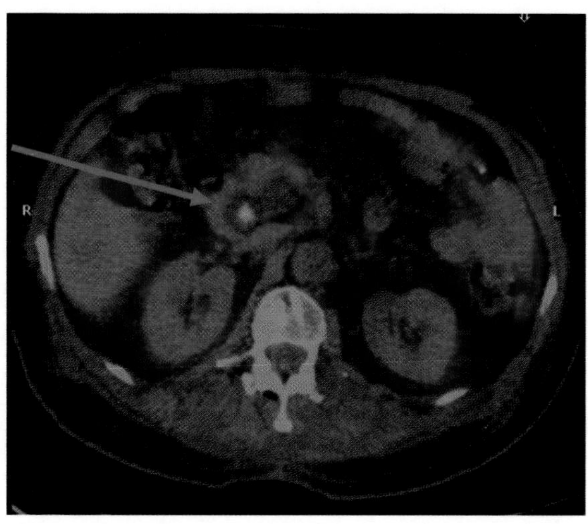

^{11}C-acetate finding

Pathologic increased uptake in a peripancreatic lymph node.

Teaching point

PET-CT enables to distinguish between pancreatic physiologic uptake and disease recurrence.

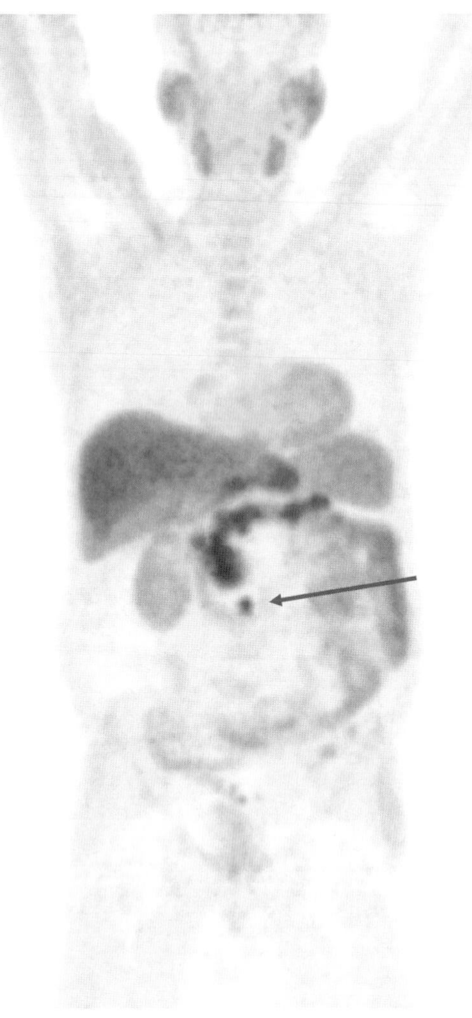

^{11}C-acetate finding

Pathologic increased uptake in a bone (L4).

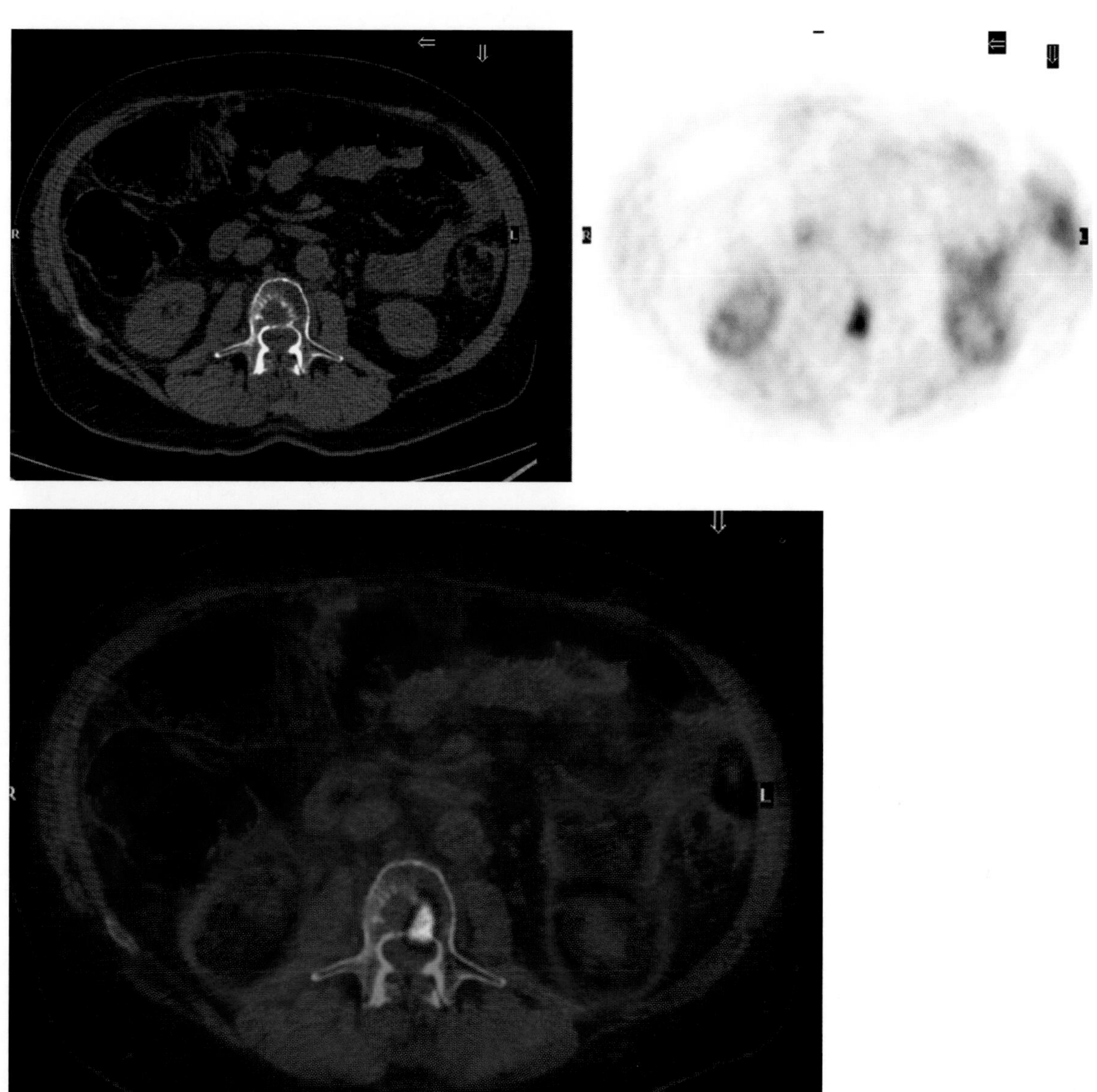

Teaching point

PET-CT with ^{11}C-acetate can be useful in selected cases of HCC after liver transplant to demonstrate relapse.

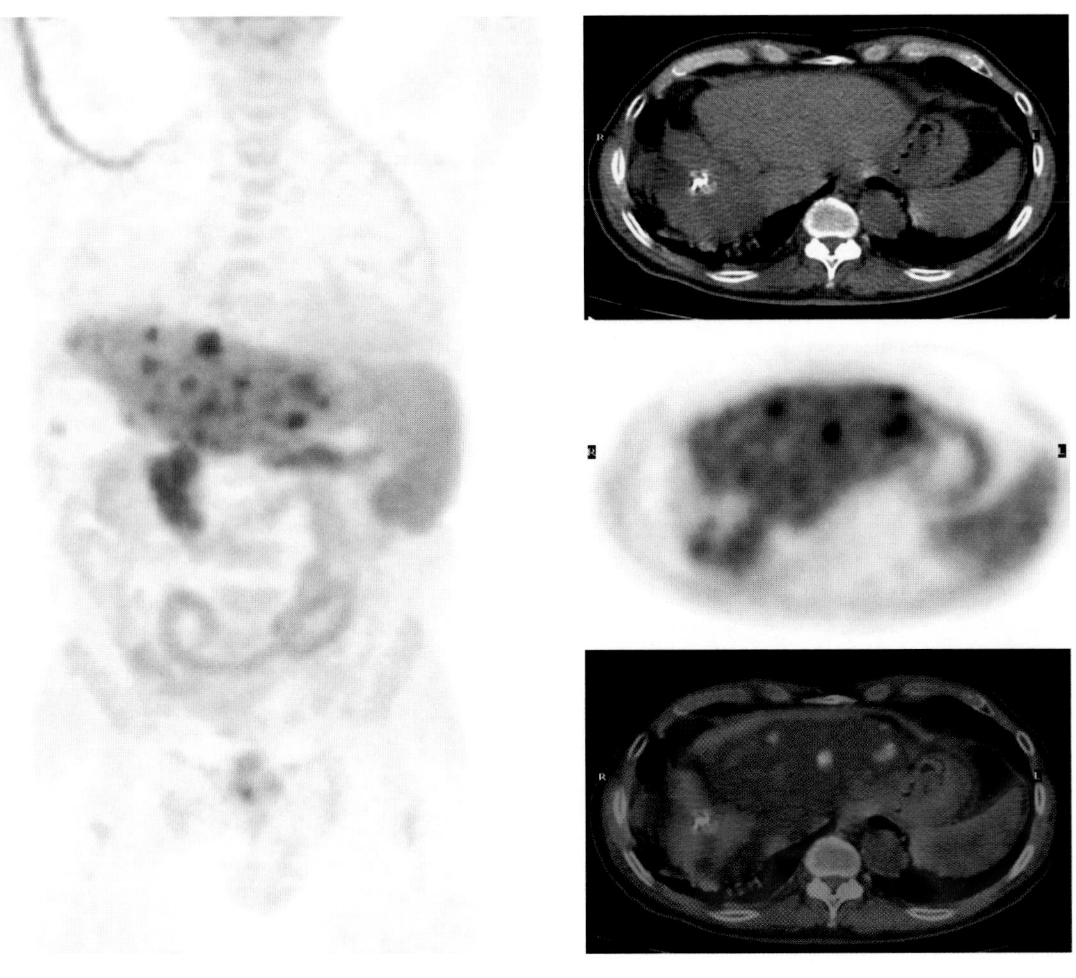

^{11}C-acetate finding

Multiple focal areas of pathologic uptake in the liver.

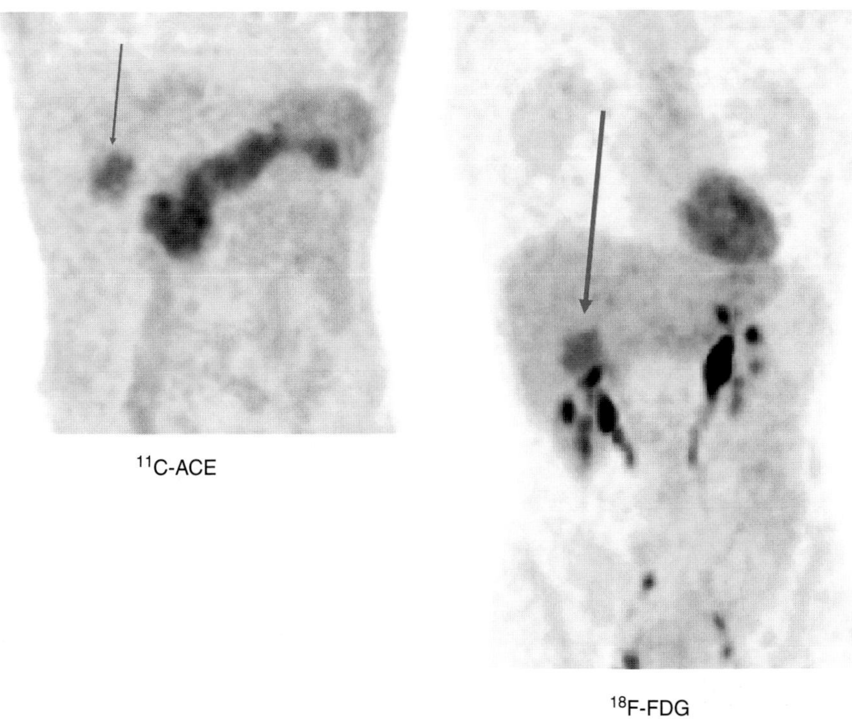

^{11}C-ACE

^{18}F-FDG

PET finding

Both ^{11}C-acetate and ^{18}F-FDG show increased uptake in the liver mass.

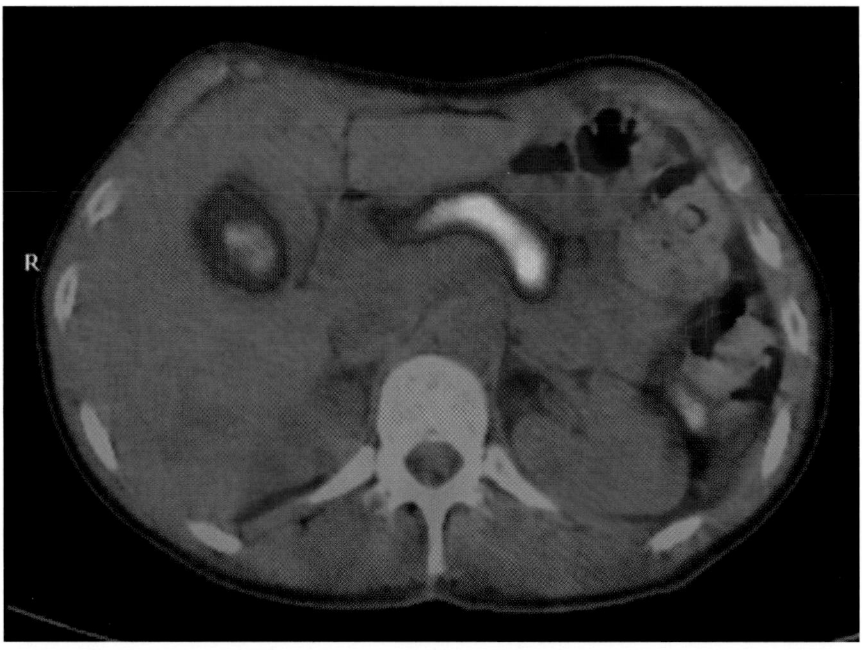

^{11}C-ACE

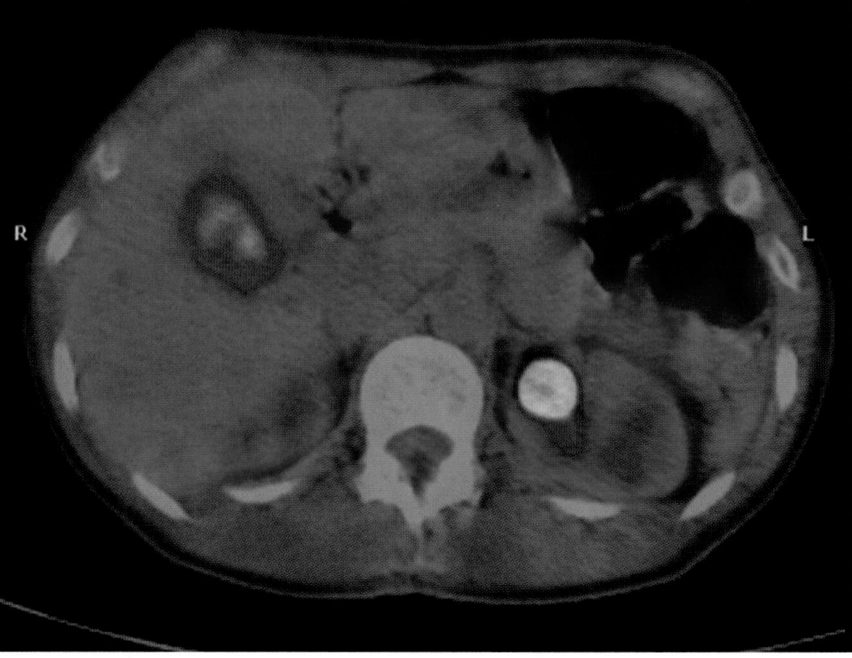

^{18}F-FDG

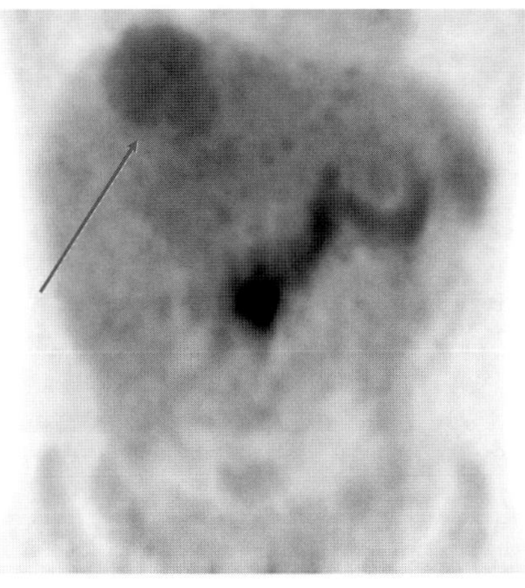

^{11}C-ACE

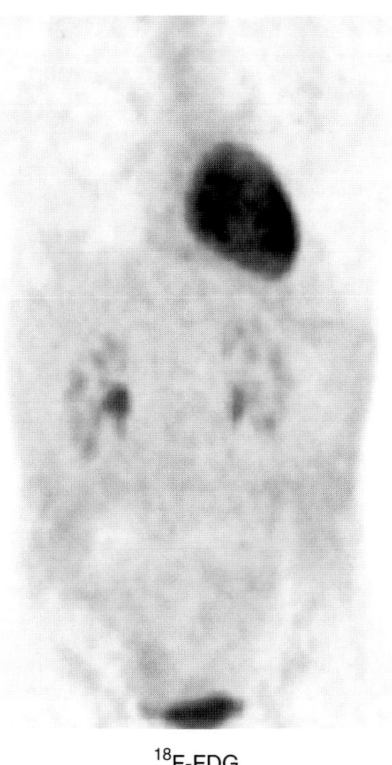

^{18}F-FDG

PET finding

Only ^{11}C-acetate shows increased uptake in the liver mass, while ^{18}F-FDG is negative.

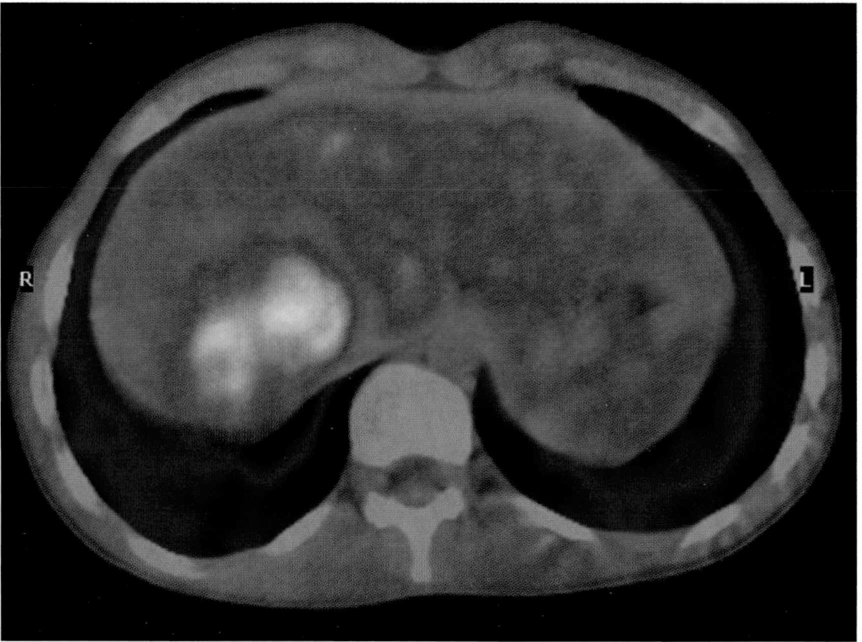

^{11}C-ACE

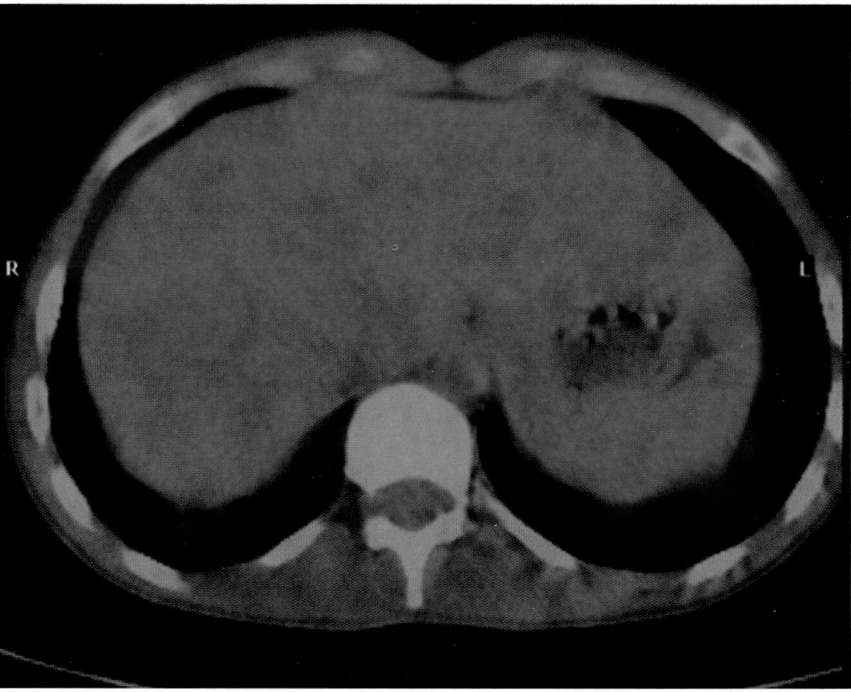

^{18}F-FDG

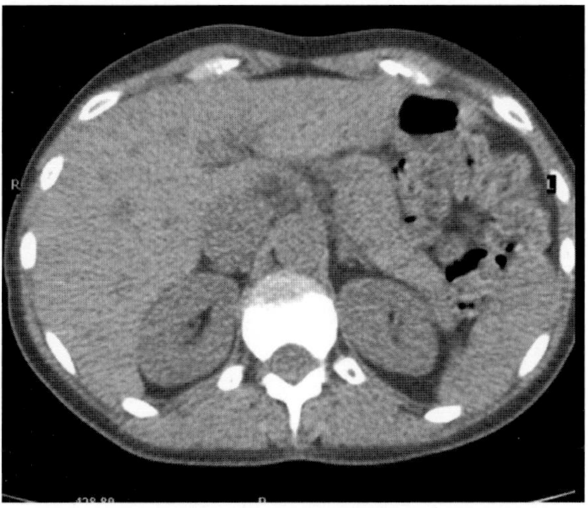

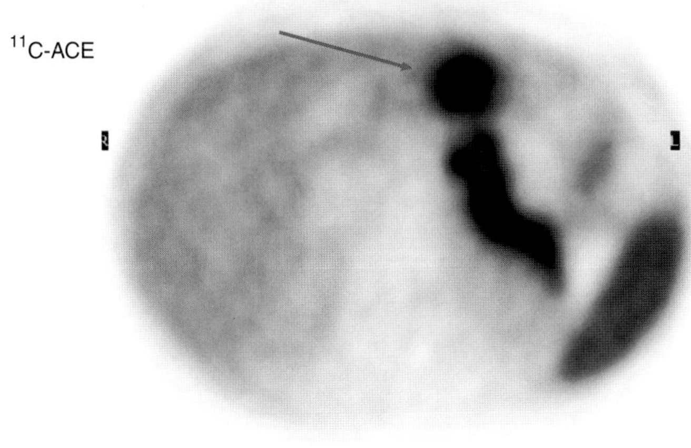

PET finding

Only ^{11}C-acetate shows increased uptake in the liver lesion, while ^{18}F-FDG is negative.

Teaching point

As compared to focal nodula hyperplasia, HCC usually shows more intense uptake of ^{11}C-acetate.

Chapter 9 Thymidine PET-CT

Ken Herrmann and Andreas Buck

As previously shown, deregulated cell cycle progression is a hallmark of cancer. Accordingly, the majority of therapeutic drugs has been designed to inhibit cell proliferation and/or to induce apoptosis. Metabolic imaging with PET and the glucose analog 2′-[^{18}F]fluoro-2′-deoxyglucose (FDG) has been demonstrated to sensitively detect malignant tumors and to identify responding tumors early in the course of anticancer treatment. [^{18}F]FDG PET is also a valuable clinical tool for predicting tumor response to therapy and patient survival.

However, tumoral uptake of FDG reflects proliferation only in part and is associated with false positive findings due to unspecific tracer retention in inflammatory processes. Therefore, to increase specificity for malignant lesions, other tracers that complement the information provided by [^{18}F]FDG are required. Measurement of tumor growth and DNA synthesis might be appropriate for assessment of proliferative activity in malignant tumors. So far, several DNA precursors have been investigated including [^{11}C]thymidine which represents the native pyrimidine base used for DNA-synthesis in vivo. Due to the short half-life of ^{11}C and rapid degradation of [^{11}C]thymidine, this tracer was considered less suitable for clinical use.

Recently, the thymidine analog 3′-deoxy-3′-[^{18}F]fluorothymidine ([^{18}F]FLT) was suggested for noninvasive assessment of proliferation and more specific tumor imaging. The effort to synthesize [^{18}F]FLT is similar to that of the standard radiotracer [^{18}F] FDG. [^{18}F]FLT which is derived from the cytostatic drug azidovudine (AZT) has been reported to be stable in vitro and to accumulate in proliferating tissues and malignant tumors. Thymidine kinase 1 was revealed as key enzyme responsible for the intracellular trapping of [^{18}F]FLT. Recently, a significant correlation of tumoral proliferation and [^{18}F]FLT uptake in various malignant tumors has been described, including breast cancer, colorectal cancer, lung cancer, gliomas, sarcoma and lymphomas. In a pilot study comprising 34 patients with malignant lymphomas, linear regression analysis indicated a significant correlation of tumoral [^{18}F]FLT uptake and proliferation fraction in biopsied tissues, as indicated by Ki-67 immunohistochemsitry ($r = 0.84$, $P < 0.0001$). All patients with indolent or aggressive lymphomas exhibited focal [^{18}F]FLT-uptake in lesions also described by routine staging procedures indicating a sensitivity of 100%. [^{18}F]FLT uptake in lymphomas was significantly lower compared to respective [^{18}F]FDG uptake (mean SUV-values 4.6 and 5.1, respectively). A reduced uptake of [^{18}F]FLT compared to [^{18}F]-FDG has also been observed in a series of nonsmall cell lung cancer (mean SUV-values 3.7 and 6.0, respectively).

[^{18}F]FLT is not or only marginally incorporated into DNA (<2%) and is therefore not a direct measure of proliferation *(17)*. In vitro studies indicated that [^{18}F]FLT uptake is closely related to thymidine kinase 1 (TK1) activity and respective protein levels. [^{18}F]FLT is therefore considered to reflect TK1 activity and, hence, S-phase fraction rather than DNA synthesis. Although being a poor substrate for type 1 equilibrative nucleoside transporters (ENT), cellular uptake of [^{18}F]FLT is further facilitated by redistribution of nucleoside transporters to the cellular membrane after inhibition of endogenous synthesis of thymidylate (TMP) (de novo synthesis of TMP). However, the detailed uptake mechanism of [^{18}F]FLT is yet unknown and the influence of membrane transporters and various nucleoside metabolizing enzymes remains to be determined.

[^{18}F]FLT PET produces images of high contrast, of both malignant tumors and proliferating tissues. Because of high physiologic tracer uptake in proliferating bone marrow, the sensitivity of [^{18}F]FLT for detecting tumor manifestations in bone marrow may be reduced. [^{18}F]FLT undergoes glucoronisation leading to enhanced liver uptake. Decreased sensitivity rates were described for liver metastases from various solid tumors. Due to negligible background uptake of [^{18}F]FLT in the brain, specific imaging of proliferation may be appropriate for detection of tumors or metastases in the central nervous system.

Recently, [^{18}F]FLT was suggested for therapeutic monitoring using various experimental settings. In an animal model of fibrosarcoma it was reported that [^{18}F] FLT uptake decreased early after antiproliferative treatment with 5-fluorouracil or cisplatin. In a mouse lymphoma xenotransplant model, significant decrease of [^{18}F]FLT uptake was already observed 48 h after chemotherapy with cyclophosphamide. An early reduction of tumoral [^{18}F]FLT uptake was further demonstrated, 48 h after treatment with tyrosine kinase inhibitors in a lung cancer xenograft model. However, data are preliminary and clinical trials are needed to further validate [^{18}F]FLT as marker for therapy response. Moreover, the lower uptake of [^{18}F]FLT compared to [^{18}F]FDG may result in a reduced sensitivity to detect residual disease after treatment. As previously reported for the standard radiotracer [^{18}F]FDG, false positive findings may also occur at [^{18}F]-FLT PET, because an increased proliferation rate is not specific for malignant tumors. Recently, reports from Troost and Yap indicated false positive findings originating from reactive cervical lymph nodes and benign lung nodules.

In conclusion, specific imaging of proliferative activity with $[^{18}F]$FLT is feasible. The use of $[^{18}F]$FLT as PET tracer showed advantages for detection of lymphomas in the central nervous system and the mediastinum. $[^{18}F]$FLT PET was suitable to differentiate indolent and aggressive tumors and to indicate progression to a more aggressive histology. However, a significantly reduced tracer uptake compared to the standard radiotracer $[^{18}F]$FDG has been observed in a variety of solid neoplasms indicating that $[^{18}F]$FDG is superior to $[^{18}F]$FLT regarding detection of tumor manifestation sites. $[^{18}F]$FLT PET has a potential, especially for early assessment of therapy response, which has to be validated in further experimental and clinical studies.

Male 58 years

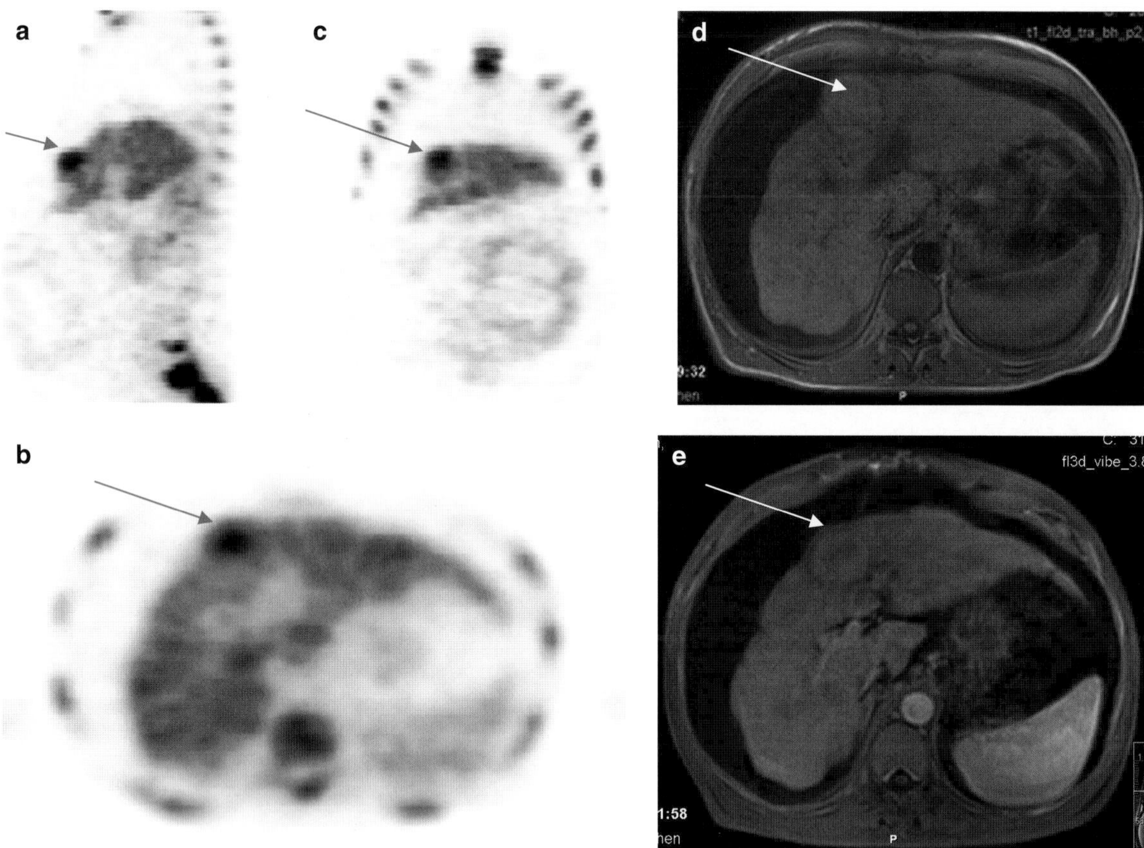

¹⁸F-FLT finding

Intense focal FLT uptake (*red arrows*) in the liver in (a) sagittal, (b) transaxial, and (c) coronal sections. MR (d, e) identifies a corresponding unifocal liver mass (*white arrows*).

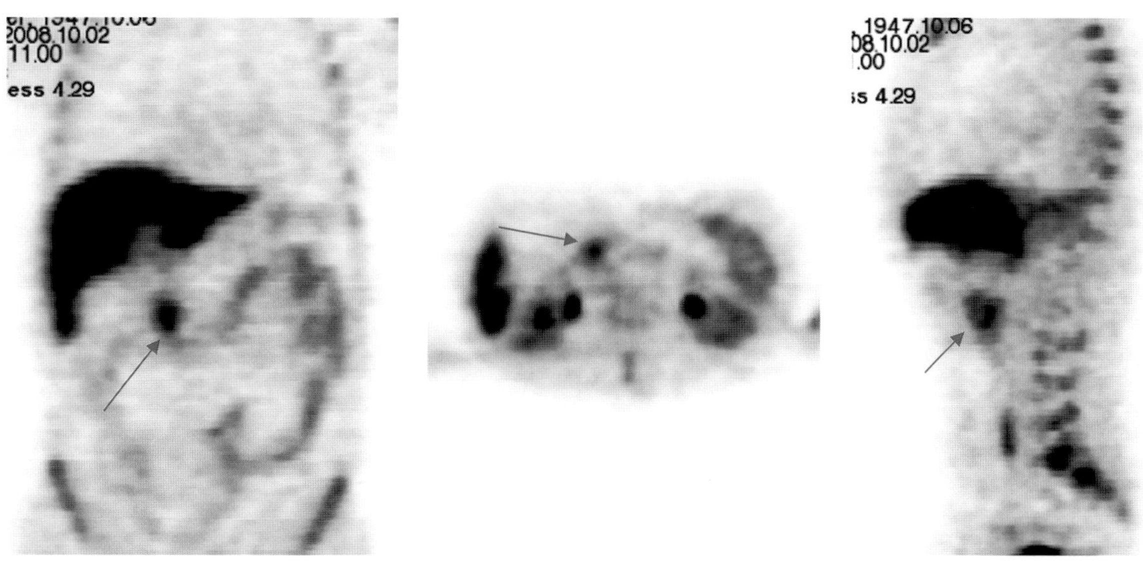

FLT

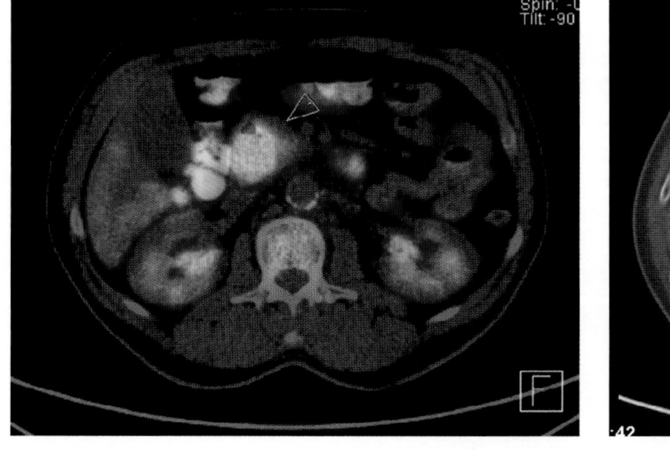

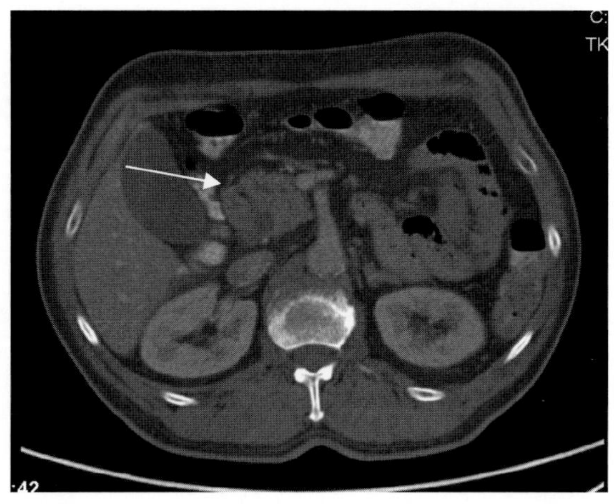

FDG

■ ^{18}F-FLT finding

Intense focal FLT uptake (*red arrows*). In the corresponding FDG PET-CT, there is also an intense uptake in the pancreatic head. Histology revealed a pT2pN1 adenocarcinoma of the pancreatic head.

Male 47 years

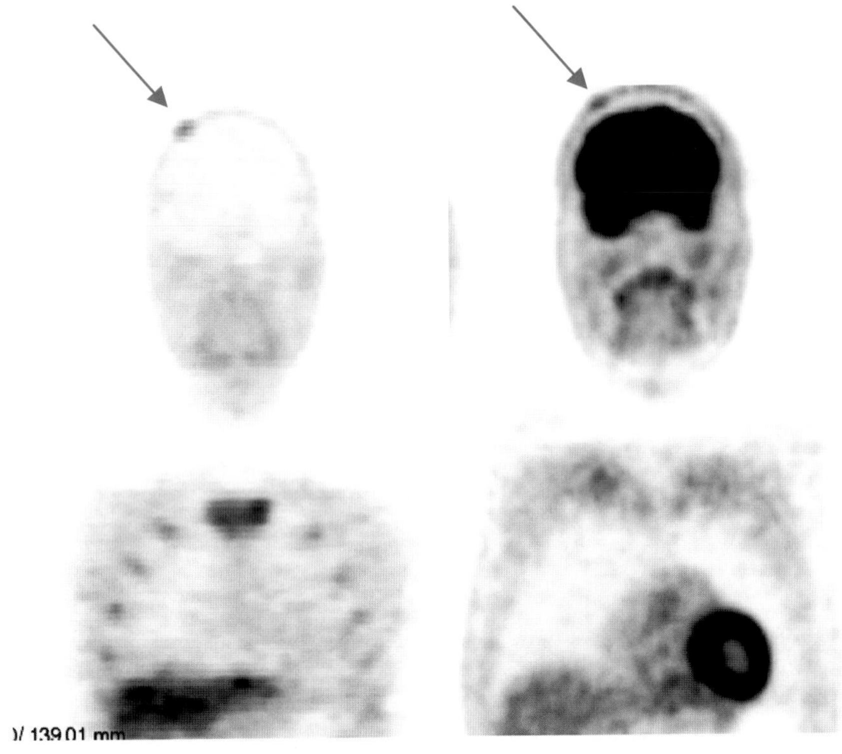

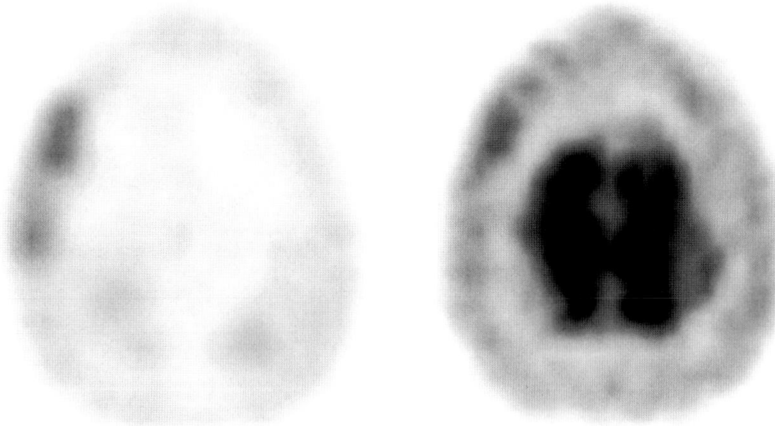

PET finding

Intense focal uptake for both FLT and FDG.

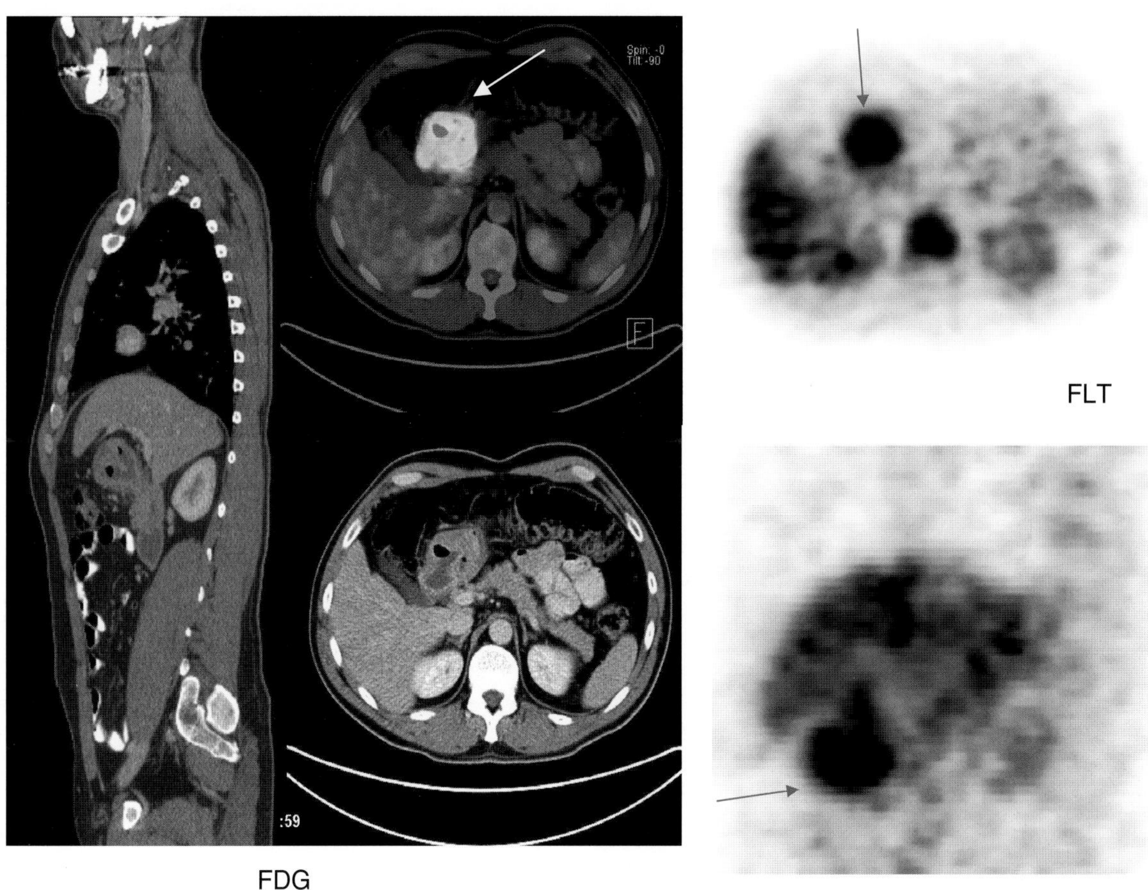

FDG

^{18}F-FDG finding

PET-CT scan shows intense focal uptake in the antrum region.

^{18}F-FLT finding

FLT PET also shows intense uptake of the tracer.

Female 71 years

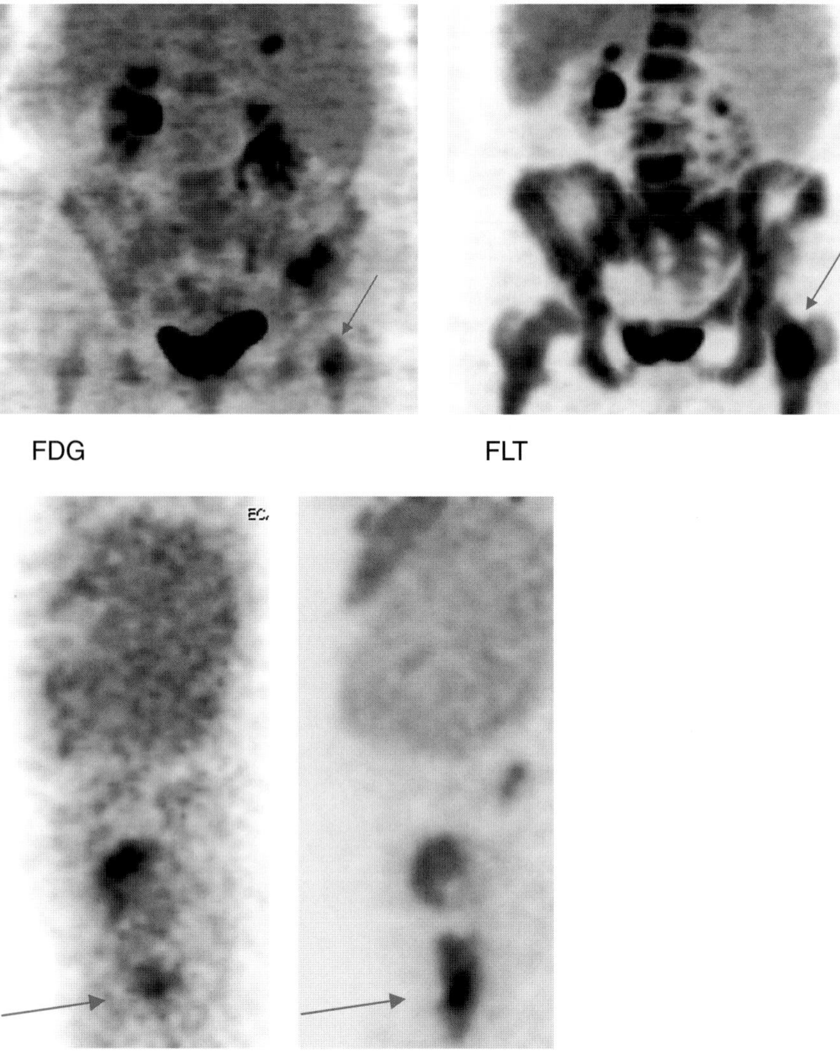

¹⁸F-FDG finding

PET scan shows intense focal uptake in the iliac bone and in the left femur (*red arrow*).

¹⁸F-FLT finding

FLT PET also shows intense uptake of the tracer.

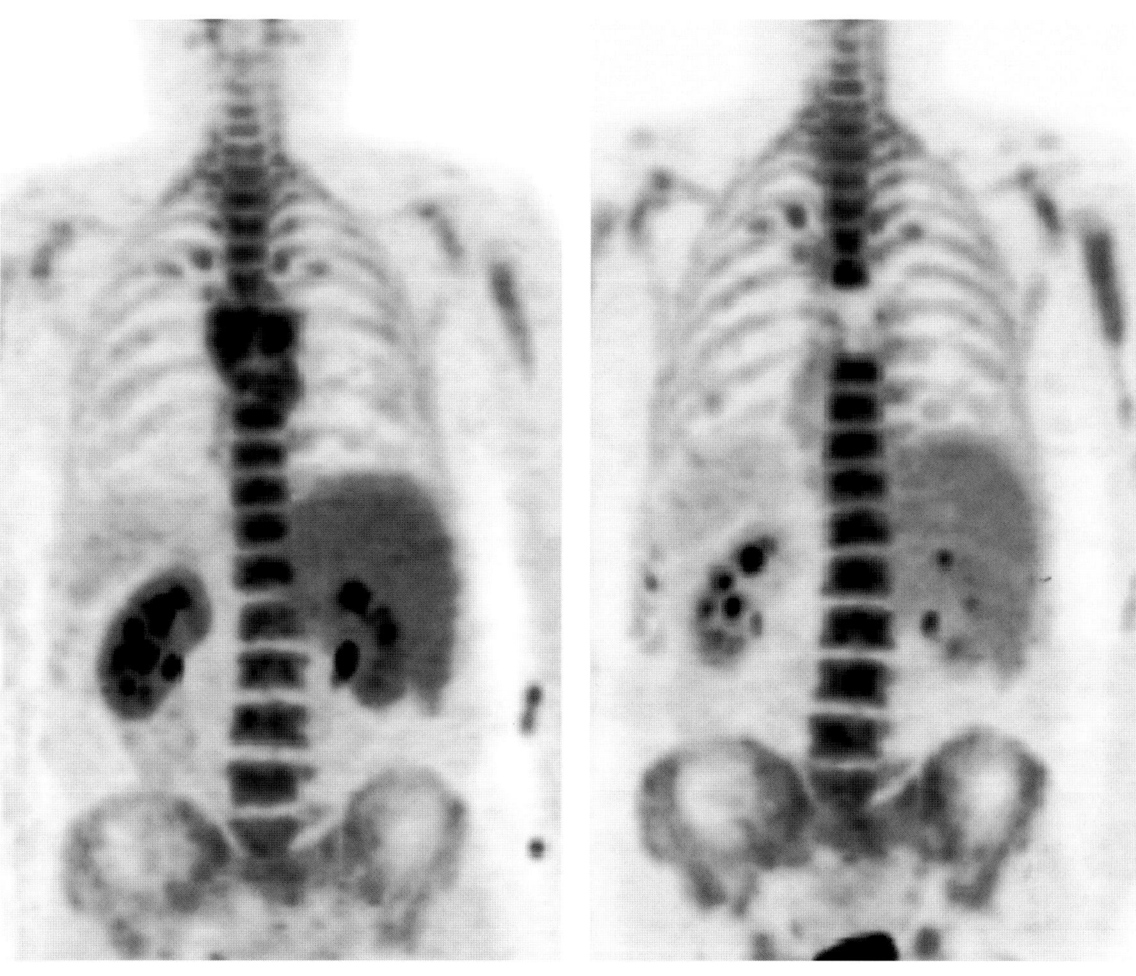

¹⁸F-FLT finding

PET scan shows intense focal uptake in the paravertebral lesion. Early during treatment (1 week after the first course of R-CHOP) a repeated PET demonstrated an evident decrease of tracer uptake.

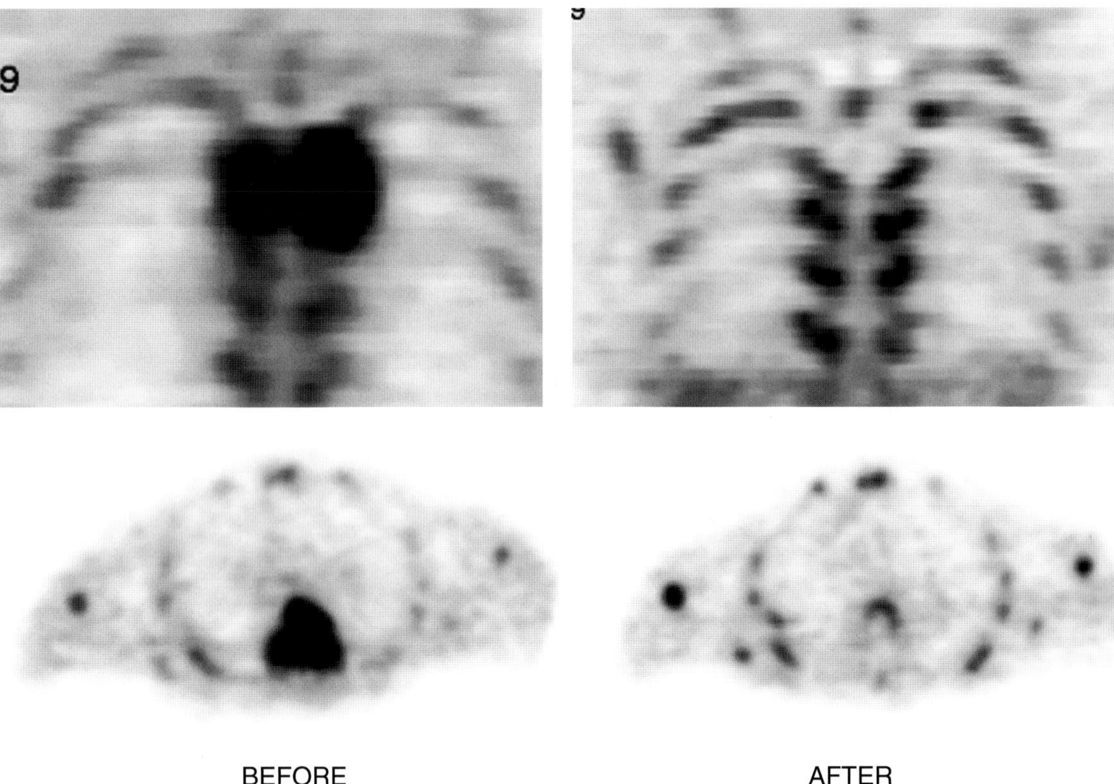
BEFORE
AFTER

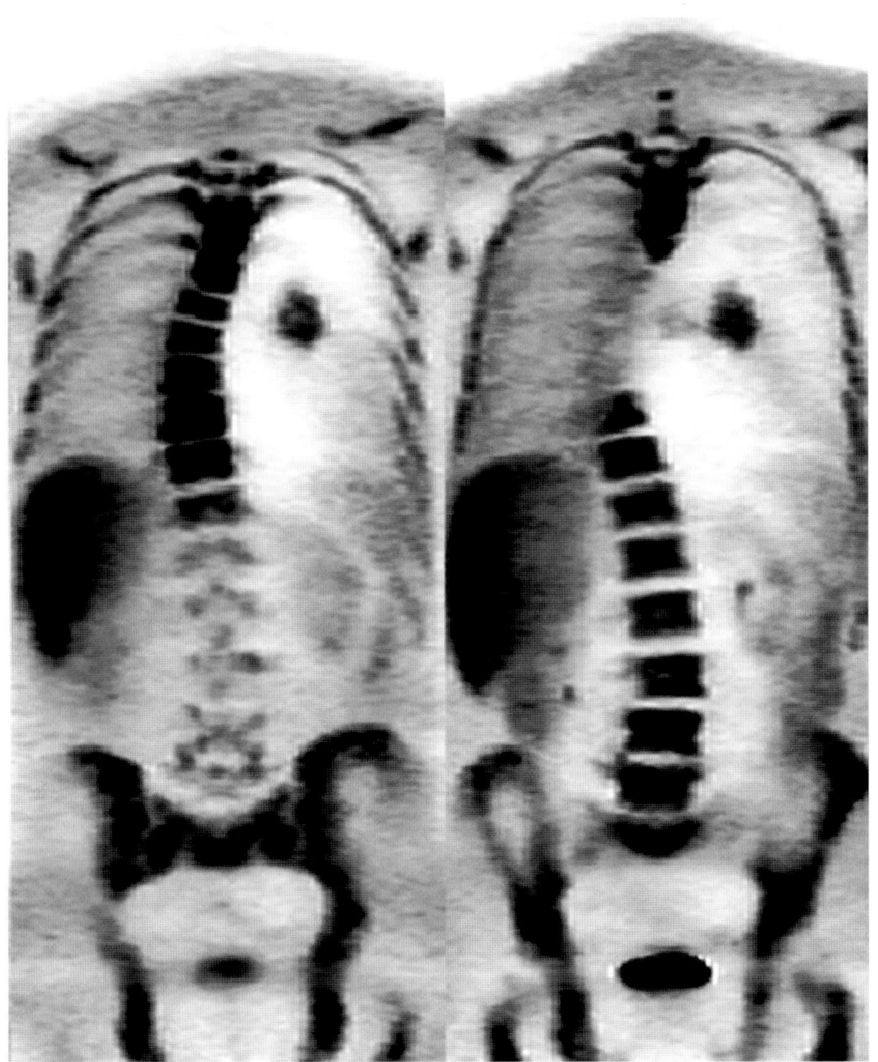

^{18}F-FLT finding

PET shows increased focal uptake in the left lung lobe, corresponding to the nodule, then resulted to be NSCLC.

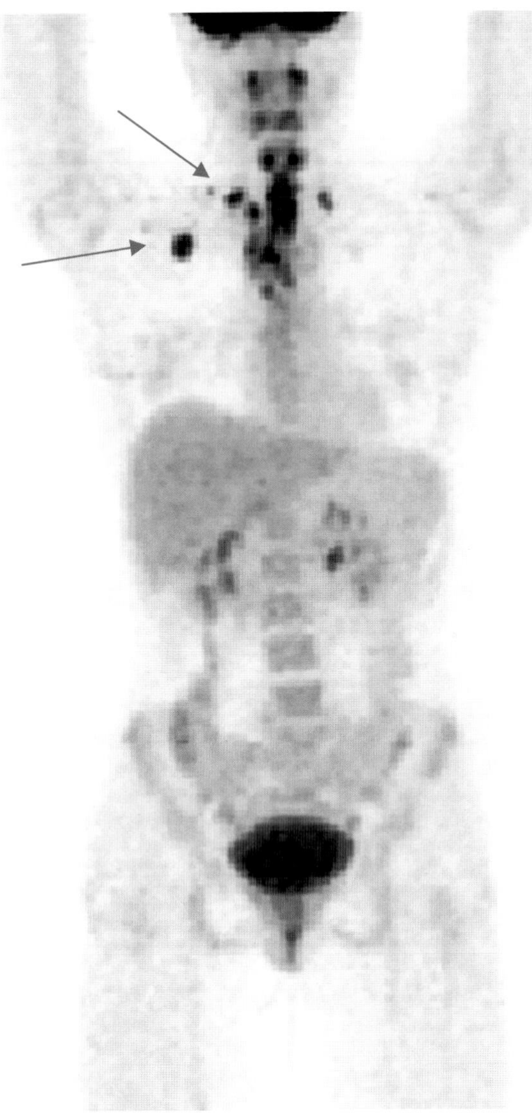

FDG

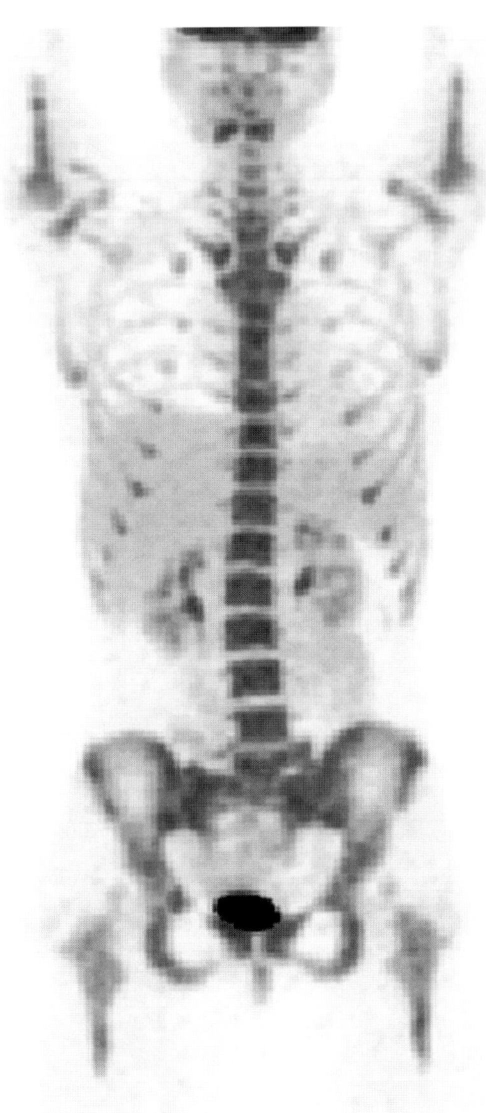

FLT

^{18}F-FDG and other findings

A patient with suspicion of lung cancer underwent FDG PET showing focal tracer uptake in the right lung lobe as well as around the trachea and mediastinal lymph nodes (*red arrows*).

^{18}F-FLT finding

No pathologically increased uptake; biopsy led to the diagnosis of laryngotracheitis.

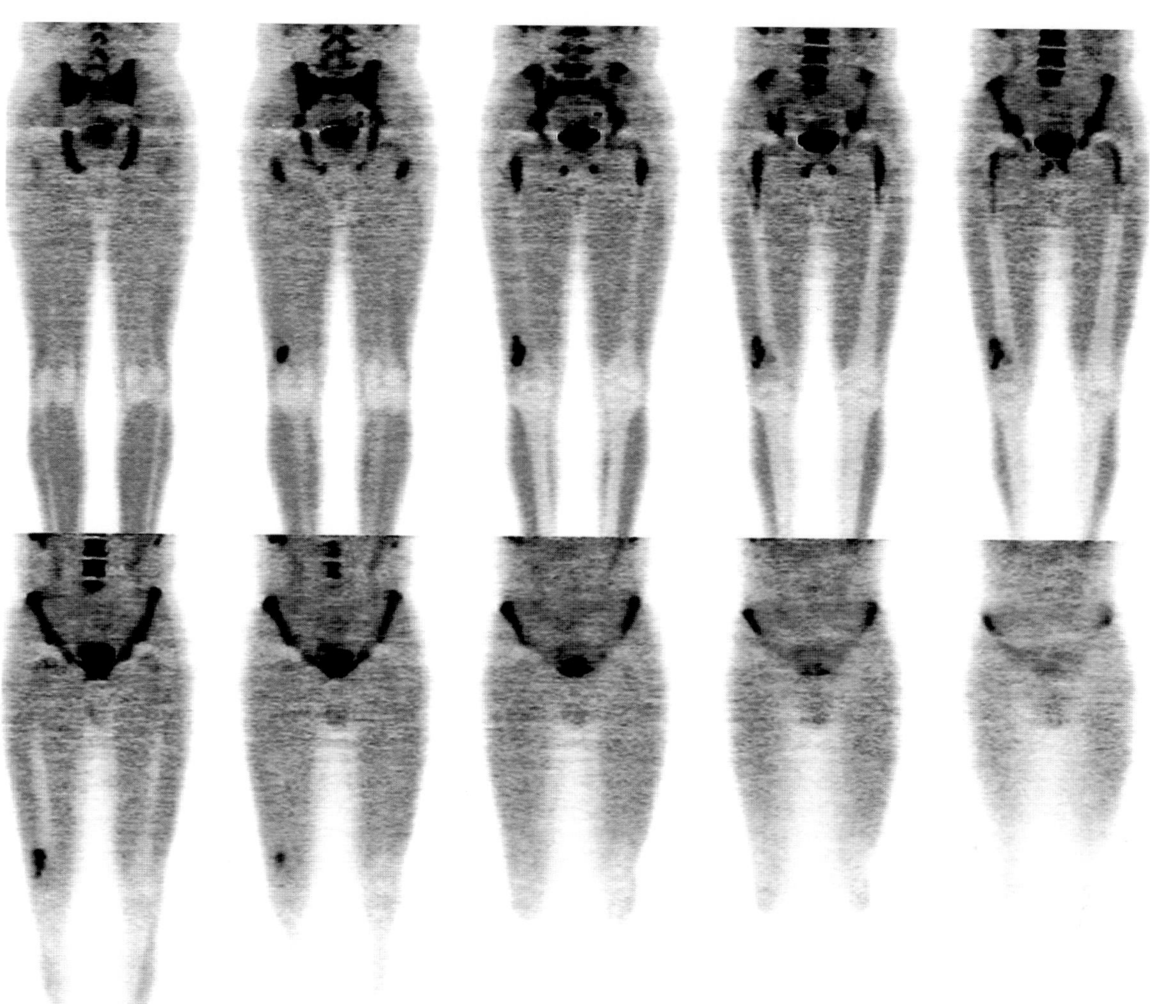

^{18}F-FLT finding

PET shows increased uptake indicating high proliferation fraction.

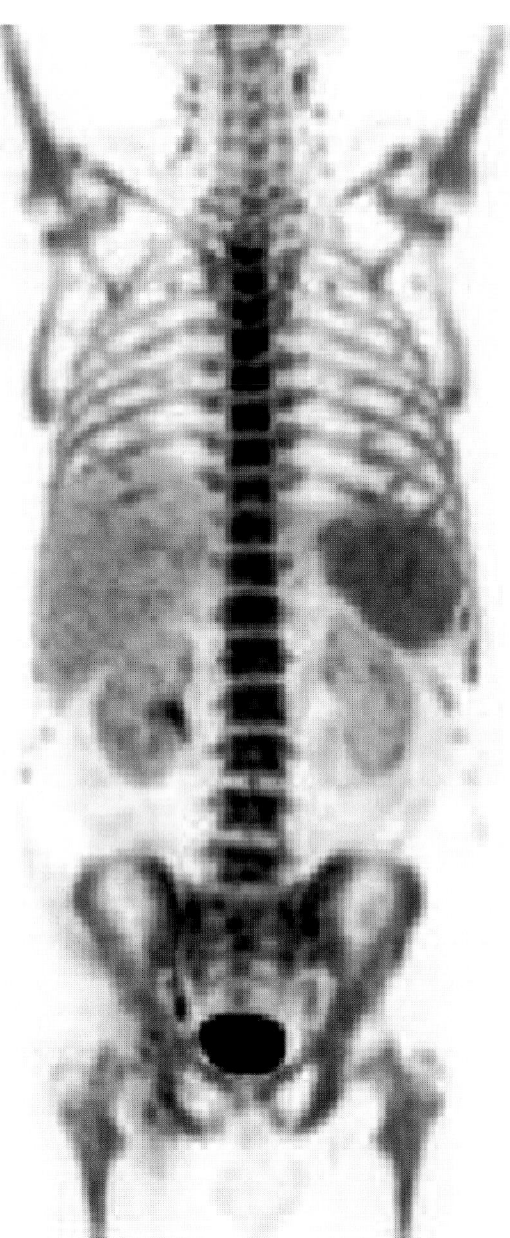

^{18}F-FLT finding

Pathologically increased FLT uptake is visible in the spleen and in the bone marrow.

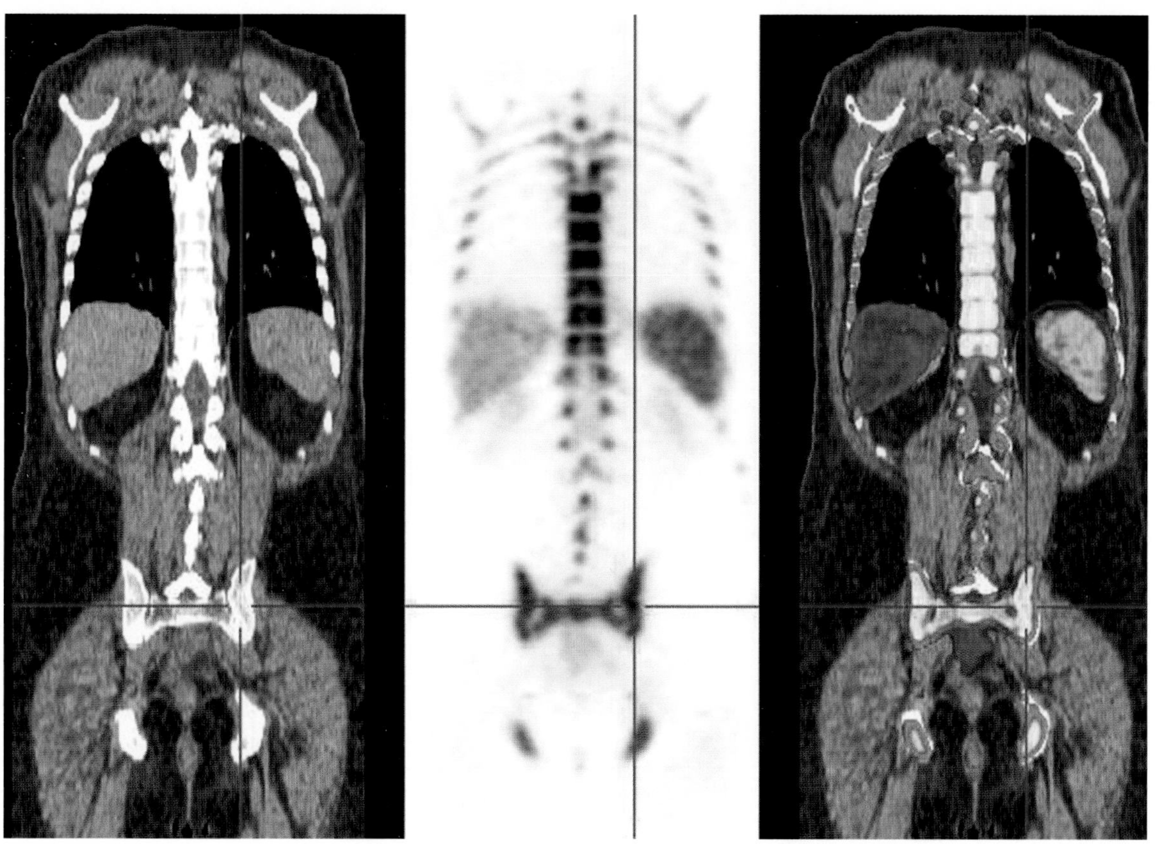

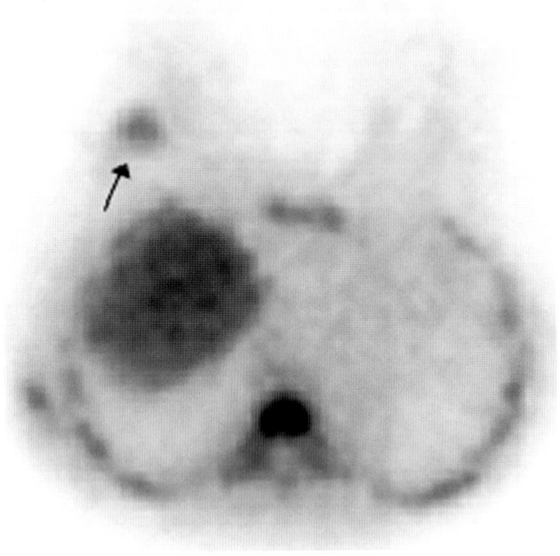

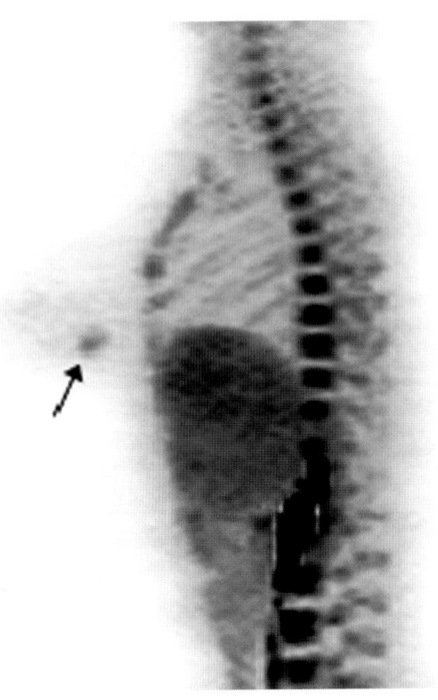

^{18}F-FLT finding

PET shows a focal area of increased uptake in the right breast.

Chapter 10 Dopa PET-CT

Adrienne H. Brouwers, Klaas P. Koopmans,
Rudi A. J. O. Dierckx, and Philip H. Elsinga

6–^{18}F –L-3,4 –dihydroxyphenylalanine (^{18}F-DOPA) is a PET tracer used for imaging neuroendocrine tumors which are derived from neuroendocrine cells. Neuroendocrine cells regulate a variety of body functions through paracrine stimulation. This is achieved via the production of a large variety of hormones, of which serotonin is the most prominent example, but the catecholamines, dopamine and (nor)adrenalin, and histamine may also be produced. The production of these hormones is accomplished via amine precursor uptake and decarboxylation. In differentiated neuroendocrine tumors, the capability to synthesize hormonal products has quite often remained. This makes imaging with amine precursors interesting in these tumors.

The catecholamine pathway is active in many neuroendocrine tumors. In this pathway, phenylalanine and intermediate products such as L-3,4 –dihydroxyphenylalanine (L-DOPA) are taken up via system L large amino acid transporters (LAT). After entering the cell, decarboxylation to dopamine takes place via the enzyme aromatic amino acid decarboxylase (AADC). Dopamine is then transported into intracellular storage vesicles through the vesicular monoamine transporter (VMAT). In these vesicles, dopamine can be further metabolized to noradrenalin and adrenalin. From these vesicles, the resulting end-products can be released in the extracellular environment. After excretion (signal transduction), these end-products can be transported back into the cells via selective transporter systems, e.g., dopamine and noradrenalin transporters. The catecholamines act as neurotransmitters, especially in the brain, or as hormones, e.g., adrenalin, when it is released from the adrenals, via α- and β-adrenergic receptors located on vessels and internal organs. Also, after release from the vesicles the catecholamines can be broken down to various degradation products. These can be measured in plasma and urine as fractionated catecholamines and metanephrines. In the serotonin pathway, the same LAT and VMAT transporter systems, and the enzyme AADC play a crucial role, resulting in the end-product serotonin. Although the exact uptake mechanism and intracellular fate of these amines and their metabolites are not precisely understood, it appears that increased LAT activity plays a role to satisfy a high precursor turnover due to an increased metabolic pathway, e.g., catecholamines or serotonin, and/or at least increased AADC activity in neuroendocrine tumors.

Nowadays, more and more PET centers are capable of producing ^{18}F-DOPA. The most widely used method for routine production is via regioselective fluorodestannylation (electrophilic fluorination). The other possible method, via nucleophilic fluorination, is a multistep, and therefore more time-consuming procedure, which on the other hand, has the advantage of having readily available large quantities of no-carrier-added ^{18}F-fluoride.

The ^{18}F-DOPA tracer has been developed during the seventies and eighties of the last century and the first injection in men was performed at Mc Master University, Hamilton, Canada. Since then, it has been widely applied for imaging of the dopaminergic system in the striatum in patients with Parkinson's disease and related disorders. More recently, the tracer has been applied as a whole-body imaging technique in patients with neuroendocrine tumors. Firstly, ^{11}C-DOPA was applied for this indication, followed by ^{18}F-DOPA.

^{18}F-DOPA PET scanning is typically performed 60 min after injection of a fixed dose (as low as 100 MBq) or a dose depending on body weight (up to 5 MBq/kg). ^{18}F-DOPA uptake at different time-points of 30 and 90 min has been described, showing no advantage of the 90-min scan over the 30-min scan with respect to interpretation, both, visual or semi-quantitative (SUV). The estimated mean radiation dose is one, 9 mSv per 100 MBq ^{18}F-DOPA. Patients are requested to fast for 2–6 h with free intake of fluids, although sometimes patients are not reported to have been fasting. Thus far, one adverse reaction after tracer injection has been reported. Especially when specific activity is low, in patients with a large tumor load fast injection of the tracer may induce a carcinoid crisis. There is debate whether or not, prior to PET scanning, patients should be pretreated with carbidopa, 2 mg/kg body weight or with a fixed dose of 100–200 mg, 1 h prior to injection. Carbidopa is a peripheral inhibitor of the enzyme AADC. It decreases the peripheral decarboxylation of ^{18}F-DOPA and also β-[^{11}C]-5-hydroxy-*L*-tryptophan (^{11}C-5-HTP), a tracer of the serotonine pathway, thus reducing renal excretion and subsequently improving tracer uptake in metastatic carcinoid tumors (well-differentiated neuroendocrine carcinomas) (^{11}C-5-HTP), and pheochromocytoma and abdominal paragangliomas (^{18}F-DOPA), most likely, due to increased tracer availability in the circulation. This resulted in better image quality due to decreased streaky image reconstruction artefacts caused by high physiological excretion of the radiotracer via kidneys and urinary bladder, and increasing SUV of tumor lesions. Why carbidopa pretreatment results in a generally decreased tracer uptake in pancreatic tissue is not quite understood but may be related to differences in

AADC activity in neuroendocrine tumor types and differences in metabolic handling of these PET tracers by exocrine and endocrine pancreatic tissue. Because of the likely strong similarities between ^{11}C-5-HTP and ^{18}F-DOPA tracer handling in patients with gastrointestinal neuroendocrine tumors, carbidopa pretreatment is also advocated for ^{18}F-DOPA PET imaging in this patient group to improve image quality especially in the region of the kidneys and bladder, and to improve lesion detectability via further increased SUV of lesions. Indeed, high accuracy rates for the detection of (metastatic) neuroendocrine tumors have been reported by the institutes that do use carbidopa pretreatment. However, pancreatic islet cell tumors may be an exception to the rule. This should be further investigated.

In the last decade, ^{18}F-DOPA PET-CT imaging has been most tested in patients with mid-gut well-differentiated neuroendocrine carcinomas (carcinoids), other gastroenteropancreatic neuroendocrine tumors, such as (non) functioning pancreatic islet cell tumors, pheochromocytomas and paragangliomas, and medullary thyroid carcinomas. In these studies, most patients had proven (recurrent) disease and ^{18}F-DOPA PET-CT has been compared with current anatomical imaging techniques, mostly CT and/or MRI, and other functional imaging techniques, such as somatostatine receptor scintigraphy with ^{111}In-octreotide (SRS), $^{123/131}$I-labeled metaiodobenzylguanidine (MIBG), ^{18}F-FDG PET, and more recently, also with ^{68}Ga-labeled PET based variants of octreotide. Regarding the anatomical imaging techniques, they are frequently found to be complementary to the functional imaging techniques under study in these patient series. In carcinoids, patient based reported sensitivities for ^{18}F-DOPA PET-CT are very high, ranging from 65–100% and seems to be an excellent staging method. However, in direct comparison to ^{11}C-5-HTP PET, on a patient based analysis, the ^{11}C-5-HTP tracer outperformed ^{18}F-DOPA (sensitivity of 100 vs. 96%, respectively), whereas per-lesion analysis showed the opposite (sensitivity of 78% for ^{11}C-5-HTP and 87% for ^{18}F-DOPA). In two smaller PET studies with mixed-type neuroendocrine tumors, the ^{68}Ga-labeled analogues of somatostatine also did better than ^{18}F-DOPA PET. This can be partly explained by the inferior imaging results of ^{18}F-DOPA in patients with (non) functioning islet cell tumors in these studies. This is in line with the study that directly compared ^{18}F-DOPA and ^{11}C-5-HTP PET, both in carcinoid and islet cell tumor patients. Metastatic tumor lesions of islet cell tumors were visualized much better with ^{11}C-5-HTP compared to ^{18}F-DOPA: patient-based sensitivity of 100 vs. 89%, respectively. Also, ^{11}C-5-HTP seems to be the tracer of choice compared to ^{18}F-DOPA, when imaging other foregut (e.g., bronchial) neuroendocrine tumors.

Also in medullary thyroid carcinoma, and pheochromocytoma and paragangliomas, ^{18}F-DOPA PET imaging has been reported to perform well or better than the reference imaging techniques. However, this seems to be also dependent on the differentiation grade of the tumor. In patients with more aggressive, and fast growing tumors, ^{18}F-FDG PET performs better than ^{18}F-DOPA PET, and vice versa. In medullary thyroid carcinoma, there is a suspicion that one may have to rely on the calcitonine doubling-time to select the optimal PET tracer for a given patient, while in malignant pheochromocytoma and paraganglioma this seems to particularly depend on the underlying germline mutation.

It is expected that the reported high detection rates of ^{18}F-DOPA PET for various types of neuroendocrine tumor lesions will be lower in clinically more difficult cases, such as when a diagnosis is only suspected and not pathologically confirmed. A recent study seems to confirm this finding. In patients ($n = 32$) with only biochemical proof of the disease, various types of neuroendocrine tumors, the diagnostic accuracy of ^{18}F-DOPA PET-CT was 88%, whereas in patients ($n = 61$) that were restaged, the overall accuracy was 92%. Likewise, specificity of the ^{18}F-DOPA tracer in the various tumor types has not been structurally studied. Furthermore, changes in therapeutic management due to initial and follow-up ^{18}F-DOPA PET-CT scans has not been documented systematically. Also, its role as a prognosticator or parameter for early response monitoring in the various neuroendocrine tumor types has not been studied to date. These are all areas in which more research is warranted.

Although ^{18}F-DOPA uptake has been reported in both functioning and nonfunctioning neuroendocrine tumors, and also independently from the type of substance produced (e.g., serotonin or catecholamine), in theory a relationship between ^{18}F-DOPA uptake and metabolic activity seems obvious. In a retrospective study analyzing the performance of ^{18}F-DOPA PET and PET-CT in patients with known or suspected feochromocytomas, no significant correlation was found between SUVmax of the lesions and plasma or urinary biochemical measurements ($n = 15$ patients available for this analysis). In a prospective analysis in feochromocytoma patients, both with benign and malignant behavior, also this relationship was studied using a PET image derived index for overall tumor activity per patient. Per patient the whole-body metabolic burden was calculated, consisting of the total sum of metabolic burden of lesions in one patient. Metabolic burden per lesion was calculated as SUV mean lesion x PET derived volume of the lesion, 40% isodensity contour. When not only SUVmax of one lesion but overall tumor activity per patient (n = 43) was taken into account, significant correlations were found with 24 h urinary excretion of total (free + conjugated) normetanephrine (r = 0.84, P < 0.001), metanephrine (r = 0.57, P < 0.01), and 3-methoxytyramine (r = 0.65, P < 0.01), as well as plasma free levels of normetanephrine (r = 0.82, P < 0.001), 3-methoxytyramine (r = 0.51, P = 0.01) and chromogranin A (r = 0.49, P < 0.01). This finding needs further confirmation in other patient groups, as well as analyzing this relationship in other situations, e.g., after therapy has been initiated, or the meaning of such a possible relationship, e.g., for prognosis and monitoring therapy response.

^{18}F-DOPA PET has been tried in other tumor types, such as small cell lung cancer, melanoma, Merkel cell tumor, prostate cancer with neuroendocrine differentiation, neuroblastoma and brain tumors. Patient numbers in these reports were often small and the performance of the ^{18}F-DOPA imaging method, compared to other anatomically or functionally imaging methods differed widely.

Furthermore, ^{18}F-DOPA whole-body PET has been tested as a tracer in various nononcological settings. In infants and children with hyperinsulinism, ^{18}F-DOPA PET has been reported to be quite successful to distinguish the histological focal from the diffuse form. In these situations, carbidopa pretreatment should not be given. Visualization of parathyroid adenomas with ^{18}F-DOPA PET does not seem to be possible. However, in search for an ectopic ACTH producing tumor, ^{18}F-DOPA PET has been reported to be helpful.

In conclusion, ^{18}F-DOPA PET is a excellent functional imaging technique in patients with proven neuroendocrine tumors, especially in carcinoids. Performance also seems to be good in feochromocytomas and medullary thyroid carcinomas, depending on the clinical context. In contrast, pancreatic islet cell tumors and more generally, foregut neuroendocrine tumors seem to perform less well compared to other functional imaging methods, e.g., somatostatine receptor based scintigraphy (SPECT and PET) and ^{11}C-5-HTP PET. Adding CT improves the detection rate even more, thus combining the ^{18}F-DOPA technique in dedicated PET-CT scanners is likely more optimal. The imaging characteristics of ^{18}F-DOPA PET-CT in complex clinical cases or in less advanced clinical stages, e.g., when there is only a suspicion of a neuroendocrine tumor, needs to be further determined. Furthermore, its role for monitoring response to therapy and predicting response to therapy needs to be further investigated. Also, how this imaging technique performs in relation to other new functional PET imaging techniques, especially the ^{68}Ga-labeled somatostatine analogues in neuroendocrine tumors, needs to be further elucidated. Potential advantages of the latter technique are that the labeling technique of the somatostatine analogues with ^{68}Ga is relatively easy to perform, and one does not need a cyclotron, since ^{68}Ga can be eluted from a commercially available generator. On the other hand, ^{18}F-DOPA PET may have a broader clinical applicability, e.g., for studying the dopaminergic system of the human brain, oncological tumors that do not usually express somatostatine receptors, nononcological settings, such as infants with hyperinsulinism, and the well-known neurological setting.

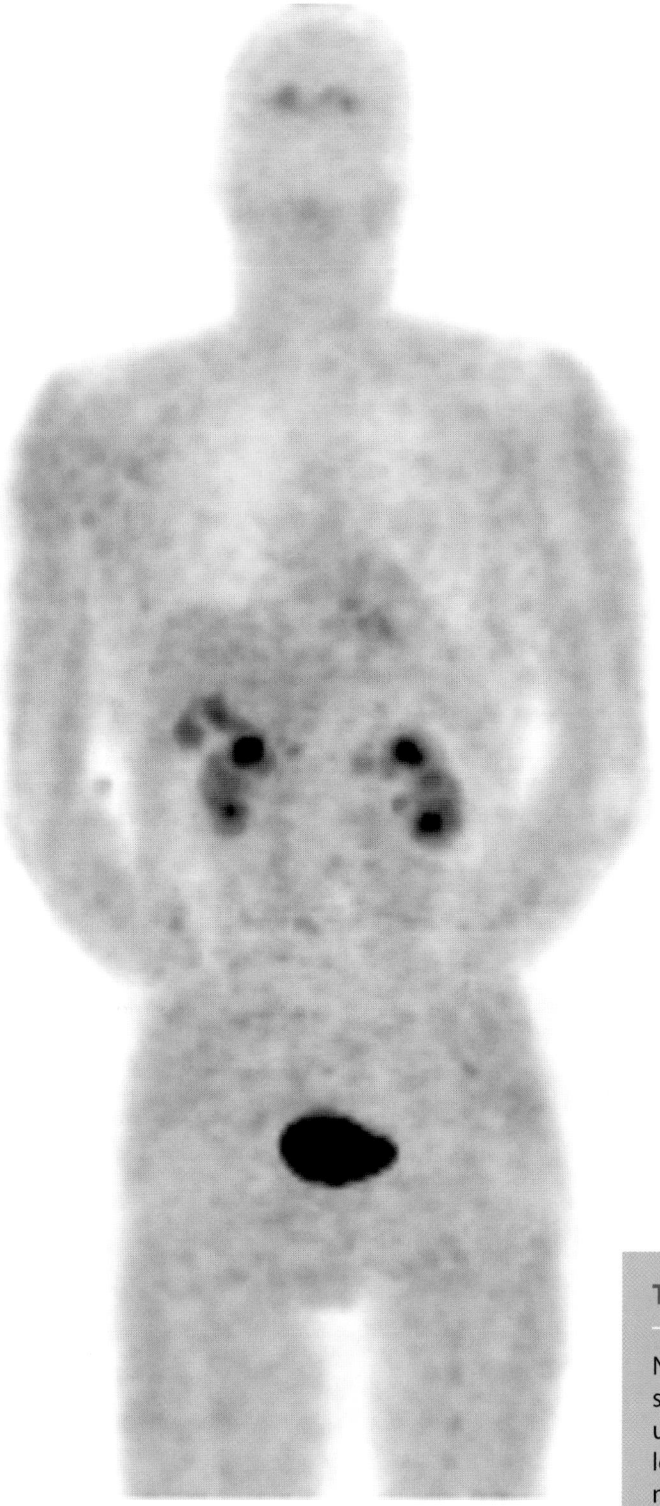

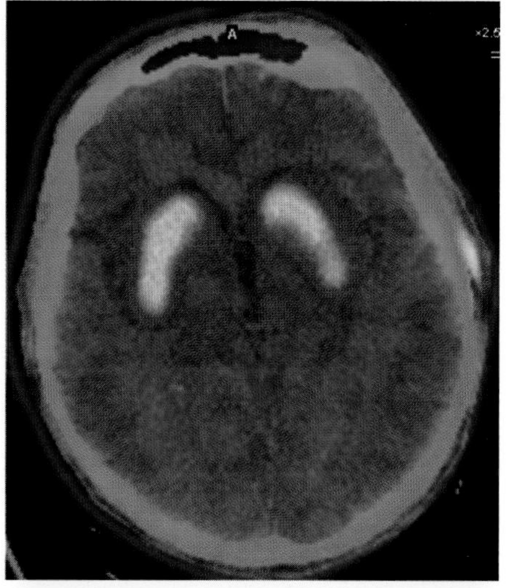

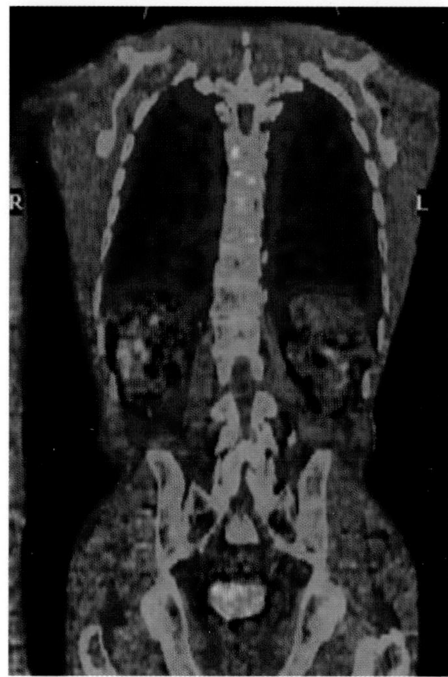

Teaching point

Note the physiological uptake in the striatum, gall bladder, kidneys, and urinary bladder. In every patient with liver lesions on ^{18}F-DOPA PET, the observer needs to be aware of the exact localization of the gall bladder in order to distinguish between physiological uptake and pathological uptake of a neuroendocrine tumor lesion.

Female 48 years

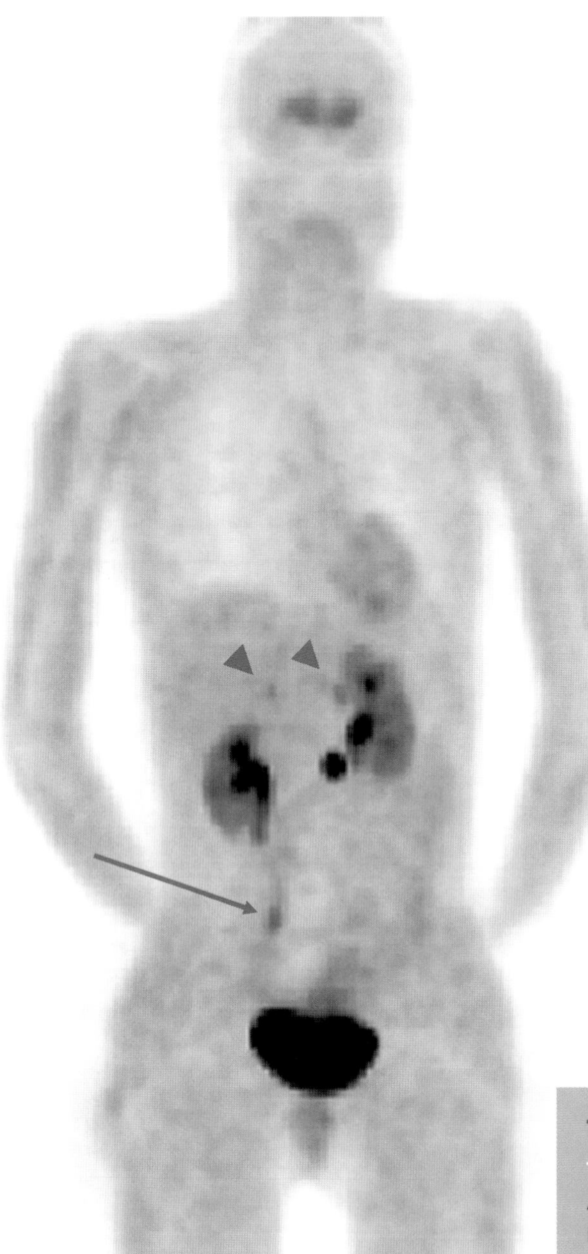

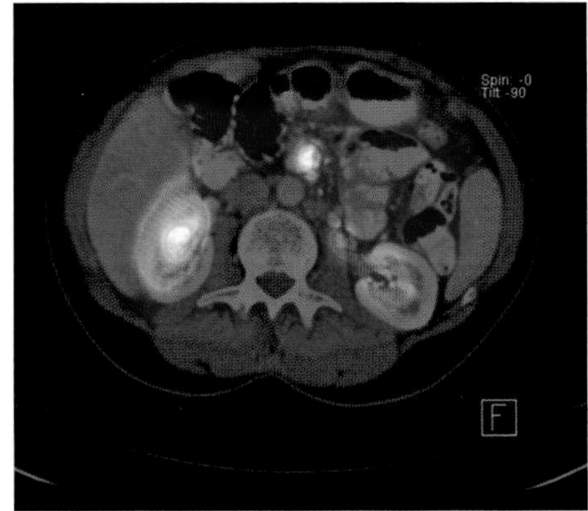

^{18}F-DOPA finding

PET shows recurrent disease in the upper abdomen, median to the left kidney.

Teaching point

Although in general for pancreatic neuroendocrine tumors ^{11}C-5-HTP PET and/or SRS is the preferred imaging technique, these tumors may also take up ^{18}F-DOPA. In case the ^{18}F-DOPA PET scan is similar to the ^{11}C-5-HTP PET scan, one can use the ^{18}F-DOPA PET scan as the PET method for follow-up, since this tracer is logistically easier to handle. Also note the physiologically faint uptake in both adrenals and in the right ureter (*arrowhead* and *arrow*, respectively).

Female 55 years

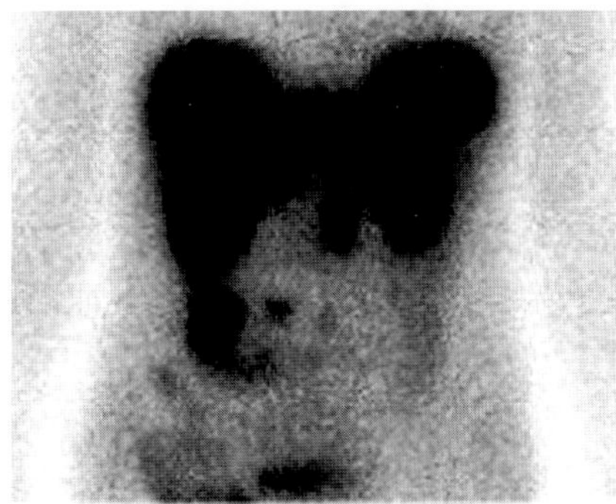

SRS

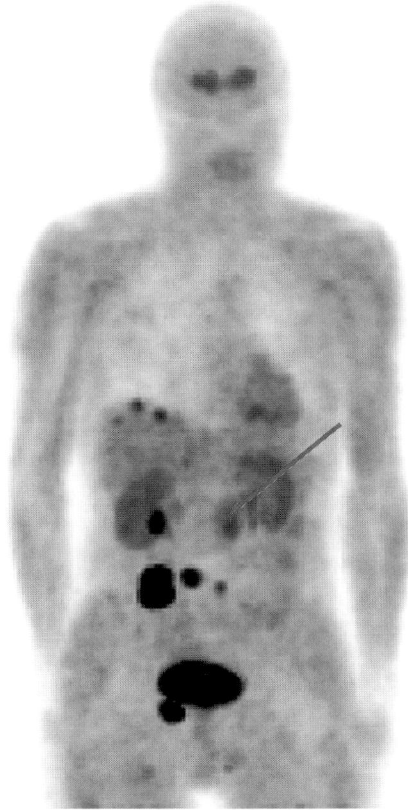

^{18}F-DOPA

Somatostatin receptors scintigraphy finding

SRS shows abdominal lesions.

^{18}F-DOPA finding

PET shows multiple lesions in the liver, abdomen, and groin, and also a faint lesion in the myocardial region. Metastatic carcinoid in the heart was later confirmed by MRI of the heart.

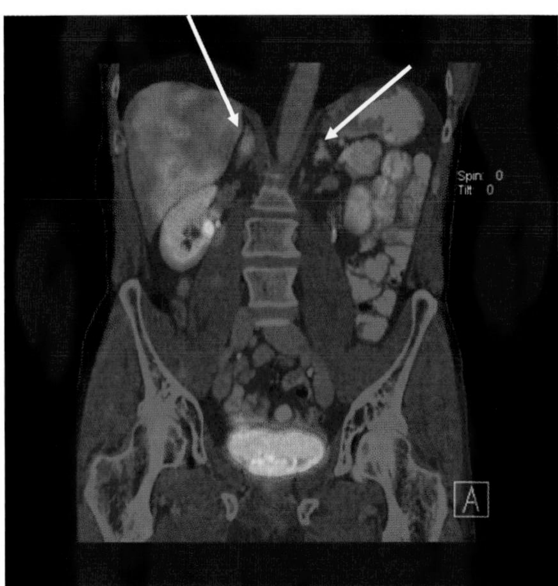

^{18}F-DOPA PET – CT fusion

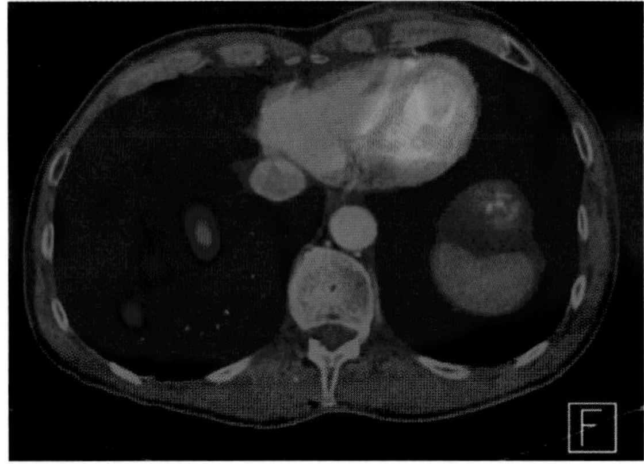

Teaching point

Note the physiological uptake in the pancreas (*red arrow*) and both adrenal glands (*white arrow*). Also, in metastasized carcinoid myocardial metastases are more frequently present than doctors are currently aware.

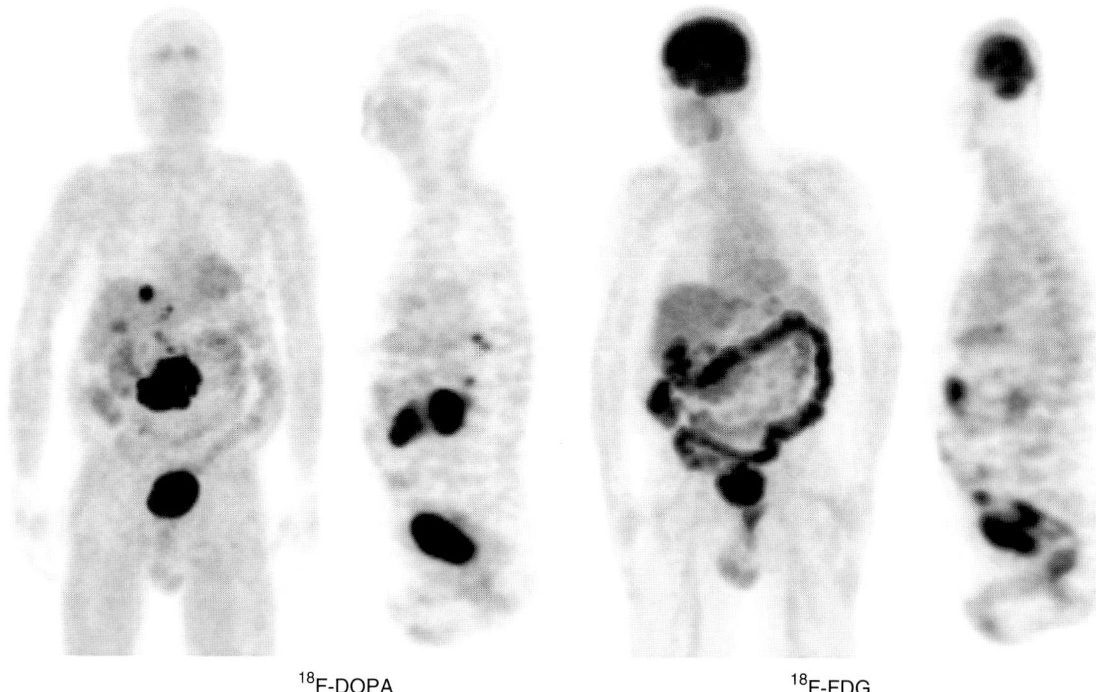

^{18}F-DOPA ^{18}F-FDG

PET findings

The abdominal mass and liver lesions corresponding to carcinoid lesions are clearly visible on the ^{18}F-DOPA scan, while the ^{18}F-FDG PET scan shows the rectal carcinoma (and a lot of physiological gut uptake).

Teaching point

These scans demonstrate that glucose metabolism in well-differentiated, slowly progressive neuroendocrine tumors is usually not increased. Therefore, these tumors often show almost no ^{18}F-FDG uptake.

Female 52 years

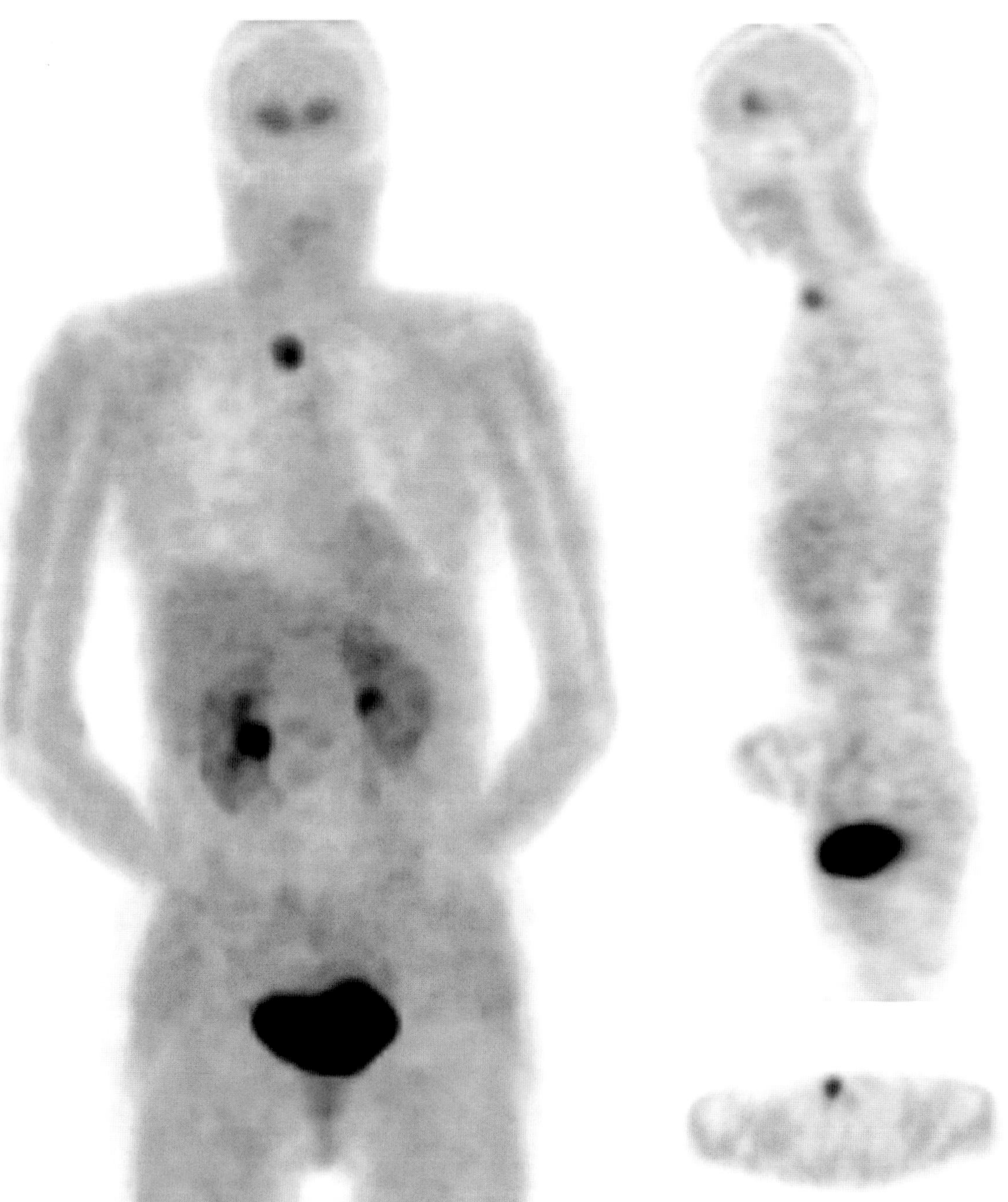

^{18}F-DOPA finding

PET shows the primary tumor in the thyroid region on the right side.

Teaching point

Also (metastatic) medullary thyroid carcinoma is often visualized with ^{18}F-DOPA. Visualization may depend on the growth pattern, and rapidly progressive patients may be better imaged with ^{18}F-FDG PET.

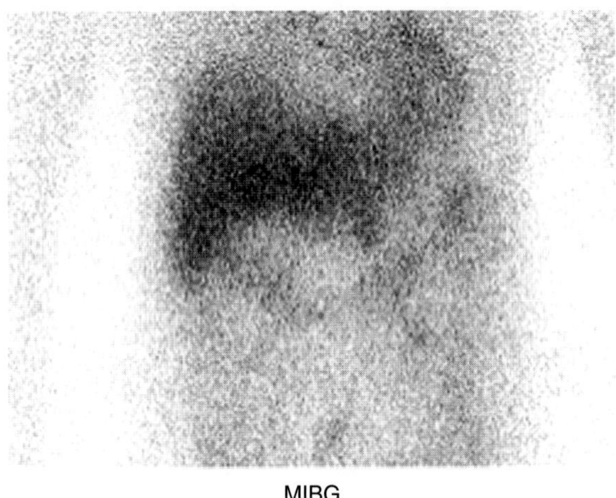

MIBG

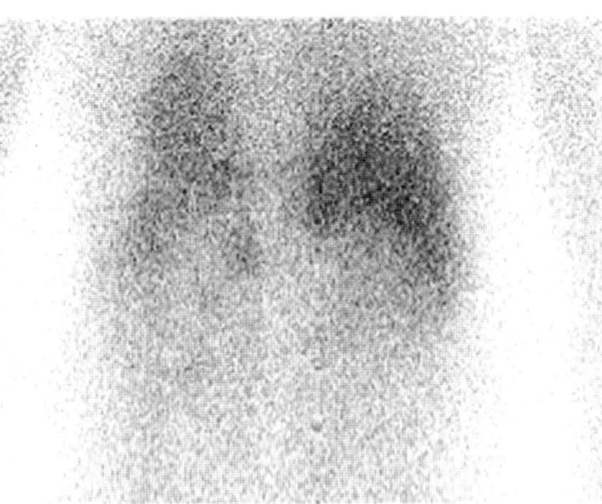

^{123}I-MIBG and other findings

Patient with MEN2a who had been previously operated upon for a medullary thyroid carcinoma. Now he presents with elevated metanephrines.
The planar abdominal images do not clearly show increased uptake in the adrenals.

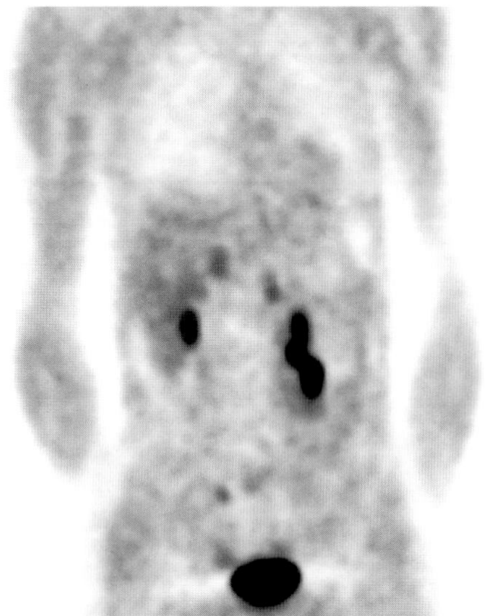

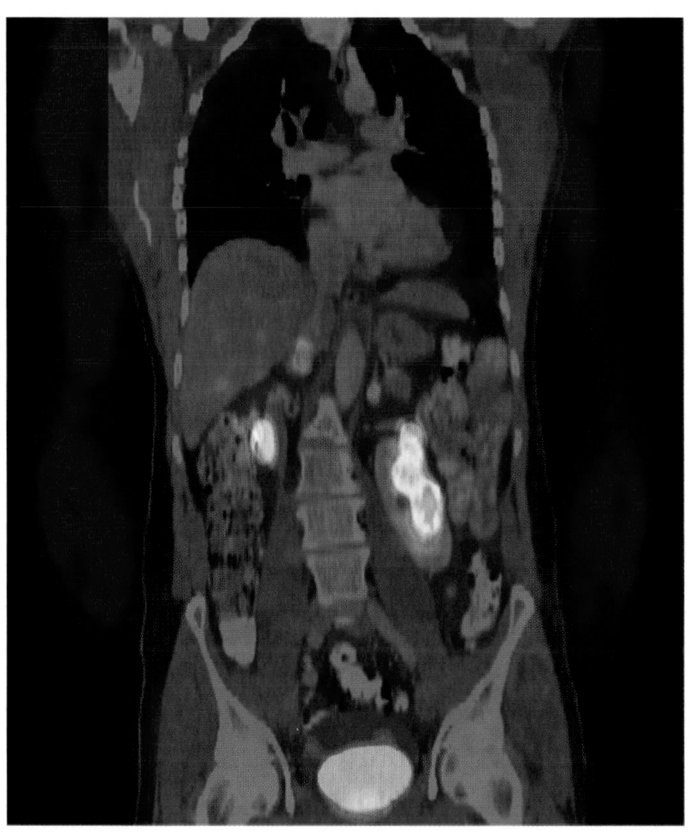

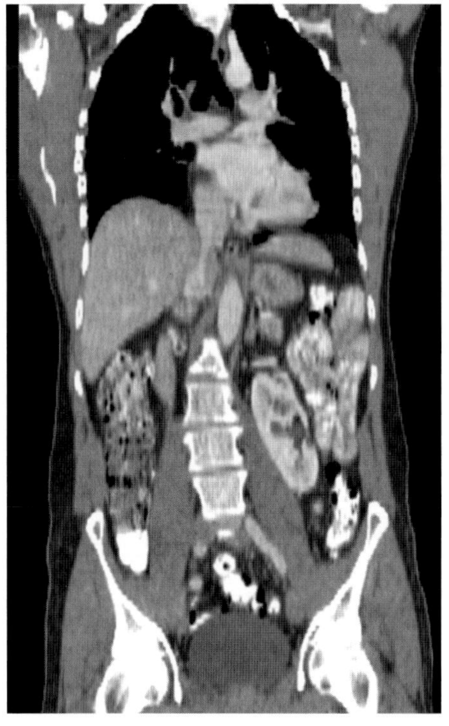

^{18}F-DOPA finding

^{18}F-DOPA PET shows slightly increased bilateral adrenal uptake, corresponding to both adrenals.

Teaching point

Sensitivity of ^{18}F-DOPA for both benign and malignant pheochromocytoma has been reported to be better compared to ^{123}I-MIBG.

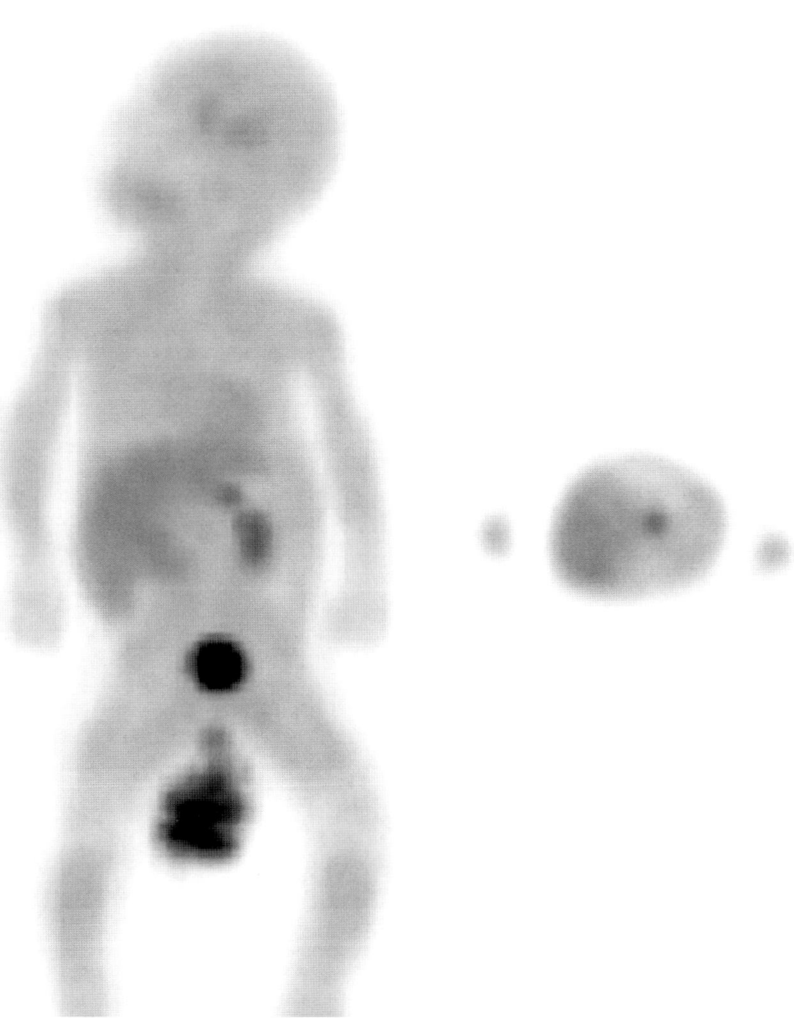

■ ^{18}F-DOPA finding

PET scan shows a focal lesion in the region of the tail of the pancreas.

Teaching point

In congenital hyperinsulinism, the ^{18}F-DOPA PET scan can be very helpful in distinguishing a focal from a diffuse form of hyperinsulinism. If a focal lesion can be demonstrated, only a partial resection of the pancreas is necessary to cure the patient.

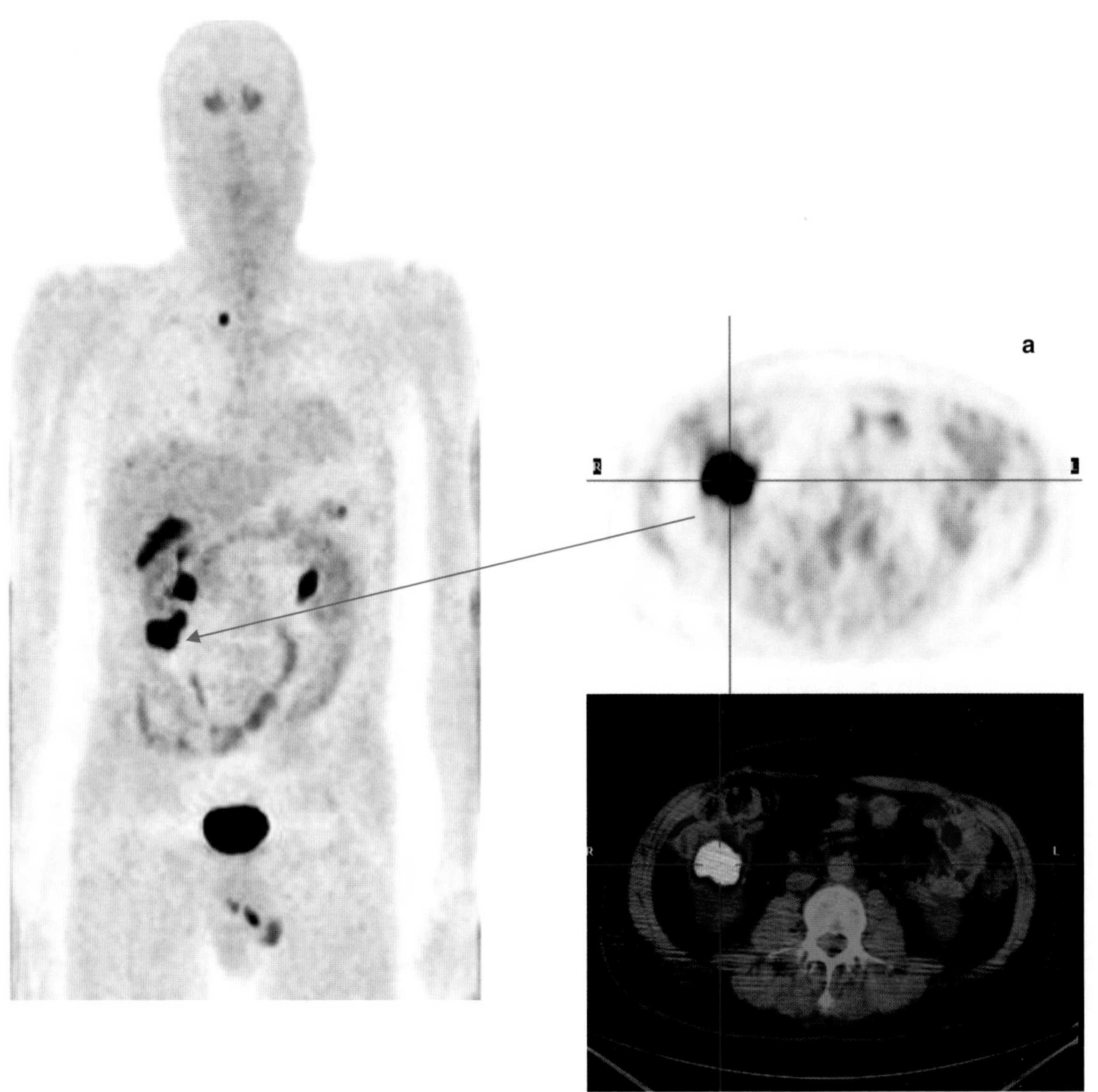

^{18}F-DOPA finding

PET scan shows the primary lesion (a) as well as secondary lesions in the liver (b) and in one lymph node (c).

b

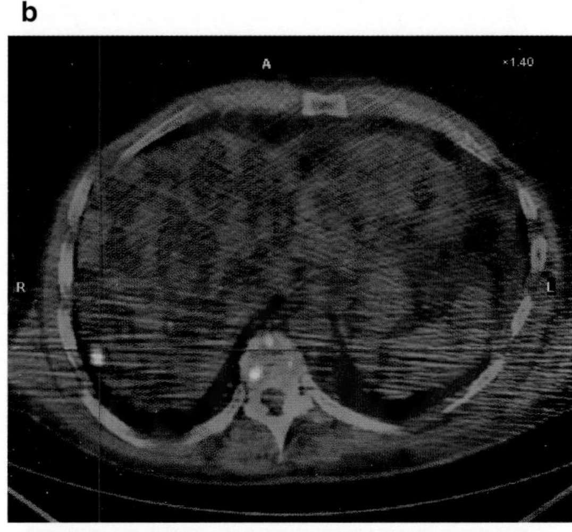

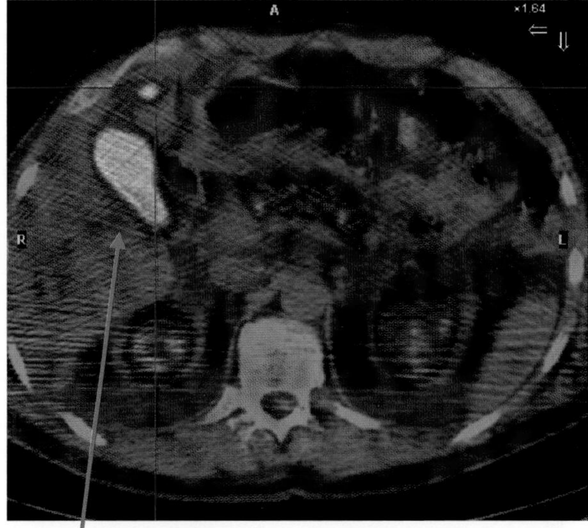

c

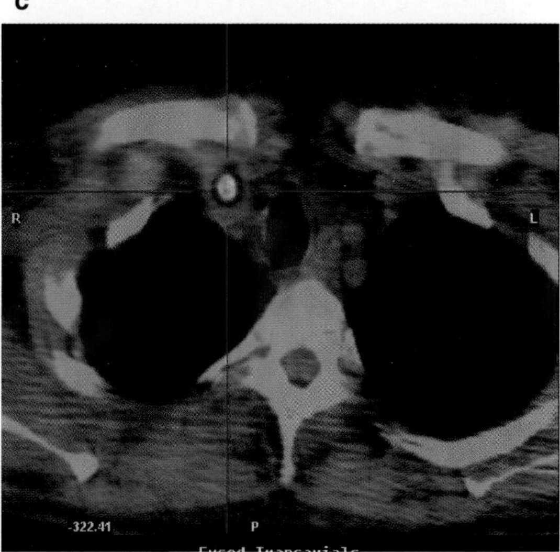

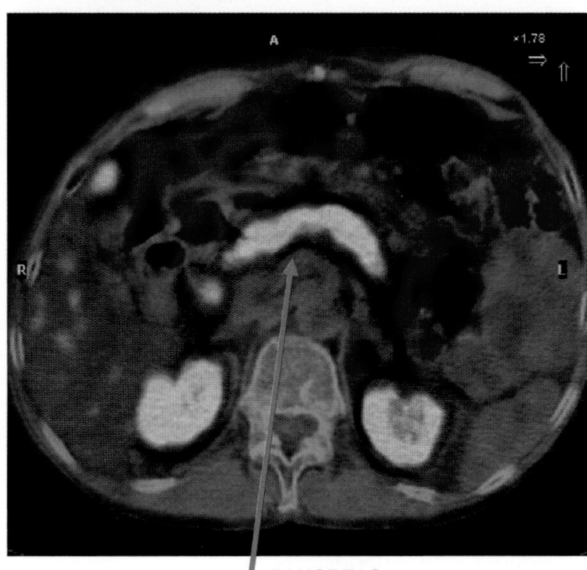

Teaching point

Note the physiological uptake in the gall bladder. There is also a major uptake in the pancreatic body, particularly intense when carbidopa pretreatment is not performed before the scan (as in this case).

Case 9 Metastatic Carcinoid

Male 75 years

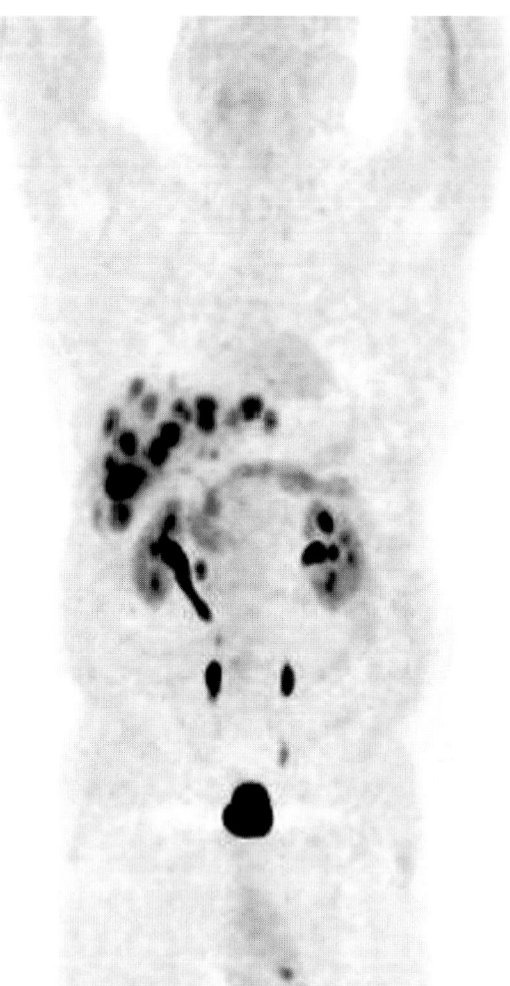

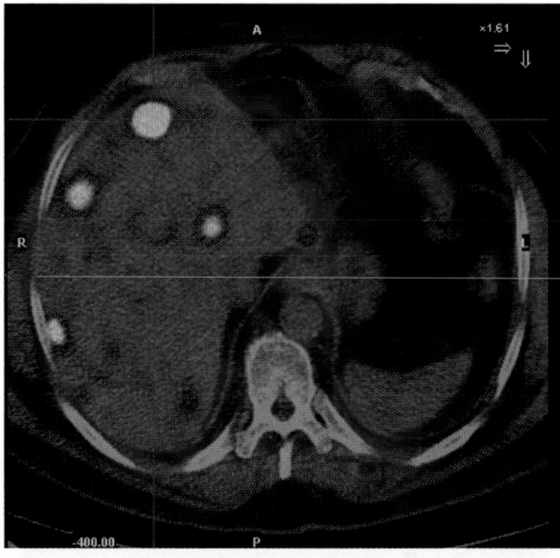

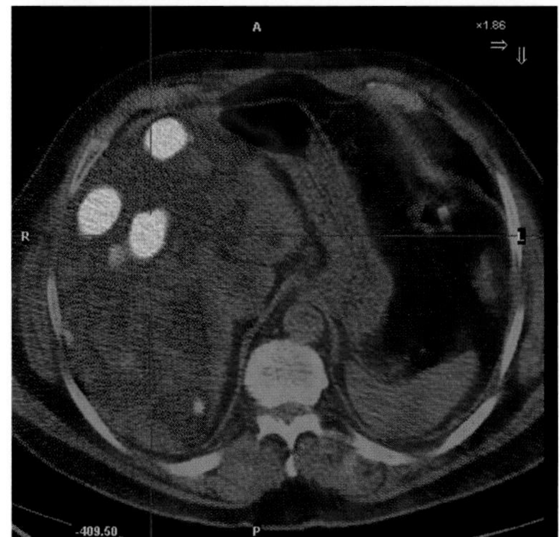

^{18}F-DOPA finding

PET scan shows multiple lesions in the liver and a mesenteric lymph node.

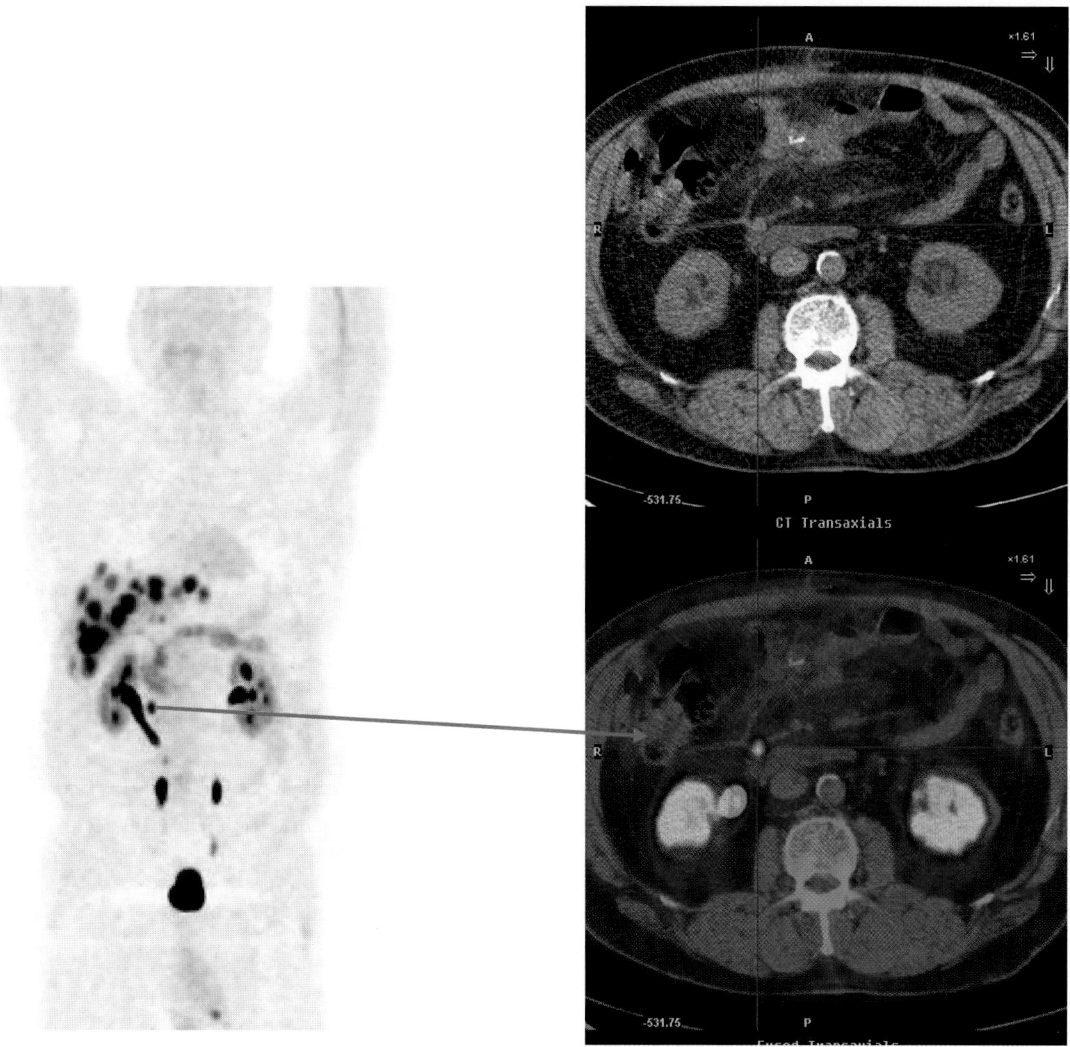

Teaching point

The use of fused or hybrid imaging with PET-CT is of great help to properly identify the exact site of tracer increased uptake.

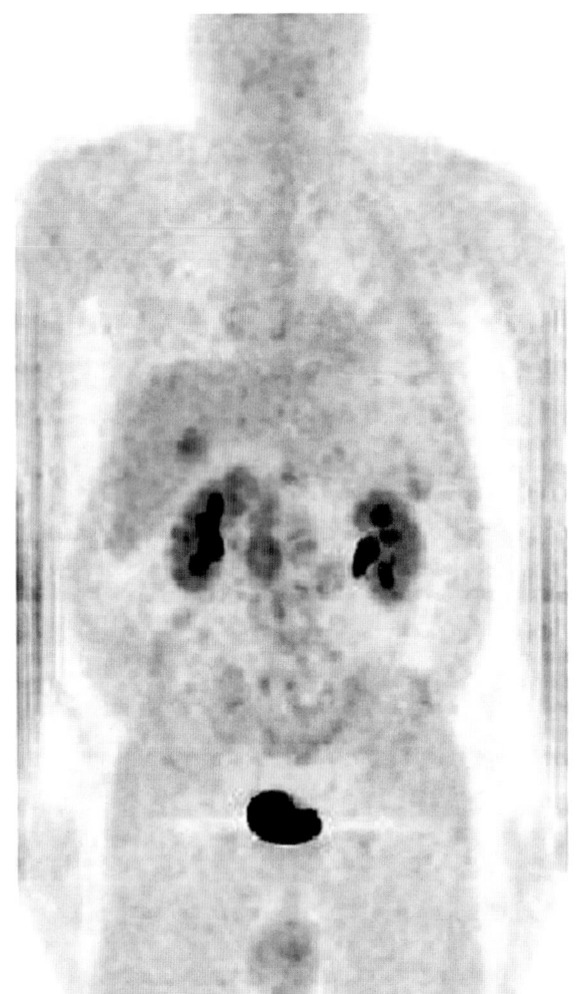

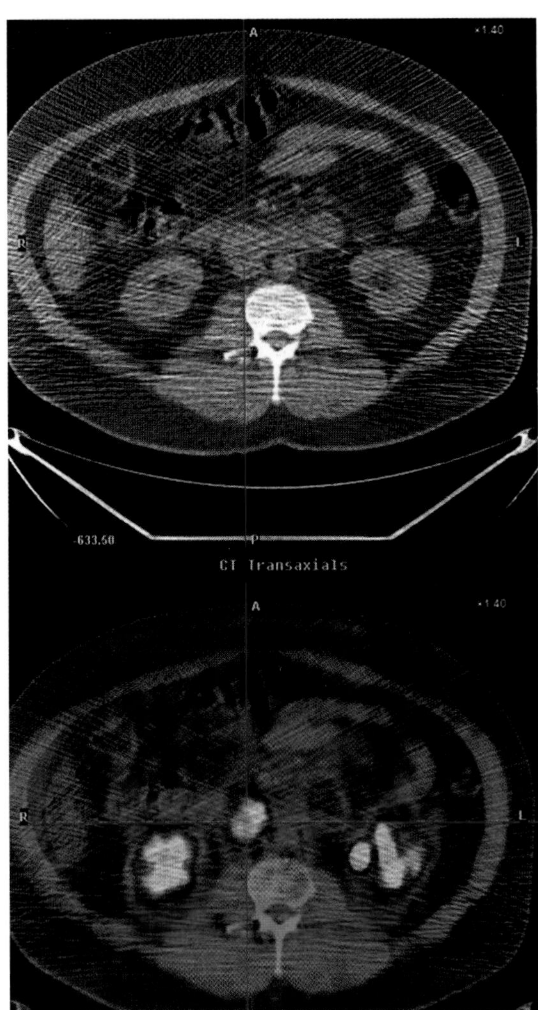

^{18}F-DOPA finding

PET-CT scan (without carbidopa pretreatment) shows single pancreatic lesion in the pancreas.

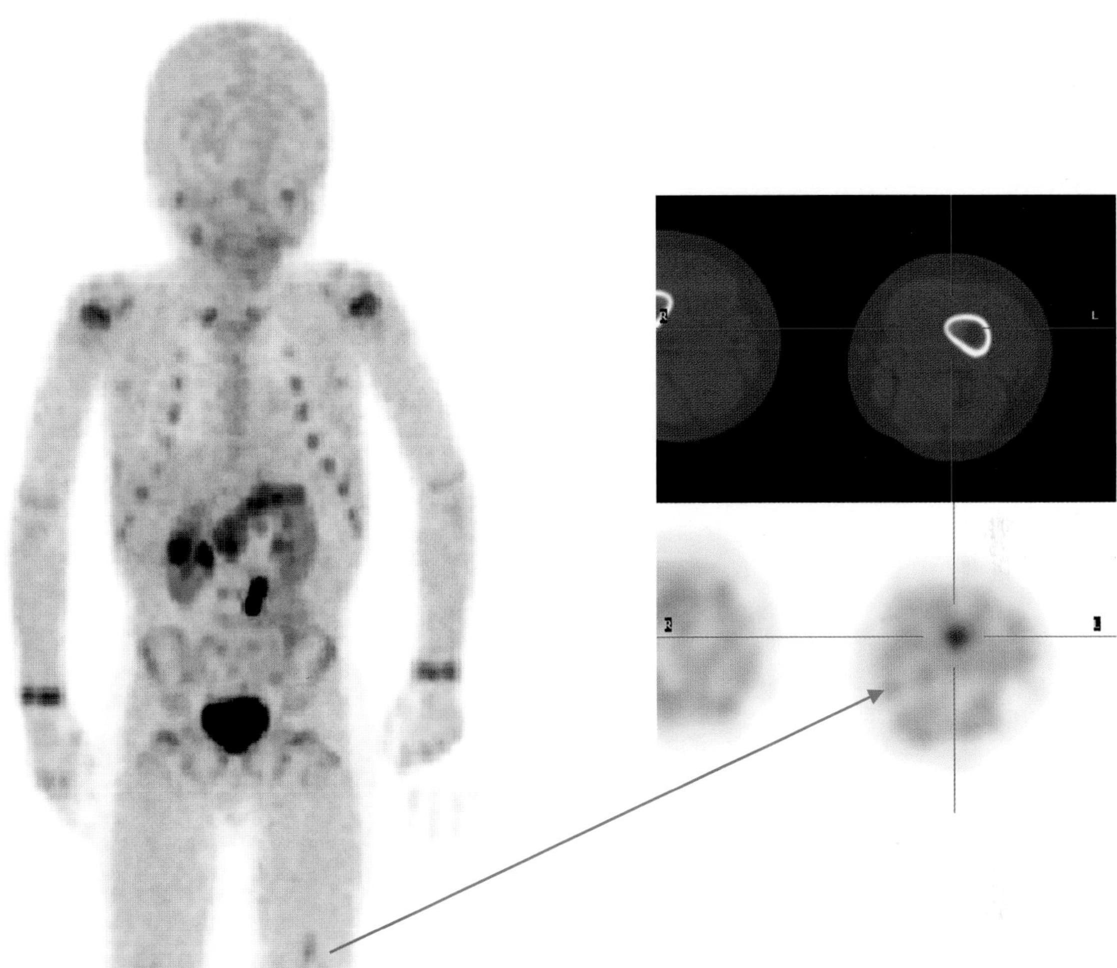

^{18}F-DOPA finding

PET-CT scan shows single lesion in the bone marrow of left tibia.

Chapter 11 Imaging of Hypoxia with PET-CT

Tove J. Grönroos, Heikki Minn, and Rodney J. Hicks

For a number of tumors, including head and neck squamous cell carcinoma (HNSCC) and cervical carcinoma, radiotherapy (RT) may fail to achieve local control due to the presence of tumor hypoxia (pO_2 < 10 mmHg), which decreases the availability of the oxygen free radicals necessary to induce sufficient DNA damage to cause cell death. The role of hypoxia in increasing tumor resistance to radiation therapy was first recognized a century ago, but it was not until 1953 that the crucial role of oxygen in radiation response was fully acknowledged and described as the oxygen enhancement effect. There is a great variability in the oxygen availability to cancer cells, and most human malignancies show microscopic hypoxic regions that are heterogeneously distributed within the tumor mass and may be located within an apparently well-vascularized lesion. Hypoxic cells are about 3 times more radioresistant than well-oxygenated cells and their presence in tumors contributes to failure of local control in RT. There is also evidence that hypoxia increases resistance to chemotherapy. This may be because hypoxia induces a decrease in proliferating cells, which constitute to target cell population of most chemotherapeutic drugs. Cells further away from a functional blood vessel may also receive a decreased concentration of drug.

Several papers have shown a clear correlation between tumor oxygenation, as measured by oxygen probes, and a poor tumor response to RT. Intratumoral hypoxia cannot be predicted by commonly used clinical prognostic variables, such as size, grade, or histology of tumor. Tumors that appear identical by clinical and radiological criteria can vary greatly in the extent of hypoxia. Thus, if tumor oxygenation is to be employed as a predictor of treatment resistance, it will have to be individually measured for each tumor and potentially at each tumor site.

Since the discovery that nitroimidazole based compounds bind to macromolecules in hypoxic cells, attempts have been made to find radiolabeled agents that could be used noninvasively with PET for assessment of hypoxia. To obtain high-contrast images, an ideal hypoxia tracer should have high affinity and specificity for cellular hypoxia and low nonspecific binding in nonhypoxic cells. Metabolic degradation of the tracer is undesirable, since the resulting labeled metabolites could bind to nontarget molecules or take part in biochemical processes unrelated to hypoxia, reducing specificity. One important property of the tracer is lipophilicity, which determines the ability of the molecule to cross cell membranes. While this capability is important to allow intra-cellular uptake, high lipophilicity increases nonspecific activity in nonhypoxic cells, particularly early after tracer administration. Finally, clearance of unbound tracer should be fast in order to discriminate between specific and nonspecific uptake. For the latter, greater hydrophilicity is desirable because this increases blood clearance through more rapid renal excretion. In reality, all these criteria are seldom fulfilled.

Hypoxia imaging with PET is for the most part based on ^{18}F-labeled 2-nitroimidazole compounds, which covalently bind to cellular macromolecules in hypoxic conditions, as a result of multistep intracellular electron reduction of the parent compound. When oxygen is present, the reoxidized reactive species exits the cell. Conversely, in hypoxia, further reductive metabolism gives rise to more or less stable intracellular hydroxylamine derivatives, which are trapped intracellularly and can be detected with PET. Most 2-nitromidazole tracers are freely diffusible and no active tissue uptake mechanism is present. The lipophilicity and peripheral metabolic properties vary amongst these tracers and lead to differences in the pharmacokinetic properties of the various 2-nitroimidazoles. These properties are mainly determined by the chemical composition of the side chain that is attached to the imidazole ring moiety. One common feature and a clear limitation of ^{18}F-labeled 2-nitroimidazoles is that they accumulate quite slowly in hypoxic tissues, showing no hypoxia-specific signal until 1.5–4 h postinjection. Most, if not all, of the 2-nitroimidazole tracers evaluated so far also show an early blood flow-dependent distribution. Although they are primarily excreted via the urinary system, leading to the bladder being the most common dose limiting organ, elimination by the hepatobiliary pathway occurs to a variable degree and can limit evaluation of the abdomen.

Enhanced tracer binding under hypoxic conditions has been convincingly shown in preclinical settings for several compounds, including [^{18}F]FMISO, [^{18}F]FETA, [^{18}F]FETNIM, [^{18}F]FAZA, [^{18}F]EF1, [^{18}F]EF3 and [^{18}F] EF5. In addition to [^{18}F]FMISO, which was the first hypoxic PET tracer to be used in humans, clinical trials have also more recently been reported using [^{18}F]FAZA, [^{18}F]FETNIM, [^{18}F]EF3 and [^{18}F]EF5. In addition to these, ^{64}Cu-labeled ATSM has also been intensively evaluated in both preclinical and clinical settings.

In this chapter, the use of [^{18}F]FMISO, [^{18}F]FAZA, and [^{18}F]EF5 in human cancer patients will be discussed with examples given in an image format.

[^{18}F]FMISO

Fluorine-18 fluoromisonidazole ([^{18}F]FMISO) has been the most widely evaluated hypoxia tracer both in preclinical and human studies up to this point in time. Results of [^{18}F]FMISO PET for evaluation of tumor hypoxia in humans have been reported by several institutions across a range of malignancies, including head and neck, cervical, nonsmall cell lung, and renal cell cancers, glioma and soft-tissue sarcoma. Most importantly, the ability of [^{18}F]FMISO to stratify prognosis in patients receiving conventional radiotherapy and targeted therapy of hypoxia has been demonstrated. These data suggest that the imaging signal may provide a noninvasive prognostic and predictive biomarker in patients receiving RT.

Despite foci hypoxia being almost universal within tumors, sites of viable malignancy, as identified on [^{18}F] FDG PET scanning, have variable uptake of hypoxia tracers like [^{18}F]FMISO. This variation occurs both between and within lesions. The extent of hypoxia-related trapping apparent on PET imaging is typically less than that of viable tumor. It is recognized that necrotic tumor areas having low reductase activity may not show retention of [^{18}F]FMISO.

Despite encouraging results with ([^{18}f]fmiso, its high lipophilicity results in slow clearance kinetics, which necessitates a delay in imaging for 4–6 h post injection to obtain optimal contrast between hypoxic and nonhypoxic tissue. By this time, count statistics are degraded by the relatively rapid decay of fluorine-18 and hence hypoxia-specific retention is typically evaluated 2 h post injection in clinical cases. However, the substantial background activity even 4 h after tracer administration interferes with the quality of the images, and generally, low contrast between putatively hypoxic tissue and normal structures makes these scans difficult to read qualitatively. It may also make it difficult to assign regions-of-interest (ROI) for lesion quantification or radiotherapy planning, although initial experience suggest feasibility of [^{18}F] FMISO PET for dose escalation beyond 80 Gy in head and neck cancer.

[^{18}F]FAZA

The low target-to-background ratios typically observed with [^{18}F]FMISO raise questions regarding its suitability as a widely applicable PET hypoxia tracer and have justified the development of related tracers that are more hydrophilic. Such tracers should allow shorter waiting time for imaging after tracer administration, potentially lower radiation exposure and greater lesion contrast, assuming similar binding to hypoxic cells. There are a number of promising agents in this regard. Encouraging results obtained with a sugar-coupled 2-nitroimidazole derivative [^{123}I]IAZA developed for SPECT imaging, initiated the development of fluorine-18 labeled 1-α-D-(5-fluoro-5-deoxy-arabinofuranosyl)-2-nitroimidazole) ([^{18}F]FAZA). This agent was first used in human subjects at the Peter MacCallum Cancer Center and the Technical University of Munich for the evaluation of head and neck cancer. Additional studies are ongoing in lung cancer and sarcoma. Even more clearly than observed with [^{18}F] FMISO, [^{18}F]FAZA demonstrates heterogeneity of hypoxic signal between and within lesions in the same individual. The Cross Cancer Institute group, which developed the tracer, recently published their own initial experience with this agent in a range of tumor types including lymphoma.

[^{18}F]EF5

EF5 (2-(2-nitro-1H-imidazol-1-yl)-N-(2,2,3,3,3-pentafluoropropyl)-acetamide) has been extensively studied as a hypoxia marker using intravenous administration followed by tumor biopsy and immunohistochemical analysis. Monoclonal antibodies conjugated with fluorescent dyes, which recognize cellular adducts of the marker have been found to be highly specific. MISO and ETA ("precursors" for FMISO and FETA) were originally developed as radiosensitizers, and later adapted as hypoxia tracers by incorporating an ^{18}F-label into the molecule. In contrast, EF5 was developed specifically for the detection of hypoxia using immunohistochemical methods, and the ^{18}F-labeled compound is identical to unlabeled EF5. EF5 has been shown to have quite a uniform biodistribution in both rodents and humans, which probably is due to the high lipophilicity of the compound. No ^{18}F-labeled metabolites have been detected in rats or humans. Noninvasive imaging of tumor hypoxia in rats using [^{18}F] EF5 was in accordance with data on EF5. The highest uptakes of the tracer were seen in the kidney, liver and in the gastrointestinal tract.

[^{18}F]EF5 has been introduced to clinical PET-CT imaging only recently. The development of an electrophilic labeling of [^{18}F]EF5 from [^{18}F]F_2 using a "post target" method has enabled high-yield tracer synthesis suitable for patient studies. Thus far, the experience is limited to head and neck cancer and glioma, with a growing interest to study other neoplasms where hypoxia is known to have importance, such as cervical cancer.

Human HNSCC is FDG-avid but uptake of [^{18}F]EF5 in line with other radiolabeled nitroimidazole analogues is variable. This is seen in patients presenting with locally advanced disease who may show differential uptake of [^{18}F]EF5 in primary tumor and lymph node metastases in the neck. For instance, one patient with multiple neck metastases from oropharyngeal carcinoma had one large [^{18}F]EF5-positive lymph node, while the other slightly smaller ipsilateral node was [^{18}F]EF5-negative. No correlation between uptake of FDG and [^{18}F]EF5 in head and neck cancer could be demonstrated, while tumors with the highest uptake of the hypoxia marker showed invariably low perfusion, measured with [^{15}O]H_2O PET-CT. [^{18}F]EF5 imaging is performed 3-h from tracer injection, and Figures x-y show representative cases of patients imaged with [^{18}F]EF5 and FDG PET-CT to demonstrate variability in uptake believed to represent hypoxia. Generally [^{18}F]EF5 shows similar pattern of uptake in head and neck cancer in comparison to related compounds such as [^{18}F]FMISO or [^{18}F]FAZA. Direct comparison between the three labeled nitroimidazole analogues has not been performed in human tumors nor is there any knowledge about relationship between uptake of [^{18}F]EF5 in tumor and outcome to treatment. One of the potential advantages of using [^{18}F]EF5 will be the potential to validate the in vivo imaging data by direct correlation with immunohistochemical examination of the same lesions *ex vivo*.

Summary

It is important for readers to acknowledge that imaging of hypoxia in a diagnostic setting has not yet emerged into routine patient management. Until now, all imaging data from human studies have been collected from research protocols in academic centers, and availability of tracers is very limited elsewhere. However, the Trans-Tasmanian chemoradiotherapy study 98.02 is an excellent example on how hypoxia imaging may change the outcome of cancer patients. This study showed that hypoxia, as detected with [^{18}F]FMISO PET is associated with locoregional failure in patients with head and neck cancer who did not receive the hypoxia-activated drug tirapazamine. Other applications such as dose painting of hypoxic tumor subvolumes detected on PET in radiotherapy planning await confirmation of clinical impact. Furthermore, which patients have most benefit from hypoxia imaging and how variable the regional tracer uptake is in the short term should be clarified.

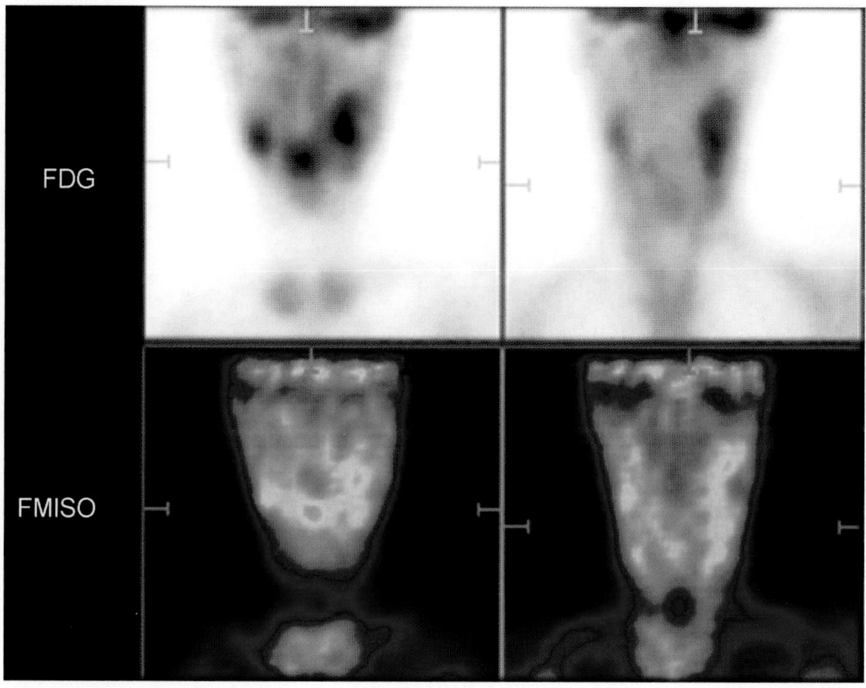

^{18}F-FMISO finding

Low tracer uptake in this patient with a primary tumor of the pyriform sinus and bilateral cervical lymph nodes.

Teaching point

[^{18}F]FMISO typically has low tumor-to-background activity ratios as demonstrated by the comparison of coronal [^{18}F]FDG performed at 1 h following tracer administration and [^{18}F] FMISO PET scans obtained 4 h after radiotracer administration. The high lipophilicity of [^{18}F] FMISO leads to relatively high non-specific uptake in muscle and the brain.

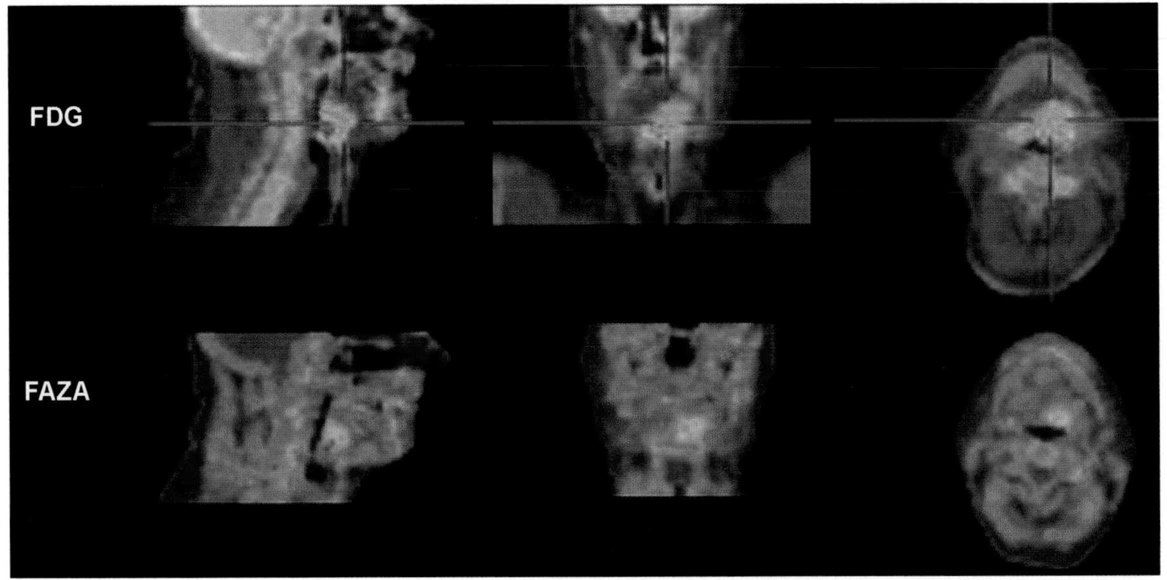

^{18}FAZA finding

Moderate tracer uptake.

Teaching point

[^{18}F]FAZA has lower lipophilicity than [^{18}F]FMISO and generally provides lower background activity. In particular, little brain uptake is apparent. This leads to good quality images within 2 h of radiotracer administration as demonstrated in this comparison of [^{18}F]FDG and [^{18}F]FAZA.

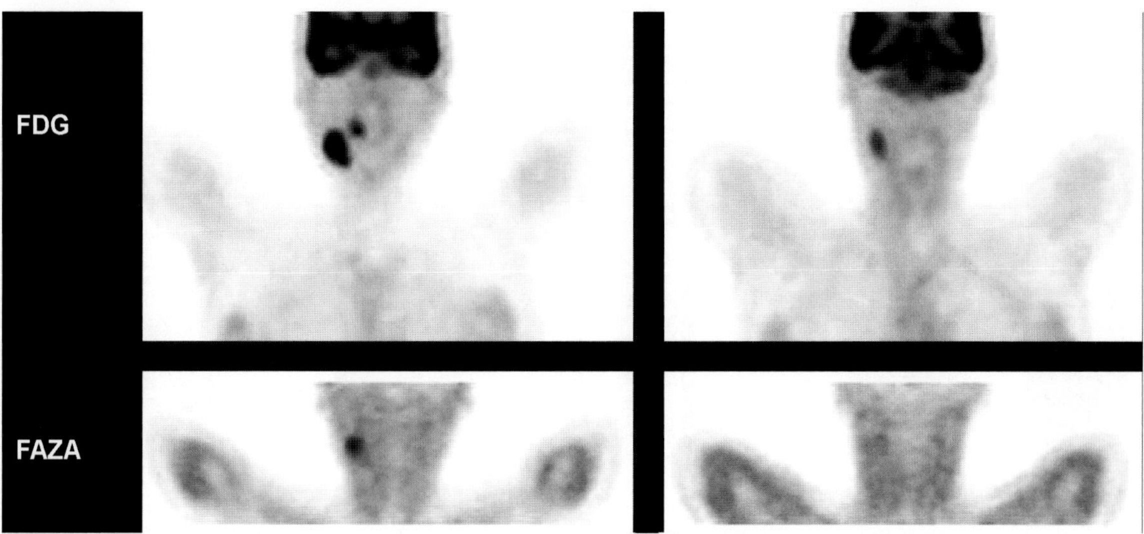

PET findings

Heterogeneity between lesions with respect to hypoxia tracer uptake is apparent in the images of this patient with a primary tumor of the vallecula, which is clearly visualized on the [^{18}F]FDG study but not on the [^{18}F]FAZA scan, and right-sided lymph node, which is visualized on both.

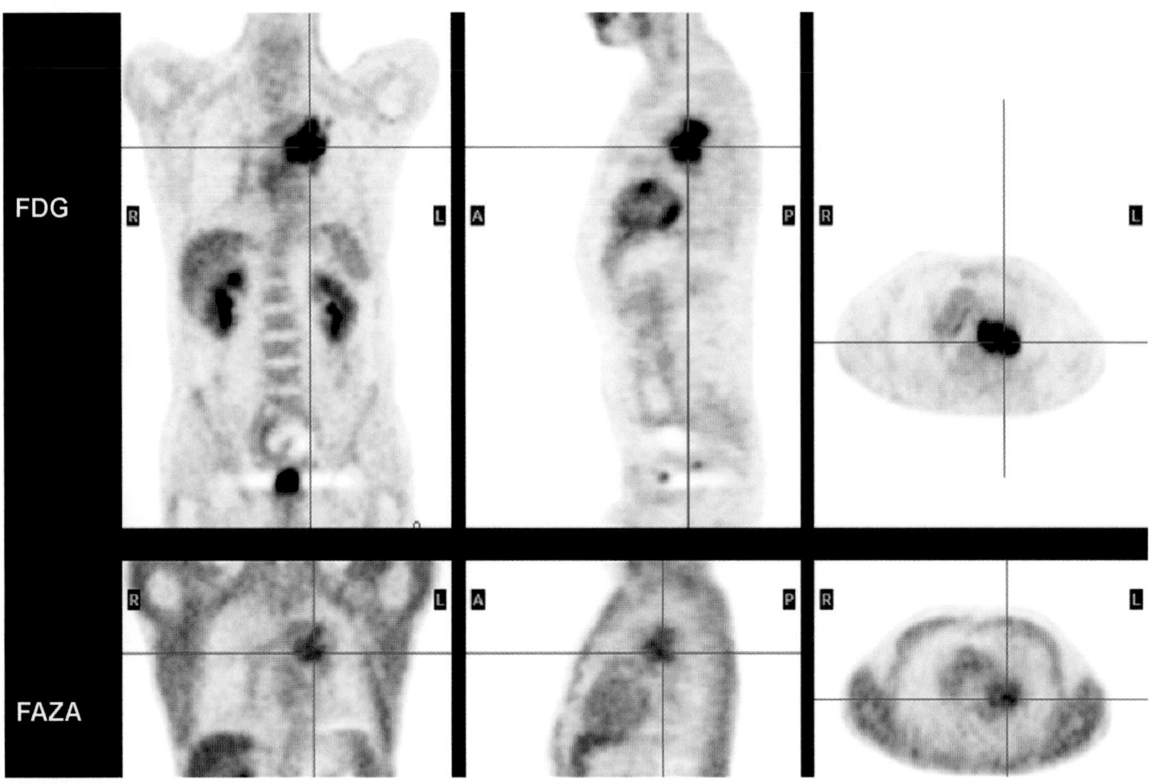

PET findings

Heterogeneity within lesions is clearly demonstrated in the images of this patient with a non-small cell lung cancer involving the left upper lobe where the extent and distribution of [^{18}F]FDG uptake differs markedly compared to that of [^{18}F]FAZA.

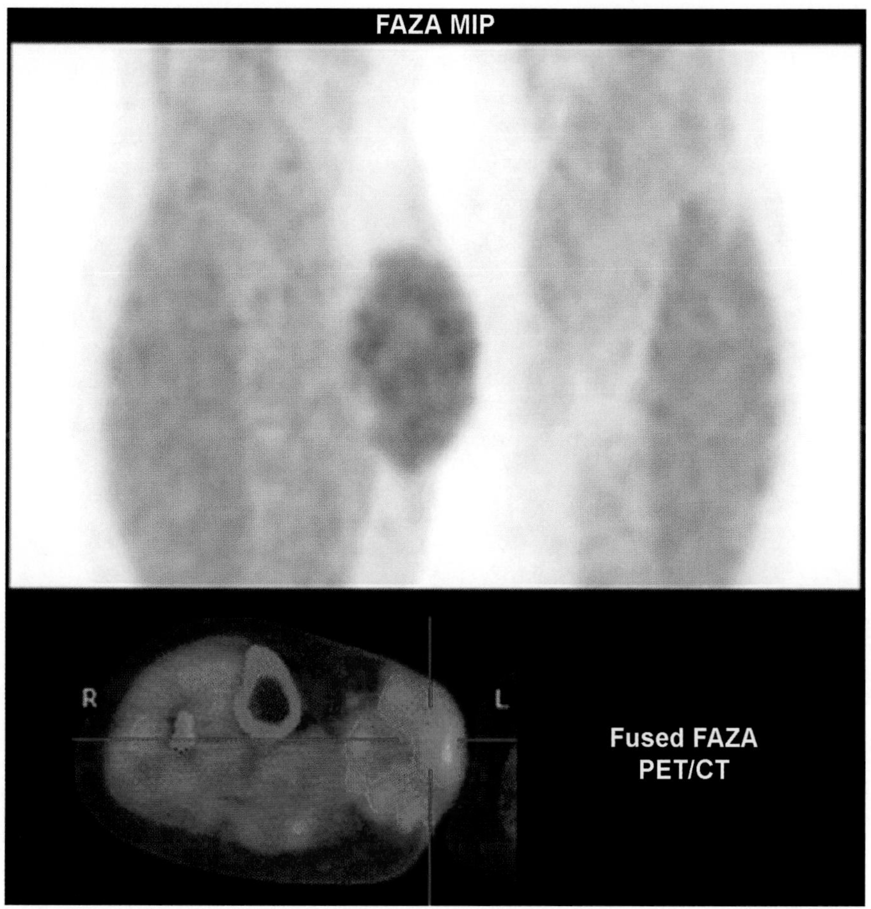

^{18}FAZA finding

Significantly higher uptake of [^{18}F]FAZA in this soft tissue sarcoma compared to adjacent skeletal muscle as observed on the maximum-intensity-projection (MIP) images (*upper row*) and fused PET-CT images (*lower row*) suggests the presence of hypoxia. Again, heterogeneity of tracer distribution is observed.

Female 39 years

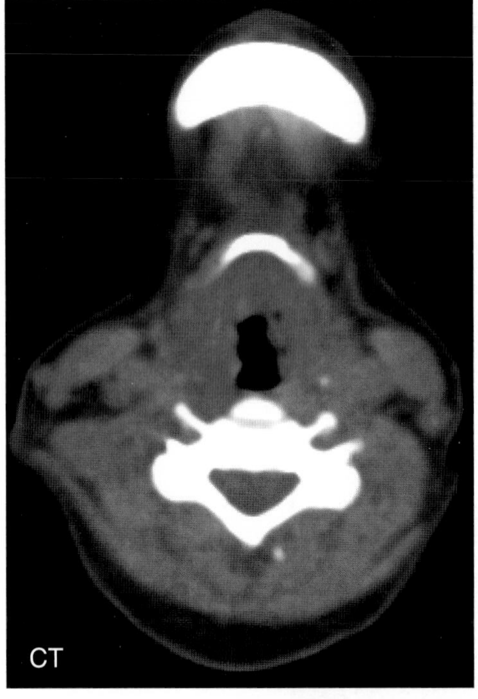

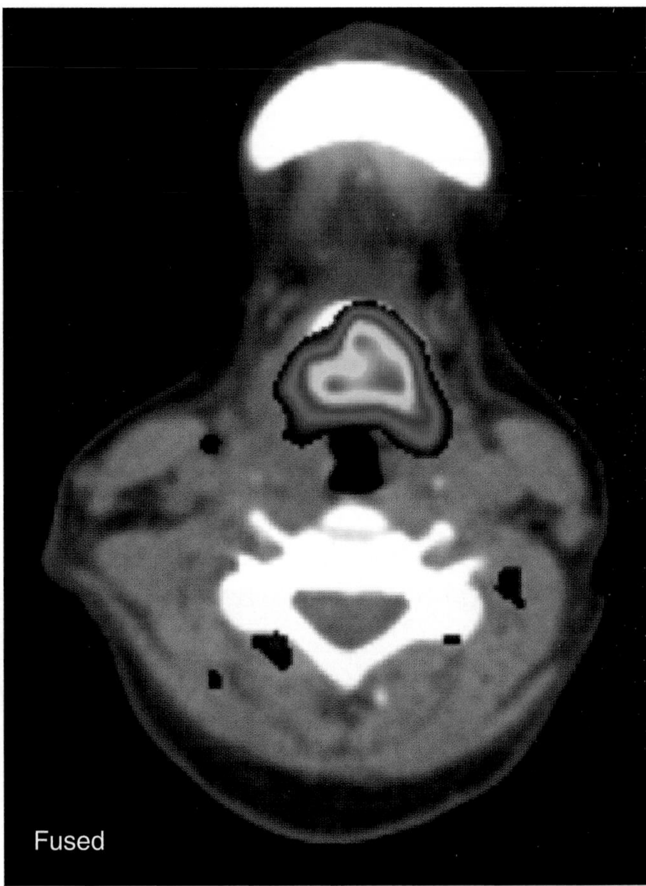

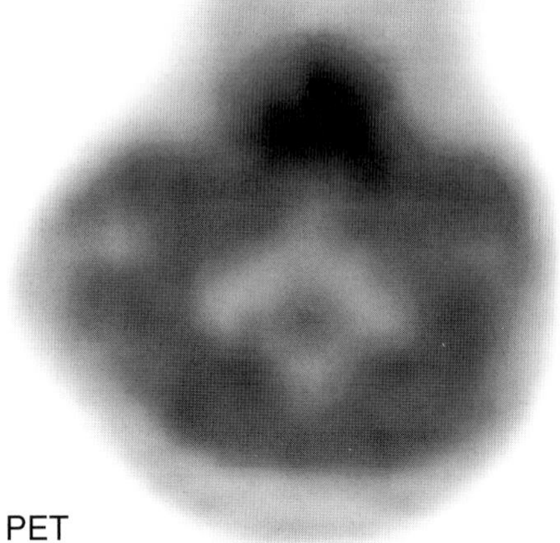

^{18}F-EF5 finding

Moderate tracer uptake (maximum tumor-to-muscle uptake ratio is 1.5 at 3-h).

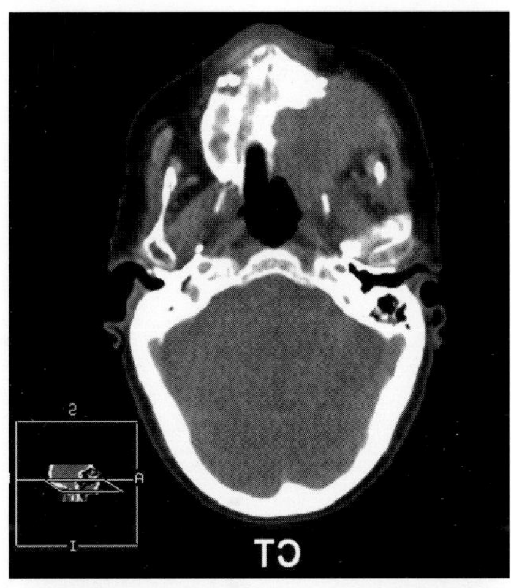

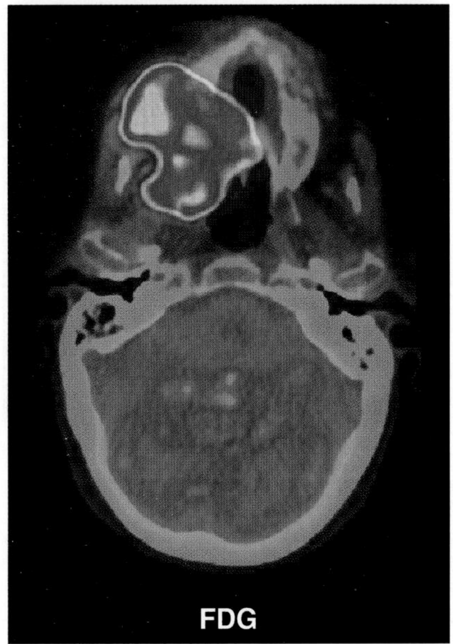

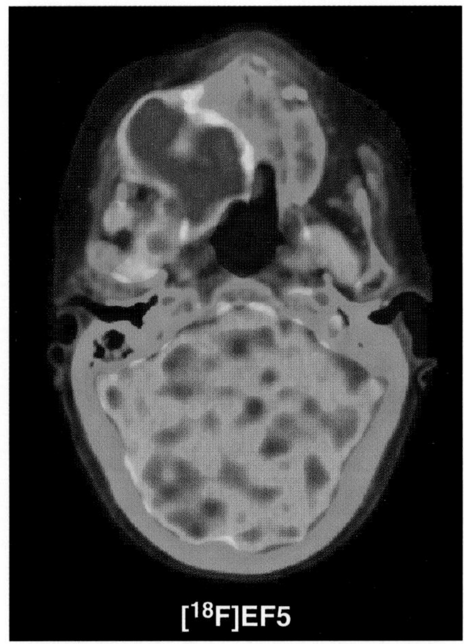

PET findings

Considerable hypoxia is seen in the large primary tumor invading the adjacent bony structures (49% of FDG-avid voxels had [^{18}F]EF5 tumor-to-muscle uptake ratio ≥1.5 at 3-h).

Male 68 years

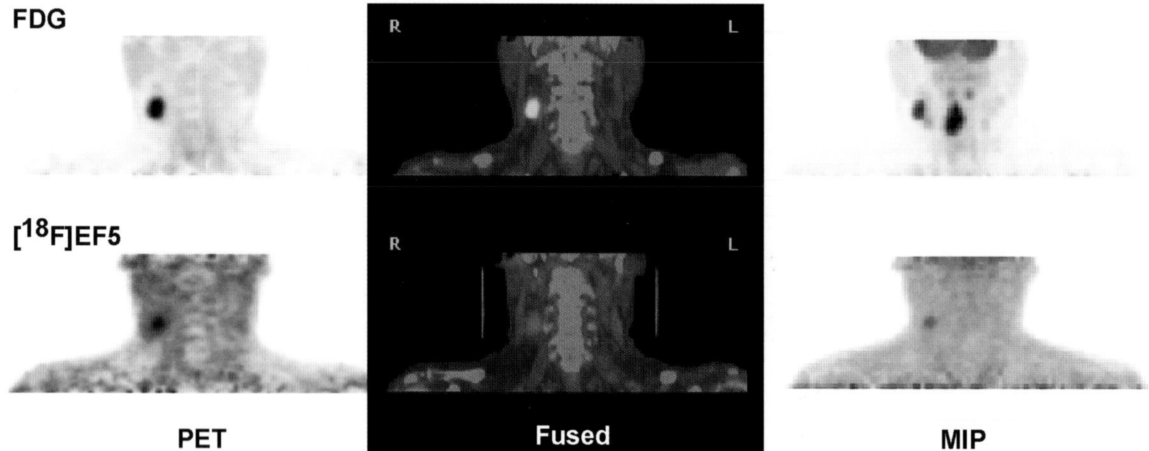

PET findings

Both primary tumor and the nodal metastasis are FDG-avid, while only the metastasis shows hypoxia (maximum [^{18}F]EF5 tumor-to-muscle uptake ratio is 2.3 at 3-h).

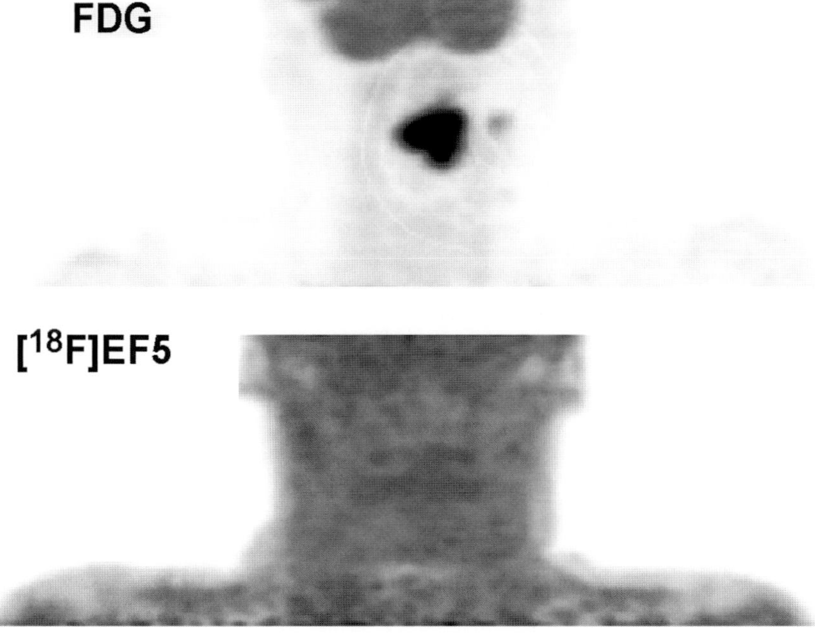

PET findings

This patient showed FDG-avid primary tumor and nodal metastases, which were [^{18}F]EF5-negative, suggesting lack of considerable hypoxia.

Chapter 12 Angiogenesis PET Using Radiolabeled RGD Peptides

Keon Wook Kang, Jae Min Jeong, and Ambros J. Beer

Angiogenesis, the process of developing a new vessel, is an essential feature of the growth of solid tumors. For decades, the targeting of tumor angiogenesis has evolved into one of the most widely pursued therapeutic strategies in cancer research. Antiangiogenic drugs like bevacizumab, sunitinib, or sorafenib, were proved to be effective in many solid cancers such as colorectal cancer, renal cell carcinoma, hepatocelluar carcinoma, etc. But, these kinds of molecular targeted therapy are responsive only in selected patient population.

Integrin αvβ3 plays an important role in tumor angiogenesis and is overexpressed on endothelial cells of newly developed vessel induced by tumors or ischemic tissues. Integrin αvβ3 is a receptor for the ligand, vitronectin, and arginine-glysine-aspartic acid (RGD) tripeptide is known to be active binding moiety to the receptor. Molecular imaging tracers containing RGD peptide have been evaluated for monitoring αvβ3 expression noninvasively using PET, SPECT, MRI, optical imaging and US. For nuclear molecular imaging, studies were done based on cyclic RGD peptides radiolabeled with ^{18}F, ^{64}Cu, ^{68}Ga for PET, or ^{99m}Tc for SPECT.

[^{18}F] Galacto-RGD has shown high tumor-to-background ratios preclinically and has been evaluated in a number of clinical studies. To improve targeting efficiency, multimeric constructs were reported revealing improved targeting properties in preclinical models. Noninvasive determination of αvβ3 expression potentially can be used to monitor treatment response to antiangiogenic drugs or to select patients likely to respond to treatment with antiangiogenic drugs.

[^{18}F]Galacto-RGD PET

Kessler and coworkers developed the pentapeptide cyclo (-Arg-Gly-Asp-DPhe-Val-), which shows high affinity and selectivity for αvβ3. For the first evaluation of this approach, Haubner et al. have synthesized radioiodinated RGD peptides which showed comparable affinity and selectivity to the lead structure. Several strategies to improve the pharmacokinetics of radiohalogenated peptides have been developed. The glycosylation approach is based on the introduction of sugar derivatives which are conjugated to the ε-amino function of a corresponding lysine in the peptide sequence. By conjugating the RGD containing cyclic pentapeptide cyclo(-Arg-Gly-Asp-DPhe-Val-) with glucose- or galactose-based sugar amino acids, [*I]Gluco-RGD and [^{18}F]Galacto-RGD have been developed for PET and SPECT imaging. Both compounds demonstrated improved pharmacokinetics with predominantly renal tracer elimination and increased uptake and retention in a murine tumor model, compared with the first generation peptides. Extensive preclinical evaluations concerning monomeric compounds were carried out using [*I]Gluco-RGD and [^{18}F]Galacto-RGD. Initial in vivo evaluation was carried out using the human melanoma M21 model, which is well characterized concerning αvβ3 expression. Using this model, [^{18}F]Galacto-RGD and [^{125}I]Gluco-RGD uptake in the tumor 120 min p.i. was 1.5 and 1.8% ID/g, respectively. Blocking experiments injecting 6 mg c(RGDfV) per kg mouse 10 min prior to tracer injection reduced tumor accumulation to approximately 15% of control for [^{125}I]Gluco-RGD and 35% of control for [^{18}F]Galacto-RGD, which demonstrates receptor specific accumulation. Furthermore, imaging studies with mice bearing melanoma tumors with increasing amounts of αvβ3-positive cells (produced by mixing M21 and M21-L cells) showed that there is a correlation between integrin expression and tracer accumulation. These data demonstrate that noninvasive determination of αvβ3 expression and quantification with radiolabelled RGD peptides is feasible with static emission scans. Moreover, animal PET study with increasing amounts of c(RGDfV) were obtained, that indicated that the dose-dependent blocking of tracer uptake in the receptor positive tumor could be monitored.

Until now, the only approach of imaging αvβ3 expression which has made the transition into the clinic is the radiotracer approach. [^{18}F]Galacto-RGD was the first PET tracer applied in patients and could successfully image αvβ3 expression in human tumors with good tumor/background ratios. In all patients, rapid, predominantly renal tracer elimination was observed, resulting in low background activity in most regions of the body. High inter and intraindividual variance in tracer accumulation in tumor lesions was noted, suggesting great diversity of αvβ3 expression. These findings emphasize the potential value of noninvasive techniques for appropriate selection of patients entering clinical trials with αvβ3-targeted therapies. Further biodistribution and dosimetry studies confirmed rapid clearance of [^{18}F] Galacto-RGD from the blood pool and primarily renal excretion. Background activity in lung and muscle tissue was low and the calculated effective dose found was approximately 19 μSv/MBq, which is very similar to an [^{18}F]FDG scan. We also studied, if [^{18}F]Galacto-RGD uptake correlates with αvβ3 expression. 19 patients with solid tumors (musculoskeletal system $n = 10$, melanoma $n = 4$, head and neck cancer $n = 2$, glioblastoma $n = 2$, breast cancer $n = 1$) were examined with PET using [18] Galacto-RGD before surgical removal of the lesions. SUVs and tumor/blood ratios were found to correlate significantly with the intensity of immunohistochemical staining as well as with the microvessel density. Moreover, immunohistochemistry confirmed lack of αvβ3 expression in normal tissue and in the two tumors without tracer uptake. We are now systematically examining different tumor entities with respect to their αvβ3 expression patterns as shown by [^{18}F]Galacto-RGD PET. In squamous cell carcinoma of the head and neck (SCCHN), we could demonstrate good tumor/background ratios with [^{18}F]Galacto-RGD PET, but again also a widely varying intensity of tracer uptake. Immunohistochemistry demonstrated predominantly vascular αvβ3 expression, thus in SCCHN, [^{18}F]Galacto-RGD PET might be used as a surrogate parameter of angiogenesis. We have also compared the tracer uptake of [^{18}F]FDG and [^{18}F]Galacto-RGD in patients with non small cell lung cancer (NSCLC, $n = 10$) and various other tumors ($n = 8$), because in case of a close correlation of the two tracers, there would probably be no need for a specific tracer like [^{18}F]Galacto-RGD. The results showed no correlation between the two tracers concerning all lesions ($r = 0.157$). For the subgroup of [^{18}F]FDG-avid lesions and lesions in patients with NSCLC, there was a slight trend toward a higher [^{18}F]Galacto-RGD uptake in more [^{18}F]FDG-avid lesions ($r = 0.337$). However, the correlation coefficient was very low. Our results suggest that αvβ3 expression and glucose metabolism are not closely correlated in tumor lesions, and that consequently [^{18}F]FDG cannot provide similar information as [^{18}F]Galacto-RGD. Recently, the SPECT tracer [^{99m}Tc]NC100692 was introduced by GE healthcare for imaging αvβ3 expression in humans and was first evaluated in breast cancer. Nineteen of twenty two tumors could be detected with this agent, which was safe and well tolerated by the patients. An αvβ3 and αvβ5 specific PET radiotracer which has recently been used in clinical trials named [^{18}F]AH111585. The chemical synthesis of the precursor for 18F-AH111585 has previously been described. Radiosynthesis was performed on an automated module (TRACERlab FX F-N; GE Healthcare) by coupling an aminooxy-functionalized precursor of [^{18}F] AH111585 with 4–18F-fluorobenzaldehyde at pH 3.5 to form the oxime [^{18}F]AH111585. The specific activity of the injectate, determined by high-performance liquid chromatography (HPLC), ranged between 76 and 170 GBq/mmol, which is substantially less compared to [^{18}F] Galacto-RGD.

[^{68}Ga]NOTA-RGD PET

^{68}Ga is a positron emitter with a short half-life of 68 min and its hydrophilic nature is adequate for the labeling of small peptides with rapid renal clearance for PET. ^{68}Ga has a great advantage for PET over other cyclotron-produced positron emitters because it can be obtained economically by use of a commercially available ^{68}Ge/^{68}Ga generator. The parent nuclide ^{68}Ge has a long half-life of 271 days, allowing its use as a generator for more than 1 year.

Cyclic Arg-Gly-Asp-D-Tyr-Lys [c(RGDyK)] was conjugated with 2-(p-isothiocyanatobenzyl)-1,4,7-triazacyclononane-1,4,7-triacetic acid (SCN-Bz-NOTA), then labeled with ^{68}Ga and finally ^{68}Ga-NOTA-RGD was produced.

Six patients with liver metastasis from colorectal cancer were enrolled. [^{18}F] FDG and ^{68}Ga-NOTA-RGD PET-CT studies were done before combination therapy with FOLFOX and bevacizumab. About 5 mCi of ^{68}Ga-NOTA-RGD was injected to the patients intravenously and PET images were acquired 30 min later. There is 1 day interval between [^{18}F] FDG and ^{68}Ga-NOTA-RGD PET-CT.

All six patients showed hypermetabolic primary and metastatic lesions on [^{18}F]FDG PET-CT. In three patients, the hypermetabolic lesions on [^{18}F] FDG PET-CT also showed mild ^{68}Ga-NOTA-RGD uptakes. However, the other three had no ^{68}Ga-NOTA-RGD uptakes. The lesions with ^{68}Ga-NOTA-RGD uptakes showed partial response to combination therapy with bevacizumab, while the lesions without ^{68}Ga-NOTA-RGD uptake showed no response or progression of disease.

^{68}Ga-NOTA-RGD PET had the potential to predict the response to combination chemotherapy with bevacizumab and might help to select appropriate patients for antiangiogenic therapy.

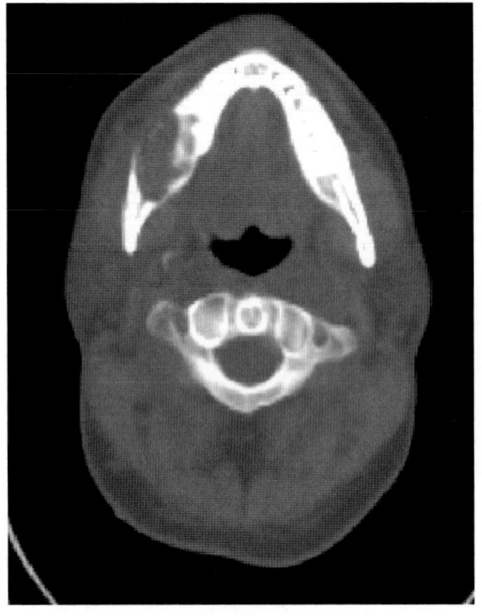

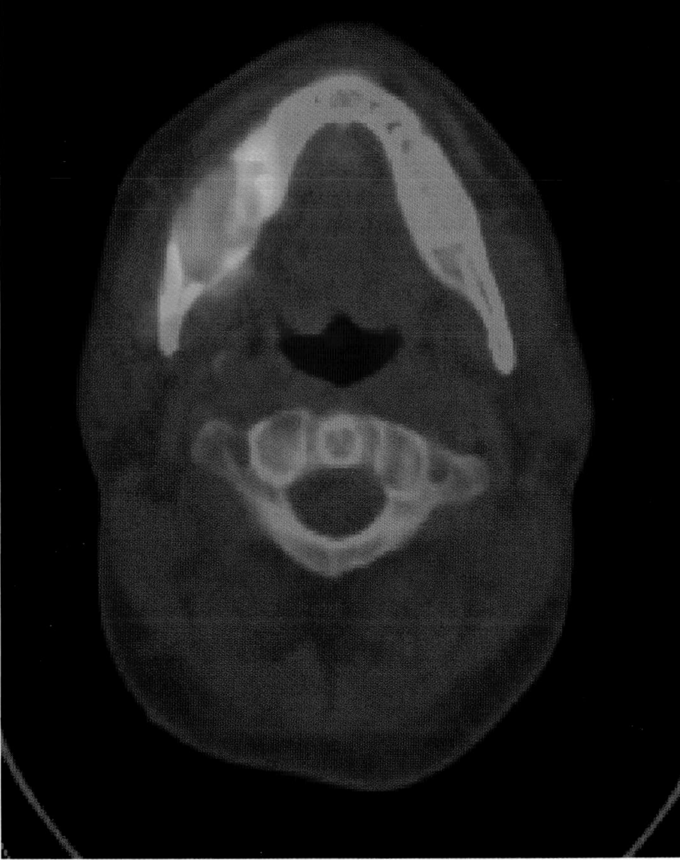

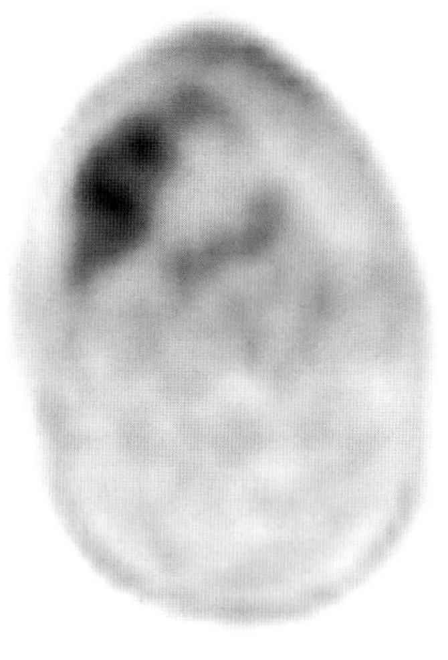

^{18}F-RGD finding

PET-CT shows heterogeneous moderate to focally intense tracer uptake in the osteolytic lesion with good tumor to background contrast.

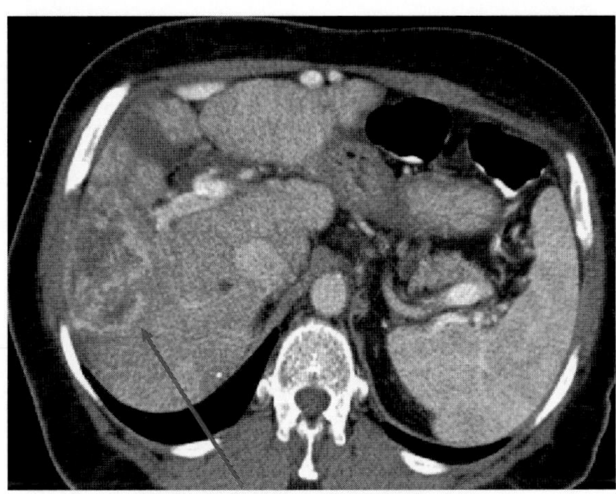

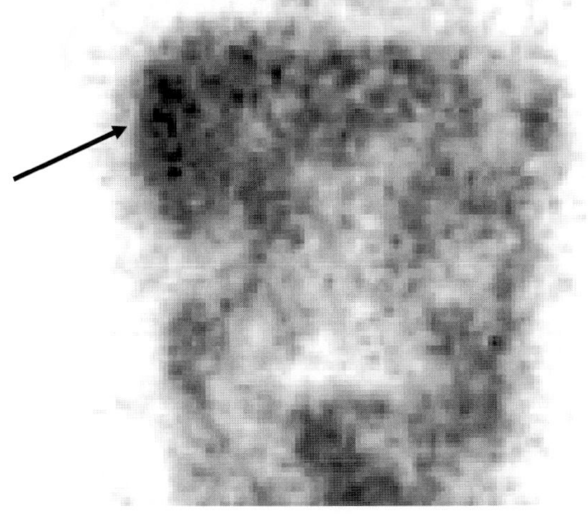

^{18}F-RGD finding

The large tumor shows contrast enhancement in the CT scan (*red arrow*); however, it can hardly be detected in the [^{18}F]Galacto-RGD PET (*black arrow*) due to the high physiological liver activity.

Teaching point

This case demonstrates that imaging of liver lesions is problematic with [^{18}F]Galacto-RGD, unless there is very high uptake.

^{99m}Tc-HDP

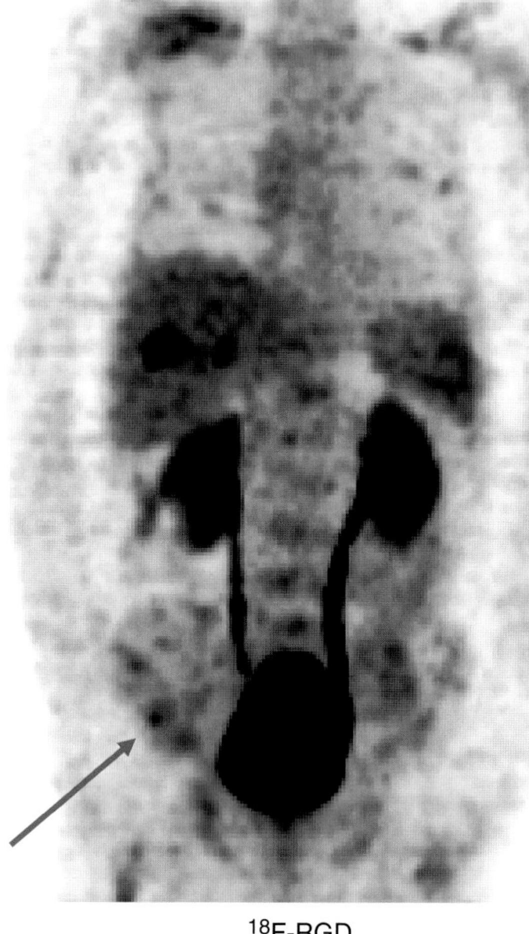

^{18}F-RGD

^{99m}Tc-HDP finding

Multiple areas with intense tracer uptake in the whole skeleton, predominantly in the right scapula and in the pelvis (*arrows*).

^{18}F-RGD finding

Multiple foci of moderate to intense tracer uptake in the whole skeleton.

Teaching point

Note that normally the skeleton is only very faintly visualized with [^{18}F]Galacto-RGD, which means that all parts of the skeleton visible in this MIP show elevated tracer uptake. Note also physiological tracer excretion via the gallbladder and urinary tract.

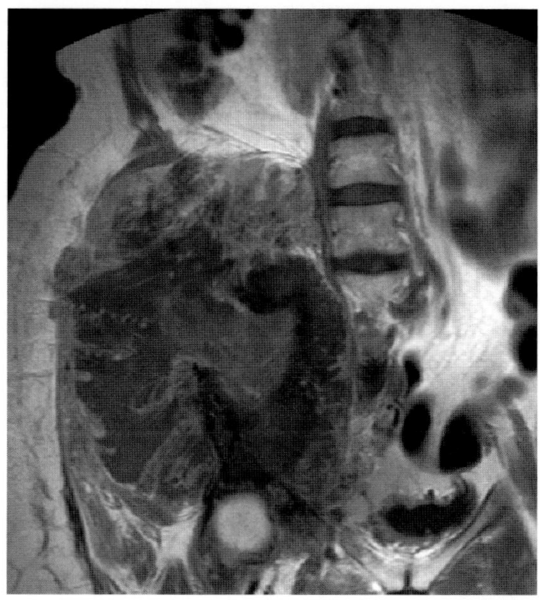

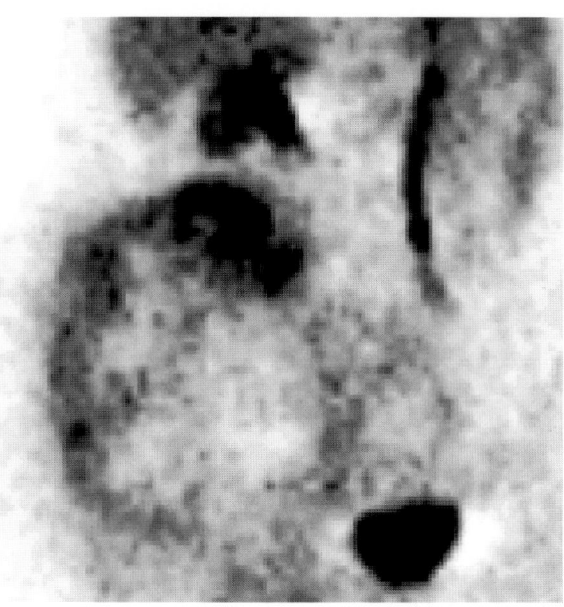

^{18}F-RGD finding

Heterogeneous peripheral tracer uptake, most pronounced in the apical parts of the lesion (corresponding MRI on the left side.

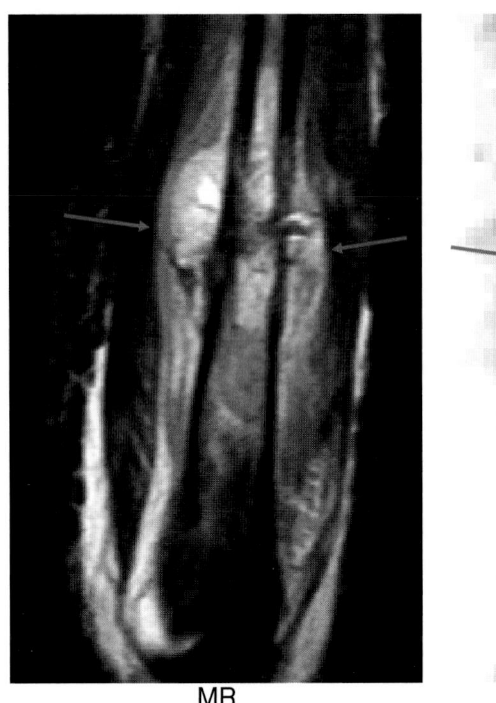

MR

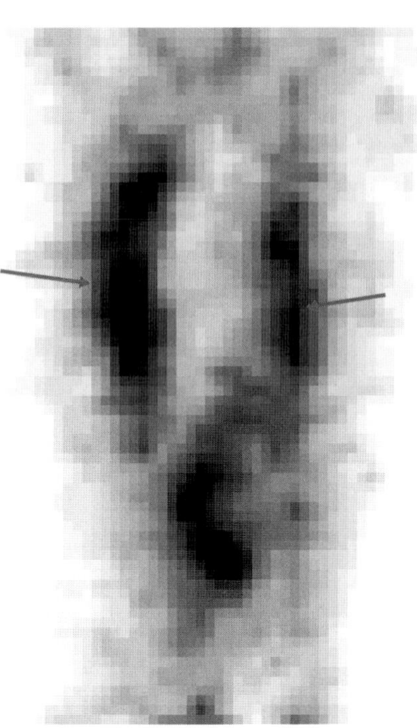

^{18}F-RGD

MR finding

Large tumor in the diaphysis with extension to the metaphysis and a large soft tissue component.

^{18}F-RGD finding

Heterogeneous predominatly peripheral tracer uptake.

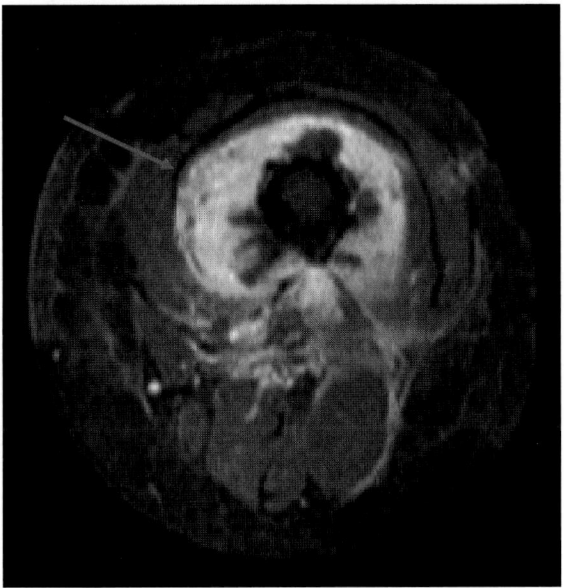

MR

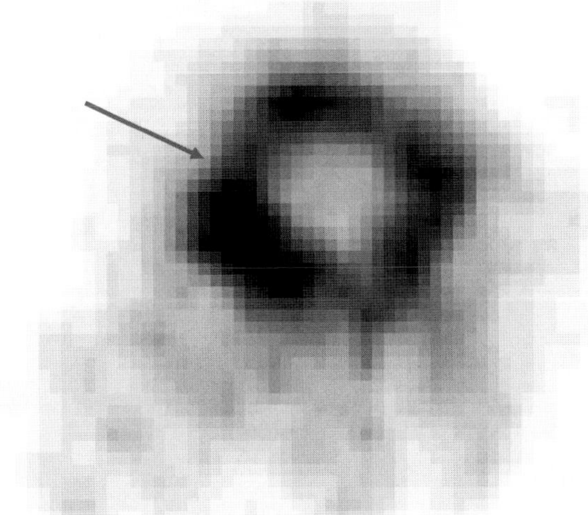

^{18}F-RGD

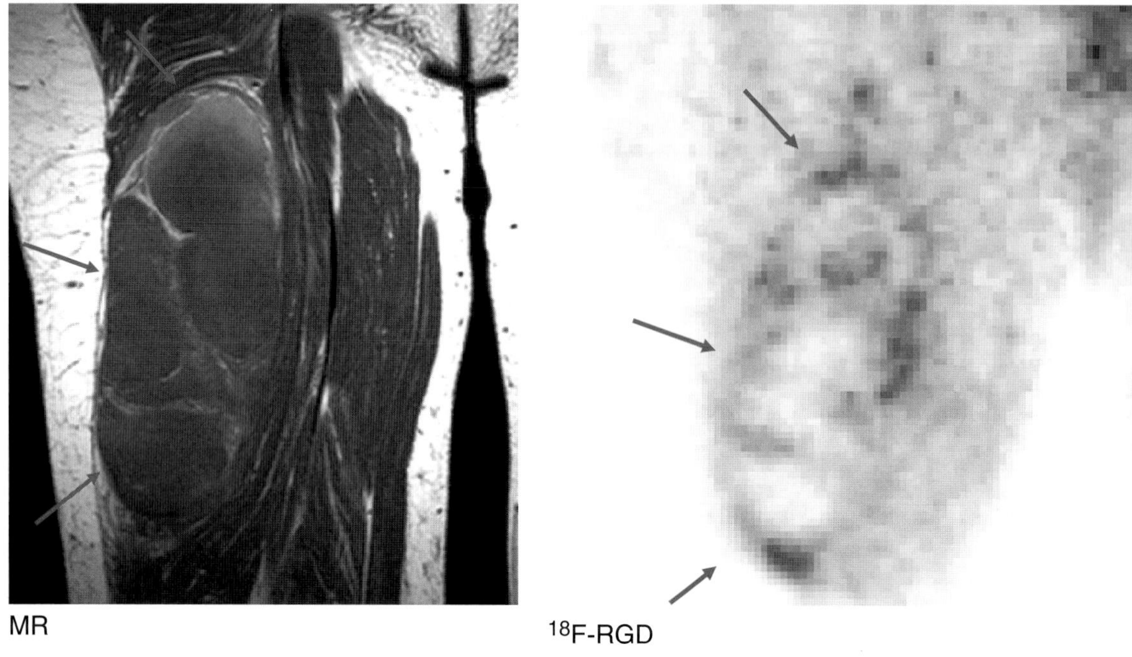

MR finding

Large tumor with contrast enhancing septa and central necrosis.

^{18}F-RGD finding

Mostly low tracer uptake in the septa of the tumor with single more intense foci.

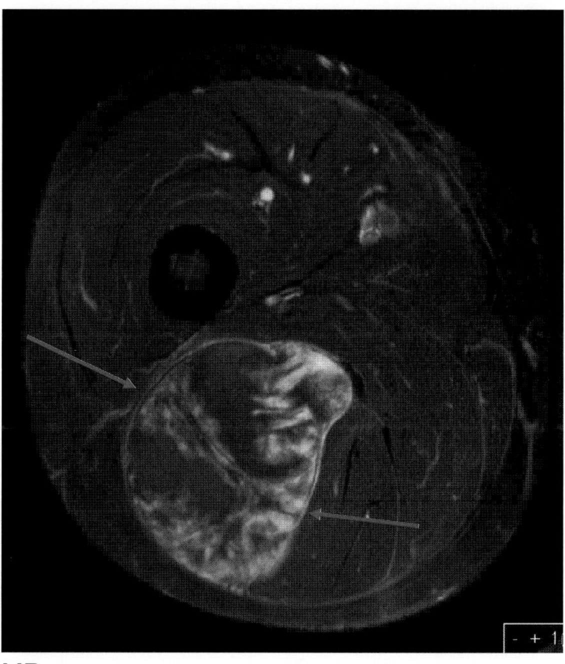

MR

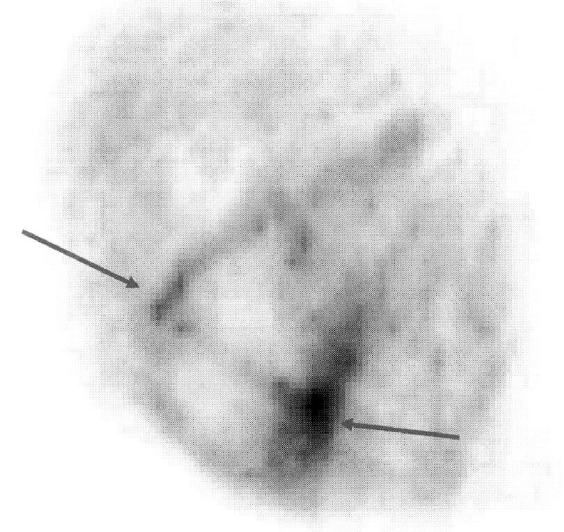

^{18}F-RGD

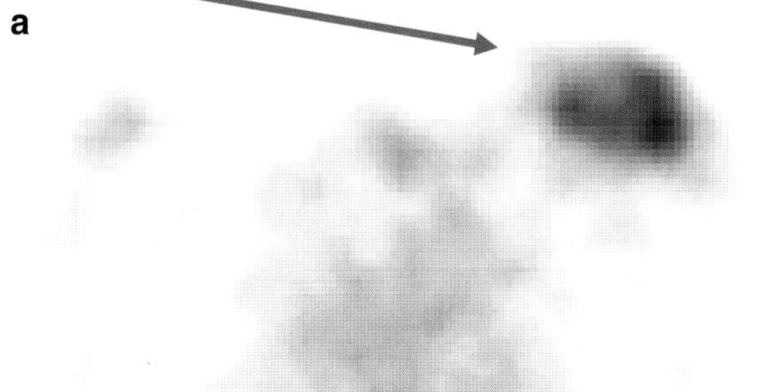

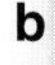

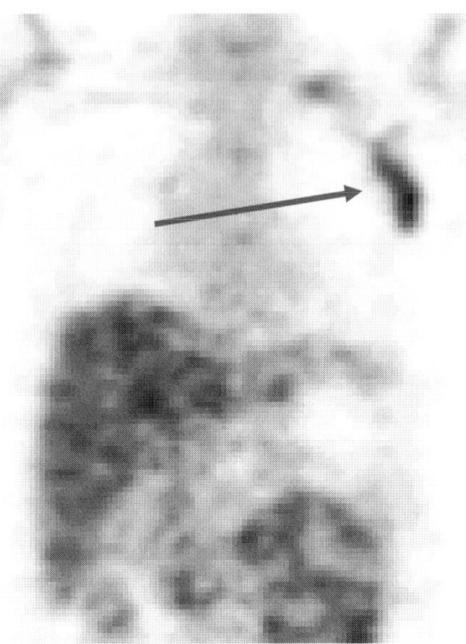

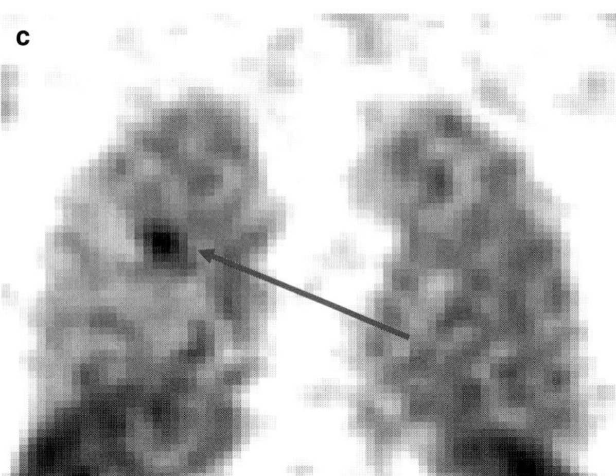

■ ^{18}F-RGD finding

PET scan allow to visualize primary tumor on the left side with heterogeneous tracer uptake (a), multiple axillary lymph node metastases on the left side with intense tracer uptake (b) and a single lung metastasis on the right side (c, non attenuation corrected image).

Teaching point

This case demonstrates that in the lungs, the review of nonattenuation corrected images can provide additional information, as with conventional [^{18}F]FDG PET.

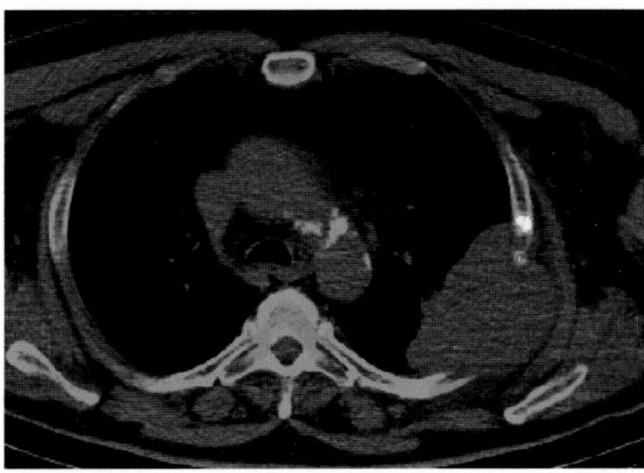

^{99m}Tc-HDP

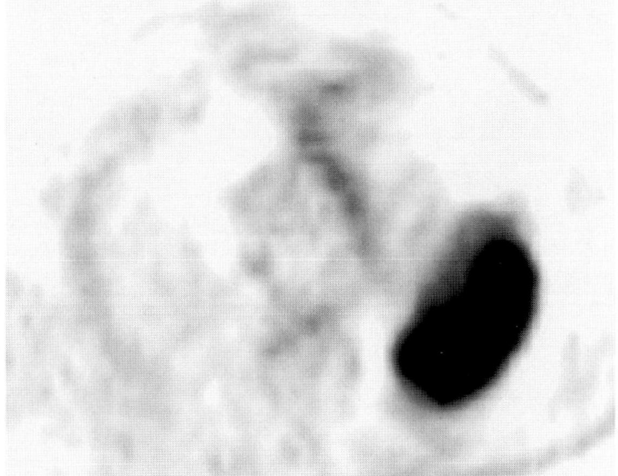

^{18}F-FGD

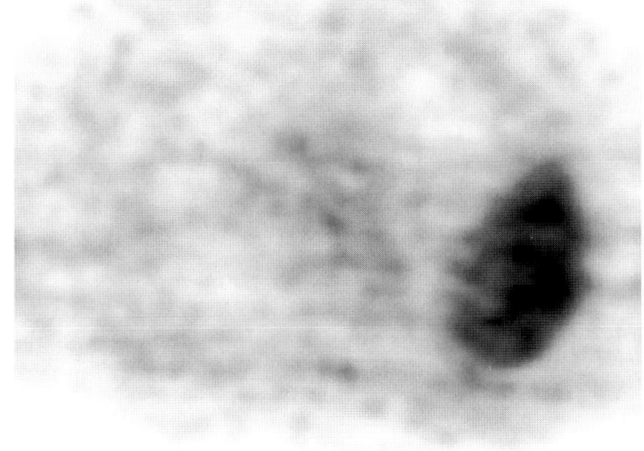

^{18}F-RGD

SPECT-CT and PET findings

In the SPECT/CT (*upper*) you see the large mass with erosion of the adjacent ribs . In the [^{18}F]FDG PET the mass shows intense tracer uptake. In the [^{18}F]Galacto-RGD PET, there is also intense tracer uptake in the lesion.

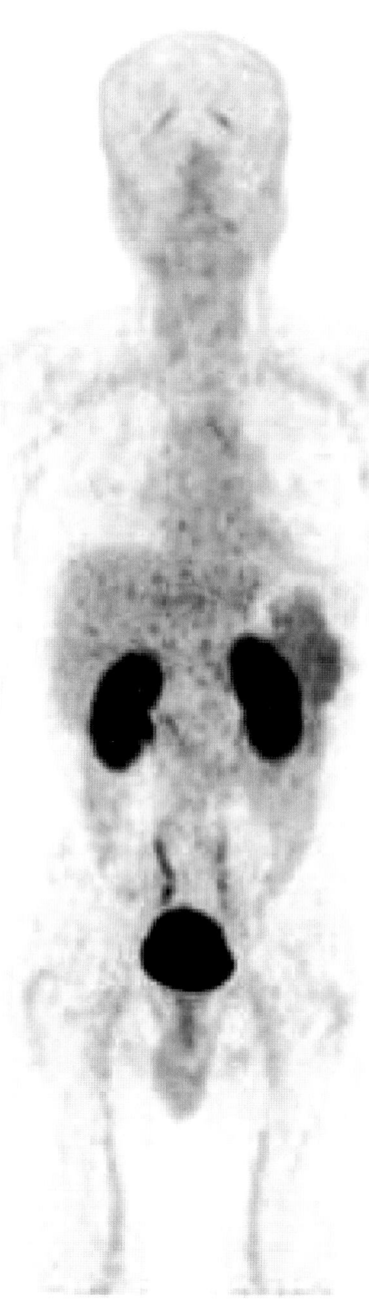

^{68}Ga-NOTA-RGD

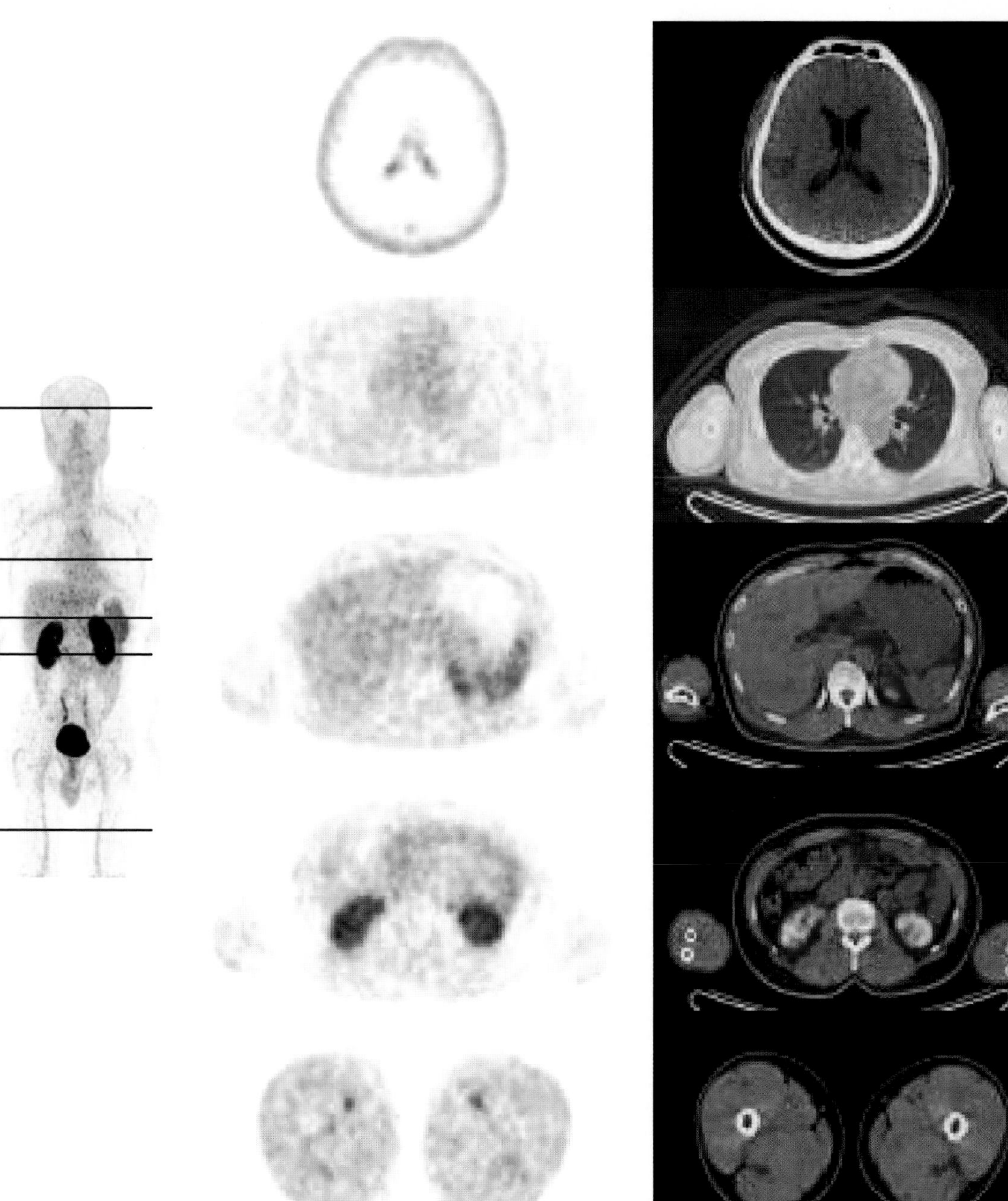

^{68}Ga-NOTA-RGD

^{68}Ga-NOTA-RGD is rapidly excreted through kidney. PET-CT images show high uptake in kidney, ureters, and urinary bladder. Mild uptake is notified in liver, spleen, large vessels, and bowel. Mild uptake in the ventricle is supposed to be choroid plexus.

Female 67 years

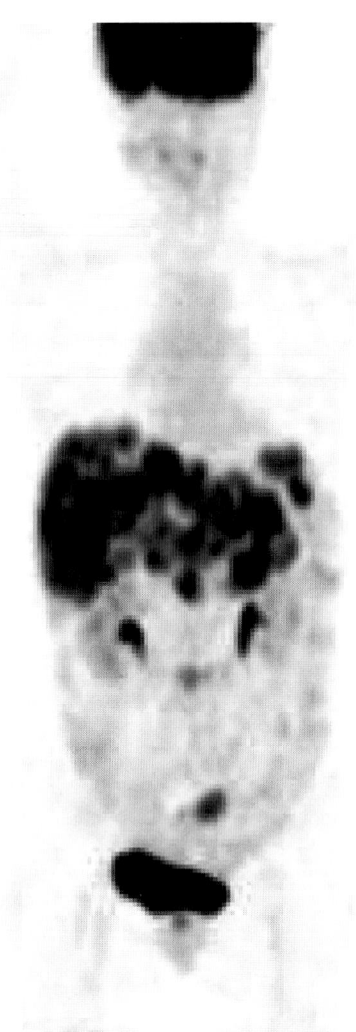

^{18}F-FDG

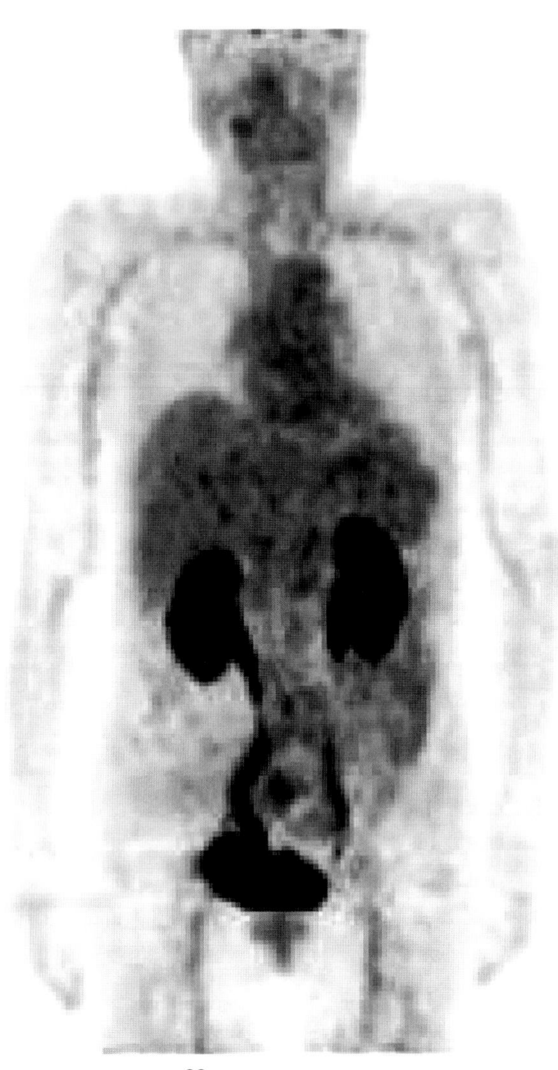

^{68}Ga-NOTA-RGD

^{18}F-FDG finding

PET reveals a hypermetabolic lesion in the sigmoid colon (SUV_{max}: 5.2) and multiple hypermetabolic lesions in the liver (SUV_{max}: 7.9).

^{68}Ga-NOTA-RGD finding

PET shows mild uptake in the sigmoid colon (SUV_{max}: 3.2) and uneven uptake in the liver (SUV_{max}: 2.3).

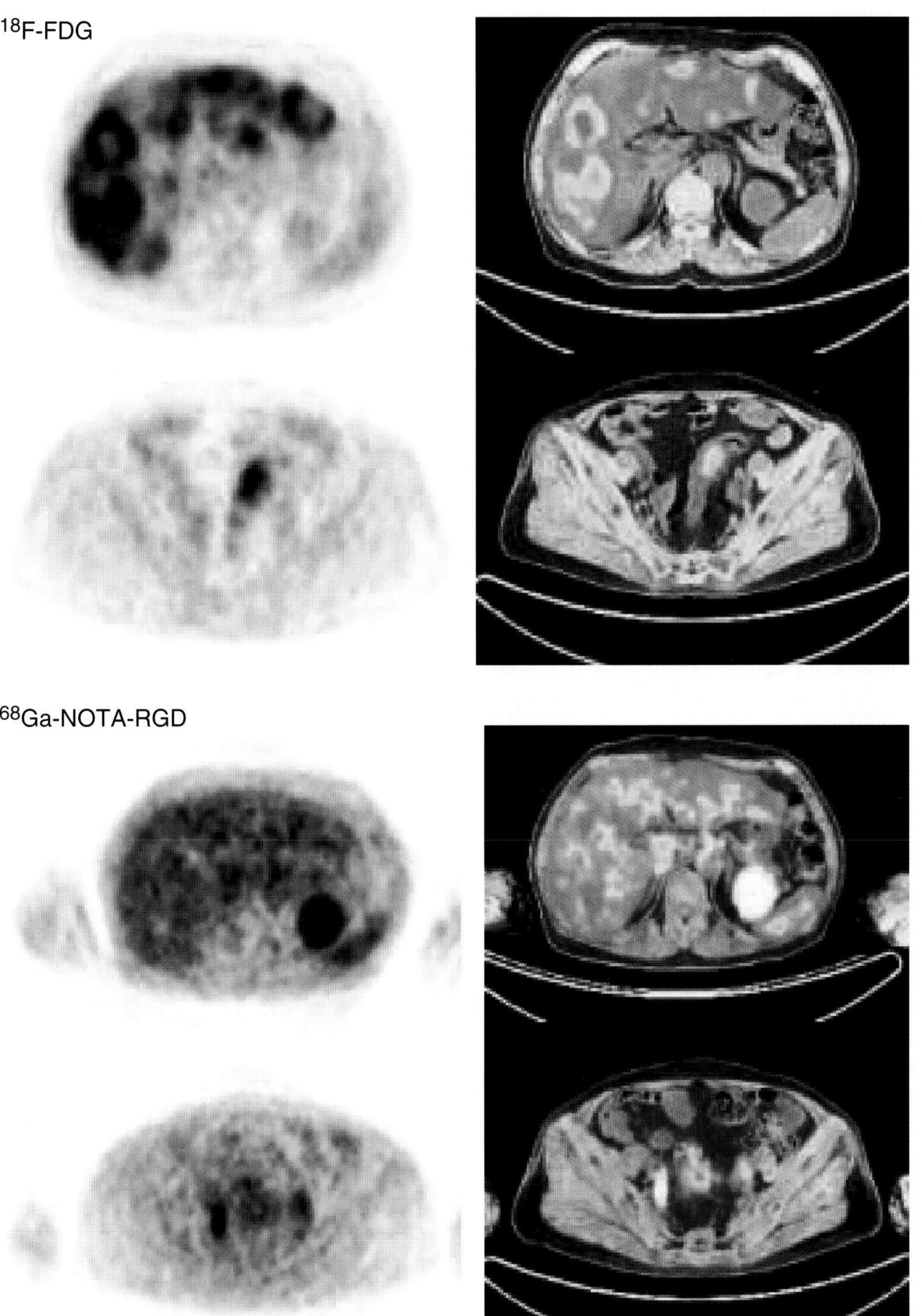
^{18}F-FDG
^{68}Ga-NOTA-RGD

Chapter 13 Hormonal Receptors PET-CT

Erik F. J. deVries, Andor W. J. M. Glaudemans,
Caroline P. Schröder,
and Geke A. P. Hospers

Sex hormones play an important role in the development and growth of cancer, especially in breast and prostate cancer. The mode of action of these sex hormones is activation of the corresponding hormone receptor in tumor cells. The hormone-bound receptor acts as a transcription factor and activates signaling pathways that induce proliferation and tumor growth. Because of the pivotal role of the sex hormones and their receptors in disease progression of breast cancer and prostate cancer, endocrine therapies are developed, that aim to interfere with hormone receptor-mediated pathways by either reducing the level of the hormone or blocking of the hormone receptor. The most important hormone receptors involved in tumor progression are estrogen and progesterone receptors in breast cancer and androgen receptors (ARs) in prostate cancer. PET allows noninvasive monitoring of receptor expression in patients with hormone-responsive tumors, and thus could potentially provide information that can support therapy management in patients. Since 1980s, many radiolabeled steroids have been evaluated as PET tracers for imaging of the hormone receptors, but most of these tracers failed in preclinical or early-clinical evaluation. So far, only 16α-[^{18}F]fluoro-17β-estradiol ([^{18}F]FES) seems to be an interesting PET tracer for estrogen receptor (ER) imaging in breast cancer patients and potentially also for endometrial cancer patients. The first clinical studies in patients with prostate cancer indicate that PET imaging of the androgen receptor (AR) with 16β-[^{18}F]fluorodihydrotestosterone ([^{18}F]FDHT) is feasible. Clinically useful PET tracers for progesterone receptor imaging are currently not available. Here, we will describe the current experience with [^{18}F]FES PET and [^{18}F]FDHT PET for imaging the ER and AR, respectively.

[^{18}F]FES PET

Methodology: [^{18}F]FES can reliably be prepared in two steps from a commercially available precursor. Practical radiochemical yields are high (several GBq) and consequently, doses for multiple patients can be obtained from a single preparation. [^{18}F]FES was shown to be stable in aqueous solution for at least 24 h. The use of [^{18}F]FES as a PET tracer was found to be safe. The radiation burden of [^{18}F]FES is 0.022 mSv/MBq, which is comparable to the radiation dose associated with other nuclear medicine procedures. The highest radiation dose is received by the liver and gall bladder. The recommended dose for [^{18}F]FES is 220 MBq (6 mCi), which typically corresponds to <5 μg of FES per injection. To date, no adverse events for a tracer dose of [^{18}F]FES have been reported.

In the literature, several acquisition protocols for [^{18}F]FES PET have been described. For research applications, dynamic imaging protocols with arterial blood sampling and metabolite analysis have been described, but for routine clinical applications, a whole body data acquisition protocol comparable to that of [^{18}F]FDG can be used. Although fasting of the patient prior to the procedure is not required, the use of medication that binds to the active site of the ER (e.g., tamoxifen, fulvestrant) should be stopped. The use of aromatase inhibitors can be continued. Usually, a dose of 220 MBq [^{18}F]FES is administered to the patient, but acceptable images can still be obtained when only 100 MBq of the tracer is injected. Data acquisition can already be performed as soon as 30 min after tracer injection, but a waiting period of 60 or 90 min is preferred to allow clearance of nonspecific uptake.

Physiological distribution: Normal physiological expression of ER is mainly located in epididymes, testes, pituitary gland, ovaries, uterus, kidneys and adrenals, but to a lesser extent also in prostate gland, bladder, liver, thymus and heart. The normal distribution of [^{18}F]FES, however, is dominated by the hepatic and renal clearance of the tracer. Consequently, [^{18}F]FES PET images show highest tracer uptake in liver, gallbladder, intestine, kidneys and bladder. Early clearance of [^{18}F]FES from blood is rapid and total blood activity remains almost constant after 10–15 min. [^{18}F]FES is rapidly converted into sulfate and glucuronide metabolites by the liver. Twenty minutes after injection, the intact tracer comprises only 20% of the total radioactivity in blood. The concentration of metabolites in blood remains almost constant between 20 and 120 min after tracer injection, because the rate of release of metabolites from the liver into the blood stream is similar to the renal clearance rate of these metabolites.

Clinical practice: The main role of [^{18}F]FES PET in clinical practice is related to detection of ER-positive breast tumors and may have also a role in endometrial carcinoma. Several studies have demonstrated that [^{18}F]FES PET can successfully detect the ER status of primary breast tumors, lymph node and distant metastases in humans. Because of the high physiological uptake of [^{18}F]FES in liver and kidneys, however, detection of lesions in these organs is difficult. Correlations between quantitative [^{18}F]FES uptake and in-vitro tests of ER density were found to be 0.96 and 0.73 in two relatively small clinical PET studies in 10 and 17 patients, respectively. By itself, [^{18}F]FES PET is not ideal for diagnosis and staging, because ER-negative tumors cannot be detected by this method and liver metastases often remain obscured.

In patients with advanced ER-positive disease, however, [^{18}F]FES PET could be a useful tool for tumor characterization, patient stratification and therapy management. [^{18}F]FES PET was able to predict responsiveness to antihormonal therapy in patients with advanced breast cancer. At baseline, PET showed significantly higher [^{18}F]FES uptake in lesions of responders ($n = 21$) to tamoxifen treatment than in those of nonresponders ($n = 19$). When a cutoff value of SUV = 2.0 was used, the positive and negative predictive values were 79 and 88%, respectively. Another study confirmed that [^{18}F]FES PET has a high negative predictive value, as none of the patients with a negative [^{18}F]FES PET (SUV <1.5) responded to tamoxifen treatment. A recent study by Dehdashti and coworkers showed comparable results for response to treatment with aromatase inhibitors. On baseline FES-PET a significantly ($P < 0.0049$) higher tumor uptake was noted in responders (SUV_{max} 3.5 ± 2.5) compared to nonresponders (SUV_{max} 2.1 ± 1.8). Based on ROC analysis with a cutoff SUV_{max} of 2.0, [^{18}F]FES PET has a positive predictive value of 50% (12/24 patients) and a negative predictive value of 81% (22/27 patients). Thus, [^{18}F]FES PET could potentially be useful to avoid unnecessary ineffective treatment.

For therapy management, it is important to realize that the ER status of the primary tumor is not always predictive for the ER status of the metastasis. Two [^{18}F]FES PET studies showed that lesions with discordant ER status are present in 15–24% of the patients with multiple metastatic foci. Obviously, the discordant ER status could affect therapy outcome and therefore should be taken into account by the leading physician.

In the clinic, [^{18}F]FES PET might also be useful in distinguishing an ER-positive tumor from a nontumor related problem in patients with metastatic disease. Cancer patients often experience complaints caused by degenerative processes and treatment-induced complications, like edema, necrosis and fibrosis. Often, a major problem for clinicians is how to discriminate whether the problem is caused by tumor activity or not, especially for bone lesions. MRI and the bone scan are often inconclusive and the sensitivity of [^{18}F]FDG PET for detection of bone metastases is rather low (lesion-based sensitivity: 69%). In addition, [^{18}F]FDG PET can give false positive results when an inflammatory response is involved or when recent treatment like radiotherapy was given. [^{18}F] FES PET, on the other hand, could provide the required information and thus guide the patient's treatment.

In conclusion, [^{18}F]FES PET may be useful for tumor characterization, particularly in metastatic breast cancer, and for distinguishing cancer from non cancer pathology. The clinical value of this technique, however, still has to be established.

[^{18}F]FDHT PET

Methodology: [^{18}F]FDHT has been developed about two decades ago, but only few clinical studies with this tracer have been reported so far. This may partly be due to the synthesis of the tracer, which requires the use of the water-sensitive reagent $LiAlH_4$ at very low temperatures (-78°C) and liquid-liquid extraction. As a result, it is difficult to automate the synthesis for routine production. The radiation burden of [^{18}F]FDHT is within acceptable limits, with an effective dose equivalent of 0.00177 mSv/MBq. The critical organ is the urinary bladder wall, which limits the recommended dose to 331 MBq. For clinical applications, a whole body data acquisition protocol with a 60–90 min delay between tracer injection and acquisition can be used.

Physiological distribution: Normal physiological uptake of [^{18}F]FDHT is found in liver, gallbladder and intestine, due to hepatic clearance of the tracer. High uptake is also observed in the blood pool, as a result of the slow clearance of radioactivity from the blood (less than 30% in 60 min). Virtually, all radioactivity in blood is due to plasma protein-bound metabolites. Approximately 80% of the [^{18}F]FDHT in plasma is metabolized within 10 min. Still, high-contrast images can be obtained, because the tracer is rapidly taken up by prostate tumors and metastases. Tracer uptake is followed by prolonged retention of the tracer in the tumor. [^{18}F]FDHT uptake in the tumor is specifically mediated by the AR, as tracer accumulation can be blocked with agonists and antagonists of the receptor, such as (dihydro)testosterone and flutamide.

Clinical practice: Two small studies in seven patients and 19 patients with metastatic prostate cancer found that the sensitivity of [^{18}F]FDHT PET was only 78% (lesion-based) and 69% (patient-based), respectively. In the latter study, 17 unexpected lesions were also observed. Discordant lesions within a single patient were found in both studies. Since no histology was performed on the lesions, it remains unclear if the lack of [^{18}F]FDHT uptake in some lesions is due to insufficient sensitivity of the imaging technique or the absence of receptor expression in the tumor.

In conclusion, it can be said that it is still too early to determine whether [^{18}F]FDHT PET may have useful clinical applications, as clinical data are scarce. The first results indicate that [^{18}F]FDHT PET by itself does not seem suitable for tumor detection and staging. However, the tracer could be further explored for tumor characterization in advanced prostate cancer.

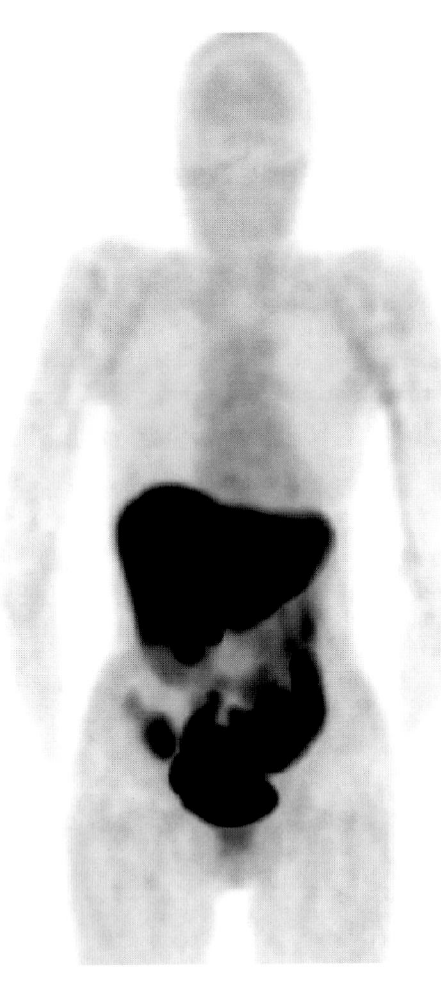

Other finding

ER-positive breast cancer and cervical trauma. The patient experienced pain in the neck. The bone scan was positive possibly due to degeneration and the MRI scan was not conclusive. Biopsy to determine tumor activity was not feasible due to the localization of the lesion.

^{18}F-FES finding

PET showed no pathological uptake.

Teaching point

Notice the very high uptake in the liver, gallbladder, and intestine, which is normal physiological uptake.

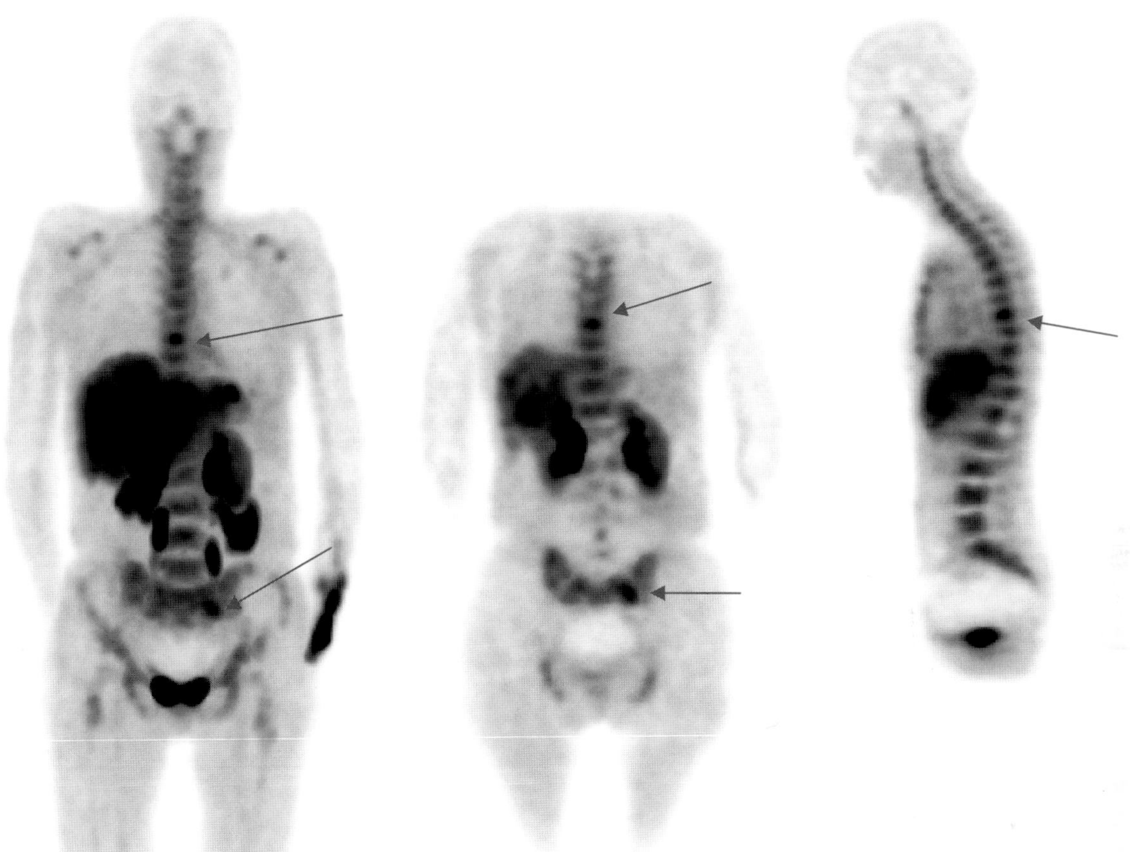

Other finding

Patient experienced heavy low back pain located at the sacroiliac joint on the left side. The bone scan showed no bone metastases and MRI detected two bone metastases in vertebras Th 7 and Th 12, but not at the location of the pain complaints.

^{18}F-FES finding

PET shows two focal lesions with high uptake at the left sacroiliac joint and in vertebra Th 8 (*red arrows*).

Teaching point

Notice the physiological uptake in liver, gallbladder, intestine, kidneys, ureters and bladder. High activity in the left wrist is due to the tracer injection. Diffuse uptake in the bone marrow.

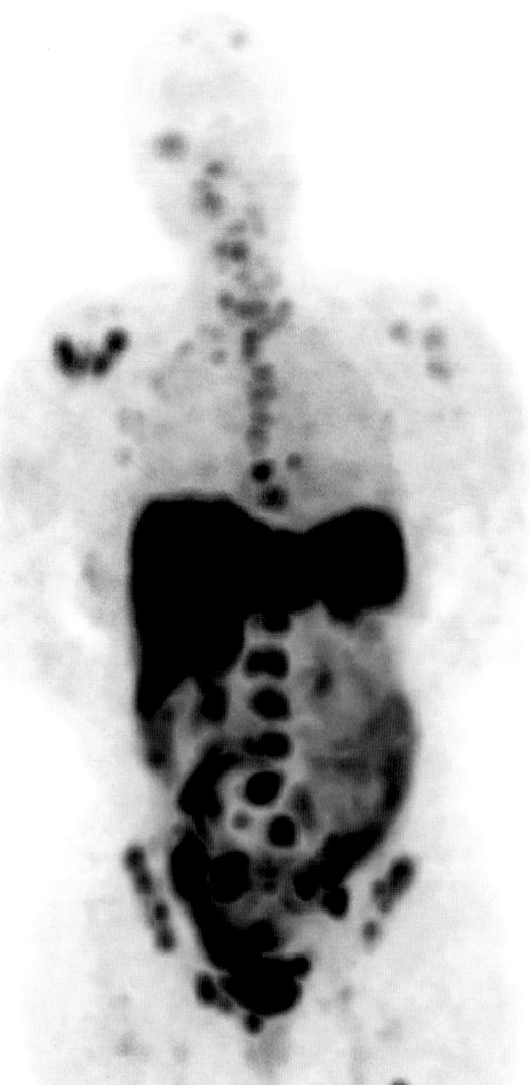

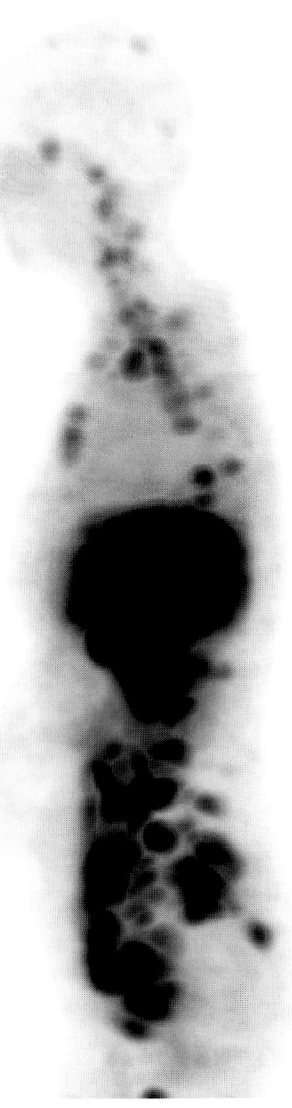

^{18}F-FES finding

Normal physiological uptake in the liver (enlarged), gallbladder, intestine, kidneys, and bladder. Notice the multiple ER-positive bone lesions, including a focal lesion in the skull, in the periorbital region, in both shoulders (right more than left), multiple lesions in the vertebral column and in the pelvis.

Teaching point

Patient with bone metastases of breast cancer with progression on third-line hormonal treatment. It was unknown whether the ER was still available in order to justify treatment with estrogen. Biopsy to determine the ER status was not easy due to the localization of the metastases. In such cases, PET was performed to determine the ER status of the lesions.

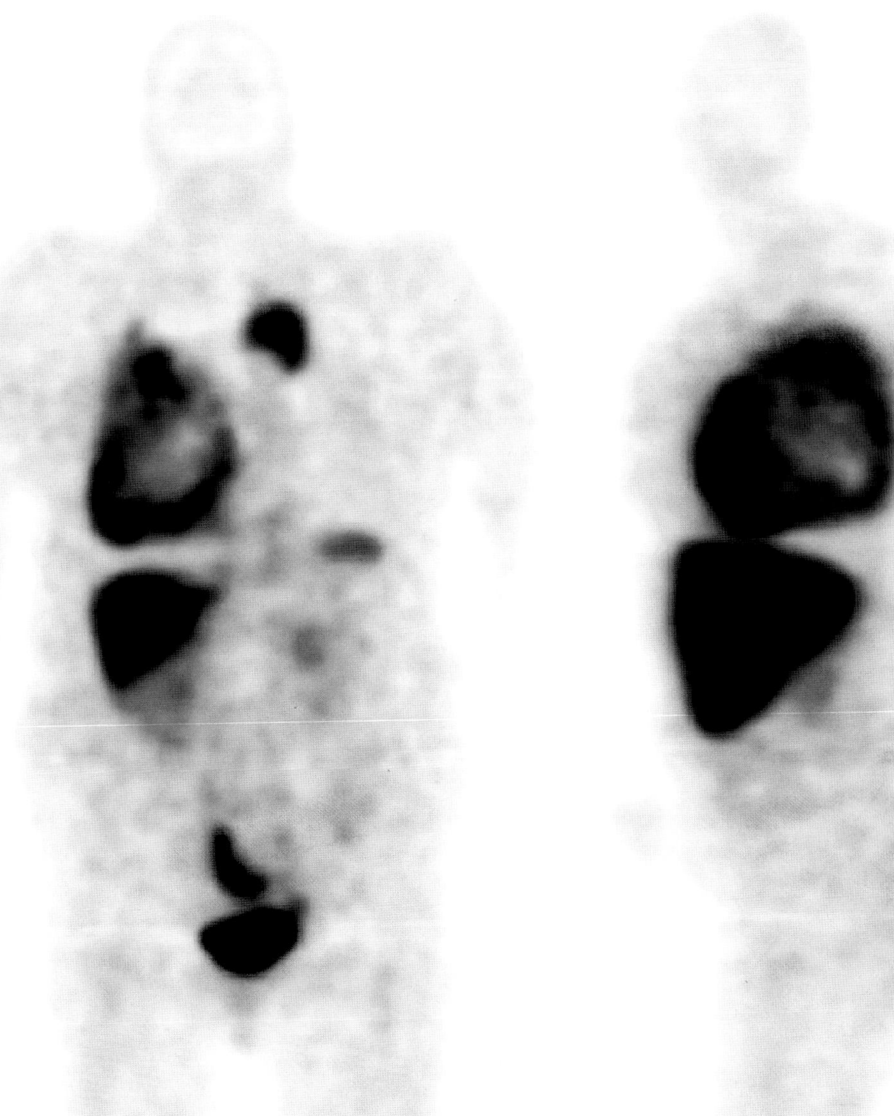

^{18}F-FES finding

Normal uptake in liver, stomach, intestine, excretion by kidneys, and bladder. Pathological uptake in almost the whole right lung with focal regions with very intense uptake. Focal uptake apicomedial in the left lung.

Teaching point

Patient with an ER positive tumor, developed lung metastases that responded well to hormonal treatment. When CT showed progression, [^{18}F]FES PET was performed to decide whether a second-line hormonal treatment could be a useful treatment. This case illustrates that FES PET could also be useful in patients with endometrium carcinoma.

Chapter 14 HTP PET-CT

Adrienne H. Brouwers, Klaas P. Koopmans, Rudi A. J. O. Dierckx, and Philip H. Elsinga

β-[^{11}C]-5-hydroxy-*L*-tryptophan (^{11}C-5-HTP) is a PET tracer used for imaging neuroendocrine tumors which are derived from neuroendocrine cells. Neuroendocrine cells regulate a variety of body functions through paracrine stimulation. This is achieved via the production of a large variety of hormones, of which serotonin and catecholamines are examples. The production of these hormones is accomplished via amine precursor uptake and decarboxylation. In many differentiated neuroendocrine tumors, the capability to synthesize hormonal products has remained. This makes imaging with amine precursors interesting in these tumors. The serotonine pathway is active in many neuroendocrine tumors. In this pathway, the naturally occurring amino acid tryptophan and 5-HTP are both precursors. Serotonin is most abundantly present in blood platelets and the intestinal wall. In the brain serotonin acts as a neurotransmitter. Both tryptophan and 5-HTP are taken up via system L large amino acid transporters (LAT). After entering the cell, decarboxylation to serotonin takes place via the enzyme aromatic amino acid decarboxylase (AADC). The resulting end-product serotonin is then transported into storage vesicles through the vesicular monoamine transporter (VMAT). From these vesicles, serotonin can be released in the extracellular environment. Serotonine is thereafter degraded and eventually excreted as urinary 5-hydroxyindole acetic acid (5-HIAA). In the catecholamine pathway, the same LAT and VMAT transporter systems, and the enzyme AADC play a crucial role, resulting in the end-products, dopamine, adrenaline and noradrenaline. Although the exact uptake mechanism and intracellular fate of these amines and their metabolites are not precisely understood, it appears that increased LAT activity plays a role to satisfy a high precursor turnover due to an increased metabolic pathway, e.g., serotonin or catecholamine, or at least increased AADC activity in neuroendocrine tumors.

^{11}C-5-HTP is only produced in a few centers worldwide. The use of this tracer is limited due to two major drawbacks. First, an on-site cyclotron is needed for the production of the ^{11}C isotope, which has a half-life of 20 min. Furthermore, the tracer synthesis is very complex since it relies on two complex multienzyme steps. However, quantities up to 1,000 MBq can be prepared reliably. Major advantages of this technique is that in one examination the whole body can be assessed for disease activity, and scans are often easy to interpret due to high uptake in tumor lesions and low background activity in normal organs. Altogether, the published clinical results using ^{11}C-5-HTP justify the use of this tracer.

The ^{11}C-5-HTP tracer has been developed during the eighties of the last century in Uppsala, Sweden. Their first clinical results with neuroendocrine tumors were published in 1993. Nowadays, ^{11}C-5-HTP PET scanning is typically performed 10–20 min after injection of 140–521 MBq ^{11}C-5-HTP with carbidopa pretreatment, 2 mg/kg body weight or with a fixed dose of 200 mg, 1 h prior to injection. The estimated mean radiation dose is 0.34 mSv per 100 MBq ^{11}C-5-HTP. Patients are requested to fast for 2–4 h with free intake of fluids. Thus far, as an endogenous compound, no adverse reactions after tracer injection have been reported.

In earlier days, PET scans were made without carbidopa. However, this resulted in lower image quality due to streaky image reconstruction artefacts caused by high physiological excretion of the radiotracer via kidneys and urinary bladder. Carbidopa, a peripheral inhibitor of AADC enzyme activity was tested for its capacity to decrease urinary activity concentration. Patients with mid-gut carcinoids (well-differentiated neuroendocrine carcinomas) were scanned with and without carbidopa pretreatment 1 h before ^{11}C-5-HTP injection. Carbidopa pretreatment significantly reduced the radioactivity concentration in the urinary collecting system, from a mean SUV of the renal pelvis of 155 ± 195–39 ± 14 SD. As a secondary effect, tumor uptake of ^{11}C-5-HTP was significantly increased after carbidopa administration, increasing from a mean SUV of 11 ± 3–14 ± 3 SD, and improving visual image interpretation. With carbidopa pretreatment in normal liver and pancreas tissue, the mean SUV was significantly increased or decreased, respectively. However, in these normal background tissues mean SUV was overall still low with mean liver SUV of 3.6 ± 0.8 and mean pancreas SUV of 4.4 ± 0.8 SD.

So far, three patient series with a reasonable number of patients have been published. In the first study, the following 18 patients with histopathologically verified neuroendocrine tumors who were referred for evaluation and medical treatment were included: mid-gut (n = 14), foregut (n = 1), hindgut carcinoid (n = 1), and endocrine pancreatic tumors (n = 2). ^{11}C-5-HTP was compared to CT. Additionally, 10 of 18 patients were monitored with PET at different intervals during treatment. Patients were not pretreated with carbidopa and fasted 4 h before start of study. Directly after injection of 110–700 MBq ^{11}C-5-HTP dynamic imaging was performed with the abdomen in the field of view, and plasma samples were taken during 45 min. Thereafter, in most patients, an additional 10 min static image with another portion of the abdomen in the field of view was recorded. All 18 patients showed increased ^{11}C-5-HTP uptake in tumor tissue; interestingly this was also the case in two patients with normal urinary 5-HIAA levels (hindgut carcinoid and a nonfunctioning endocrine pancreatic tumor). Fifteen baseline PET scans could be compared with contrast-enhanced CT scans. ^{11}C-5-HTP PET detected more tumor lesions than CT in ten patients, and was equal in five patients (four mid-gut, one foregut), with missing data in three patients with mid-gut neuroendocrine tumors. In the ten patients that were on treatment (interferon-α ± octreotide, or somatostatin analog only), a close correlation between the changes in ^{11}C-5-HTP transport rate constant in the tumors and urinary 5-HIAA was noted. It was suggested that ^{11}C-5-HTP PET may serve as a means to monitor therapy. However, it is still unknown whether these biochemical changes in the tumor, while on medical treatment, reflect changes in tumor metabolism or primarily amine processing.

In another patient series 38 patients were evaluated, again with a variety of neuroendocrine tumors, but among others, consisting of mid-gut carcinoids ($n = 13$), lung carcinoids ($n = 7$), and nonfunctioning endocrine pancreatic tumors ($n = 5$). Whole-body ^{11}C-5-HTP PET imaging was compared to both CT and the functional imaging technique, somatostatin receptor scintigraphy (SRS), which is often used in clinical routine in neuroendocrine tumors, and more widely available. Whole-body PET scanning with a mean dose of 381 MBq ^{11}C-5-HTP was started 20 min after tracer injection in carbidopa pretreated patients. ^{11}C-5-HTP PET detected tumor lesions in 36 of 38 (95%) patients. In 84% of patients SRS was positive, whereas CT was positive in 79%. More lesions were detected with ^{11}C-5-HTP PET in 22 of 38 (58%) patients compared to SRS and CT, whereas the imaging modalities showed equal number of lesions in 13 of 38 patients (34%). In three patients, SRS or CT showed more lesions; patients with a nonfunctioning endocrine pancreatic tumor, and a pancreatic carcinoma with some endocrine differentiation on immunohistochemistry were PET negative. A patient with metastasized thymus carcinoma only showed the primary tumor on ^{11}C-5-HTP PET and SRS, while CT scan also detected metastases. From these patients, it was speculated that in case of high proliferation rate and dedifferentiation of neuroendocrine tumors, ^{18}FDG PET is probably the imaging modality of choice. In the 17 patients who had their primary tumor still in situ, ^{11}C-5-HTP PET was positive in 16, compared to SRS in nine, and CT in eight patients. PET could detect surgically removed lesions as small as six mm. The main conclusion of this study was that PET imaging with ^{11}C-5-HTP can be universally applied in neuroendocrine tumors, also in patients without elevated 5-HIAA excretion in urine, as long as the tumor is not highly proliferating and/or dedifferentiating.

Another study confirmed that the information obtained with ^{11}C-5-HTP PET considerably contributes to the information regarding tumor status in patients with neuroendocrine tumors. In this study, carcinoid ($n = 24$) or pancreatic islet cell tumor ($n = 23$) patients with at least one lesion visible on conventional imaging (e.g., CT, SRS) underwent a ^{11}C-5-HTP and a 6-[F-18]- fluoro-L-dihydroxy-phenylalanin (^{18}F-DOPA) PET scan. ^{18}F-DOPA PET images the catecholamine metabolic pathway. Whole-body PET images with carbidopa pre-treatment were recorded 10 min after intravenous injection of 200 ± 50 SD MBq ^{11}C-5-HTP, or 60 min after i.v. administration of 180 ± 50 SD MBq ^{18}F-DOPA. The PET findings were compared, per-patient and per-lesion, with a composite reference standard derived from all available imaging data along with clinical and cytological/histological information. Results indicated that indeed, ^{11}C-5-HTP PET can be seen as a universal imaging agent for carcinoid and pancreatic islet cell tumor patients. It was the only imaging modality that was positive in all patients (100% sensitivity). Especially in islet cell tumor patients, more tumor-positive patients and lesions were found with ^{11}C-5-HTP (100 and 67%) compared to ^{18}F-DOPA (89 and 41%), and SRS (78 and 46%), and CT (87 and 68%). In carcinoid patients, the per-lesion analysis showed that ^{18}F-DOPA PET outperformed all other imaging techniques. Adding CT to both imaging techniques resulted in a further improvement in sensitivity in a per-lesion analysis, since both types of imaging techniques were complementary to each other. Therefore, for pancreatic islet cell patients, ^{11}C-5-HTP PET-CT was considered the optimal imaging technique, whereas for carcinoid patients, it was ^{18}F-DOPA PET-CT. Furthermore, it was stated that in carcinoid patients SRS scanning can be omitted without missing any lesions. However, in a minority of islet cell patients, (8%) SRS performed better than both PET techniques and therefore remains of additional value. In this regard, direct comparison of ^{11}C-5-HTP (and ^{18}F-DOPA) to the recently developed ^{68}Ga-labeled somatostatin analogs for PET imaging in various subtypes of neuroendocrine tumors would be much of interest.

Besides application in neuroendocrine tumors, ^{11}C-5-HTP has also been tested in a few patients with hormone-refractory prostate cancer, after it became known that hormone-refractory prostate cancer may undergo neuroendocrine differentiation. In nononcological studies ^{11}C-5-HTP uptake has been studied in brains of healthy volunteers and patients with major depression. Also, another labeled variant of tryptophan, α-[^{11}C]methyl-*L*-tryptophan (α-[^{11}C]MTrp), has been tested in the normal and diseased brains, both neurologically and psychiatrically.

In conclusion, ^{11}C-5-HTP PET is a excellent functional imaging technique in patients with proven neuroendocrine tumors, especially in pancreatic islet cell tumors and carcinoids. Adding CT improves the detection rate even more; thus, combining these techniques in dedicated PET-CT scanners is likely more optimal. The imaging characteristics of ^{11}C-5-HTP PET-CT in complex clinical cases or in less advanced clinical stages, e.g., when there is only a suspicion of a neuroendocrine tumor, needs to be determined. Furthermore, its role in monitoring response to therapy and predicting response to therapy needs to be further investigated. Also, how this imaging technique performs in relation to other new functional PET imaging techniques in neuroendocrine tumors needs to be further elucidated. ^{11}C-5-HTP PET has also been proven useful in neuroendocrine tumors that do not produce bioactive amines and metabolites of the serotonine or catecholamine pathways. More research should be directed in elucidating the exact uptake mechanisms and intracellular fate of these amines and their metabolites, since these are not precisely understood. The major drawback of ^{11}C-5-HTP PET is the difficult and laborious synthesis of ^{11}C-5-HTP, and the need for a cyclotron to produce ^{11}C on-site. Thus, the development of a more straightforward synthesis of ^{18}F-labeled 5-HTP could be much helpful, provided this newly developed tracer has the same imaging capacities as ^{11}C-5-HTP.

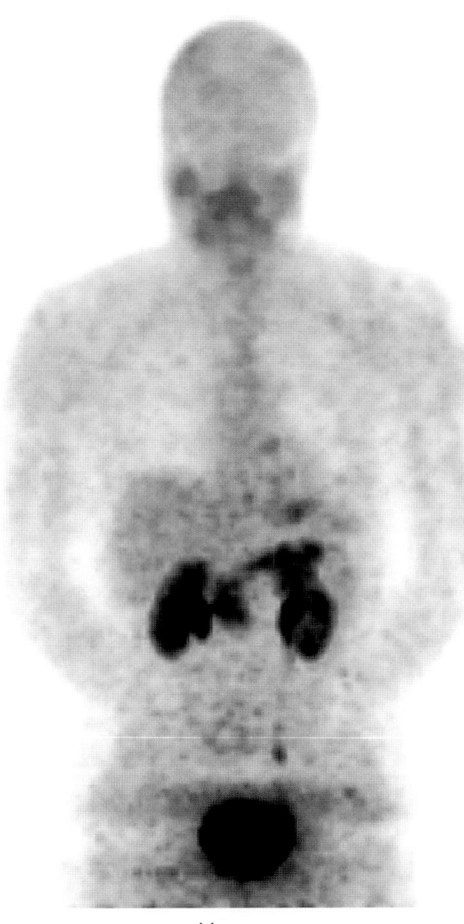

^{11}C-HTP

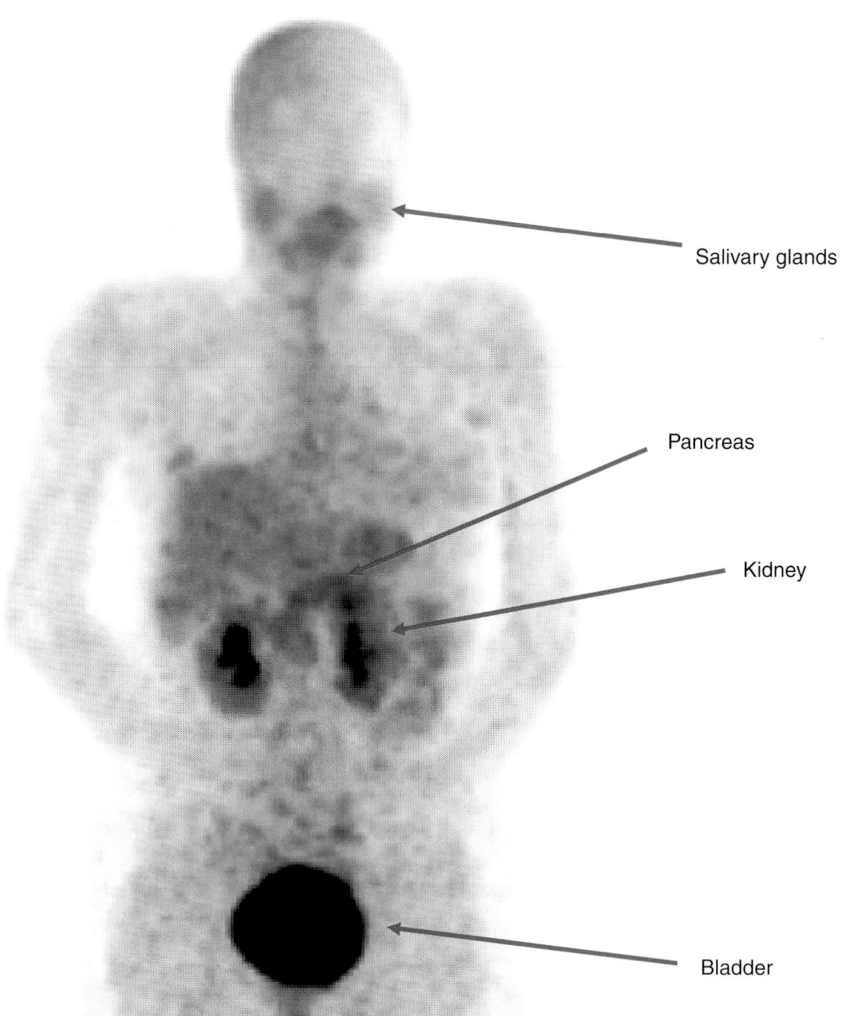

Teaching point

Normal HTP PET scans showing physiological uptake in the pancreas, kidneys, and urinary bladder. As with many amino acid tracers, there is some tracer uptake in the salivary glands, the myocardium, stomach, and esophagus. Note that the pancreatic uptake is variable between patients (patient was pretreated with carbidopa).

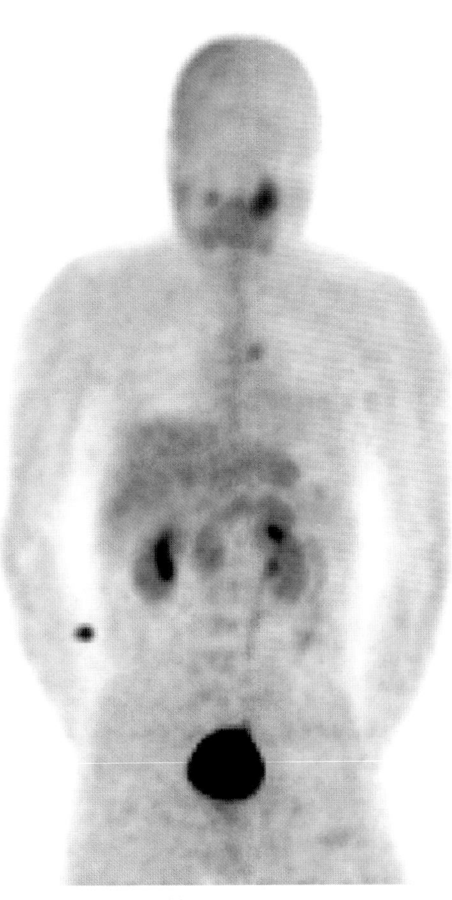

^{11}C-5-HTP

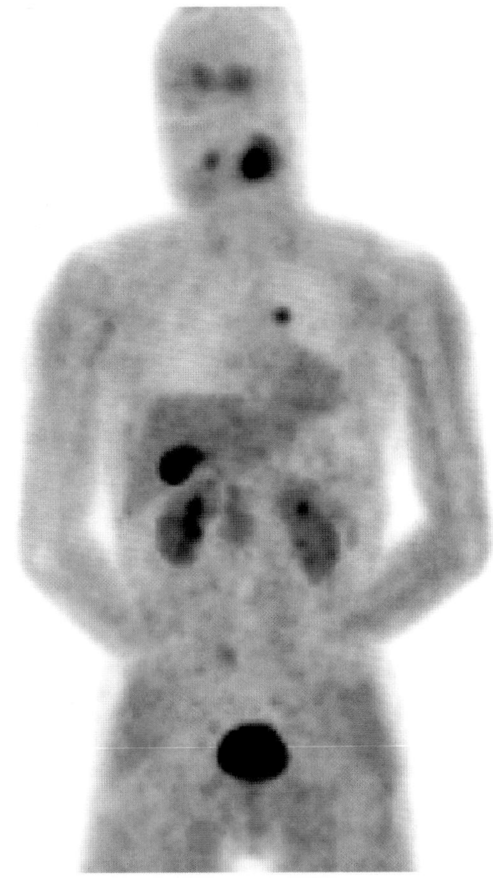

^{18}F-DOPA

PET findings

Both ^{11}C-5-HTP PET and ^{18}F-DOPA PET show increased tracer uptake in the left > right carotid region, and also in the hilar region of the left lung, due to paragangliomas.

Teaching point

Although both scans show intense uptake in the paragangliomas, these lesions show a slightly better ^{18}F-DOPA uptake. This could be related to the active catecholamine pathway in these tumors. Furthermore, note the physiologic ^{18}F-DOPA uptake in the gall bladder, which is a potential pitfall as it can be mistaken for a tumor lesion.

Female 59 years

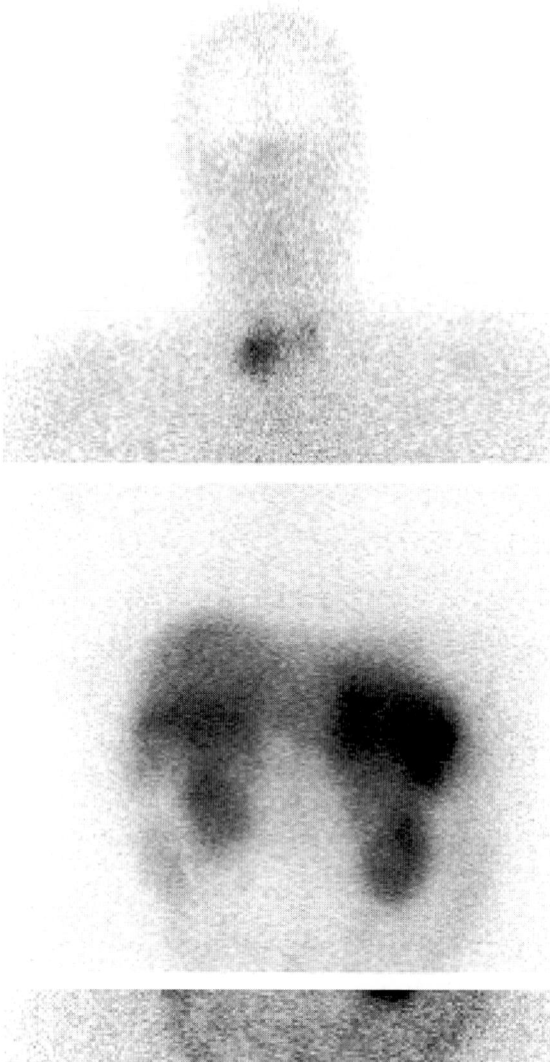

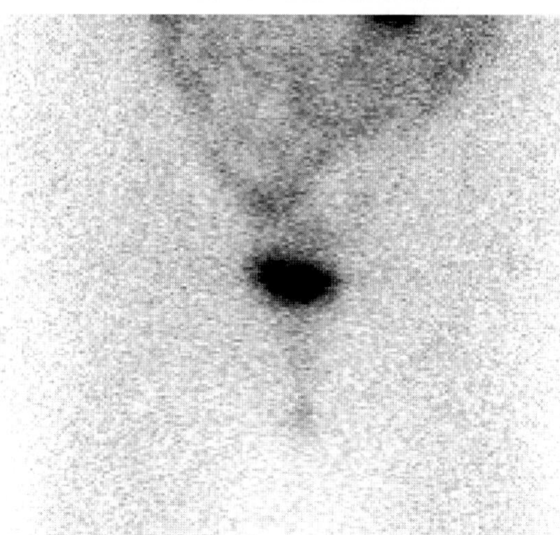

SRS and other findings

Patient presenting with abdominal pain, changed defecational pattern, and weight loss. A biopsy of the pancreatic process revealed a neuroendocrine tumor.

Somatostatin receptor scintigraphy only shows a lesion in the region of the tail of the pancreas.

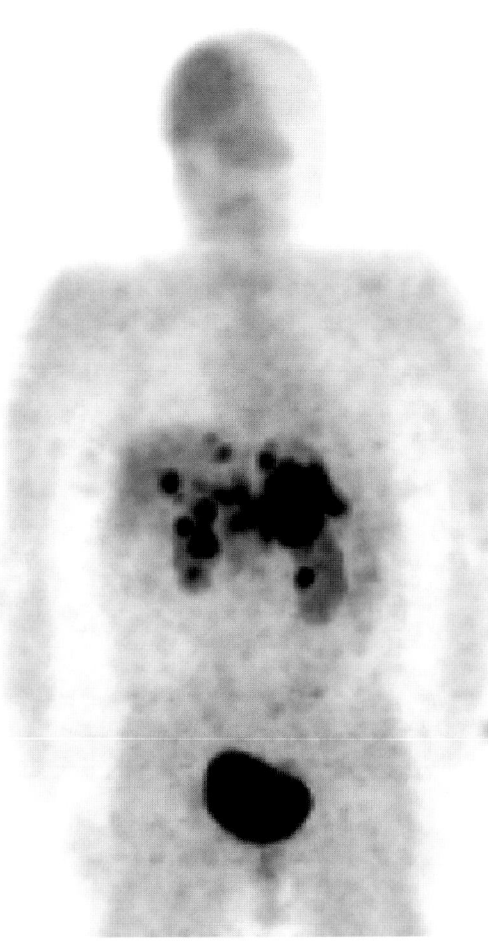

^{11}C-HTP

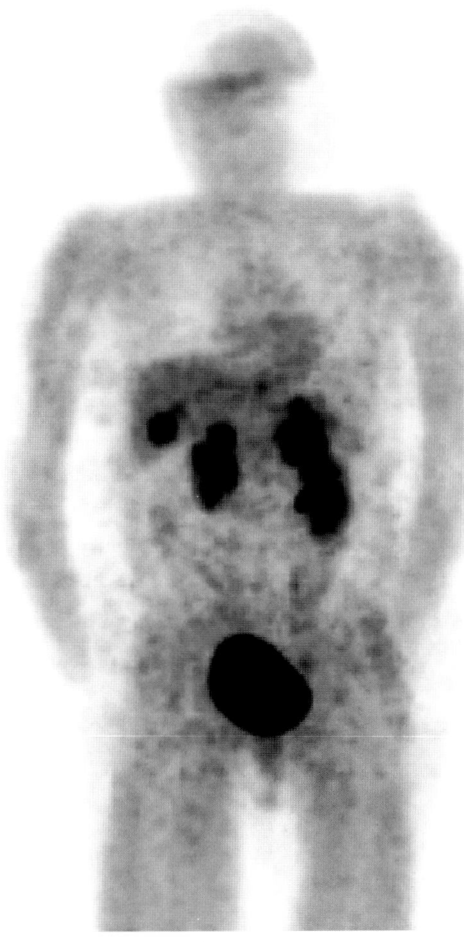

^{18}F-DOPA

PET findings

The ^{11}C-5-HTP PET and ^{18}F-DOPA PET show a large mass in the region of the pancreatic tail, consistent with the SRS scintigraphy. However, ^{11}C-5-HTP PET shows numerous lesions in the liver and abdomen, which were not present on either ^{18}F-DOPA PET or the octreotide scintigraphy.

Teaching point

Neuroendocrine tumors of the pancreas are very heterogeneous in their biochemical behavior. In these patients, often a combination of several imaging types (anatomical imaging, PET, somatostatin receptor scintigraphy) will reveal the true extent of the disease.

Chapter 15 References

Choline

Breeuwsma AJ, Pruim J, Jongen MM. In vivo uptake of [11C] choline does not correlate with cell proliferation in human prostate cancer. Eur J Nucl Med Mol Imaging. 32(6):668–73

DeGrado TR, Coleman RE, Wang S. Synthesis and evaluation of 18F-labeled choline as an oncologic tracer for positron emission tomography: initial findings in prostate cancer. Cancer Res. 2001;61:110–7

Giovacchini G, Fallanca F, Landoni C, et al F. C-11 choline versus F-18 fluorodeoxyglucose for imaging meningiomas: an initial experience. Clin Nucl Med. 2009;34(1):7–10

Hara T. 11C-choline and 2-deoxy-2-[18F]fluoro-D-glucose in tumor imaging with positron emission tomography. Mol Imaging Biol. 2002;4(4):267–73

Hara T, Kosaka N, Kishi H. PET imaging of prostate cancer using carbon-11-choline. J Nucl Med. 1998;39:990–5

Husarik DB, Miralbell R, Dubs M, et al Evaluation of [(18)F]-choline PET/CT for staging and restaging of prostate cancer. Eur J Nucl Med Mol Imaging. 2008;35(2):253–63

Kwee SA, Ko JP, Jiang CS, Watters MR, Coel MN. Solitary brain lesions enhancing at MR imaging: evaluation with fluorine 18 fluorocholine PET. Radiology. 2007;244(2):557–65

Nanni C, Zamagni E, Cavo M, et al 11C-choline vs. 18F-FDG PET/CT in assessing bone involvement in patients with multiple myeloma. World J Surg Oncol. 2007;5:68

Picchio M, Messa C, Bandoni C, et al Value of [11C]coline positron emission tomography for re-staging prostate cancer: a comparison with [18F]fluorodeoxyglucose positron emission tomography. J Urol. 2003;169:1337–40

Picchio M, Treiber U, Beer AJ, et al Value of 11C-choline PET and contrast-enhanced CT for staging of bladder cancer: correlation with histopathologic findings. J Nucl Med. 2006;47(6):938–44

Schiavina R, Scattoni V, Castellucci P, et al 11C-choline positron emission tomography/computerized tomography for preoperative lymph-node staging in intermediate-risk and high-risk prostate cancer: comparison with clinical staging nomograms. Eur Urol. 2008;54(2):392–401

Sofue K, Tateishi U, Sawada M, et al Role of carbon-11 choline PET/CT in the management of uterine carcinoma: initial experience. Ann Nucl Med. 2009;23(3):235–43

Methionine

Galldiks N, Kracht LW, Burghaus L, et al Use of 11C-methionine PET to monitor the effects of temozolomide chemotherapy in malignant gliomas. Eur J Nucl Med Mol Imaging. 2006;33(5):516–24

Kato T, Shinoda J, Nakayama N, et al Metabolic assessment of gliomas using 11C-methionine, [18F] fluorodeoxyglucose, and 11C-choline positron-emission tomography. AJNR Am J Neuroradiol. 2008;29(6):1176–82

Kracht LW, Friese M, Herholz K, et al Methyl-[11C]- l-methionine uptake as measured by positron emission tomography correlates to microvessel density in patients with glioma. Eur J Nucl Med Mol Imaging. 2003;30(6):868–73

Moulin-Romsée G, D'Hondt E, de Groot T, et al Non-invasive grading of brain tumours using dynamic amino acid PET imaging: does it work for 11C-methionine? Eur J Nucl Med Mol Imaging. 2007;34(12):2082–7

Price SJ. The role of advanced MR imaging in understanding brain tumour pathology. Br J Neurosurg. 2007;21(6):562–75

Pirotte B, Goldman S, Massager N, et al Comparison of 18F-FDG and 11C-methionine for PET-guided stereotactic brain biopsy of gliomas. J Nucl Med. 2004;45(8):1293–8

Scott JN, Brasher PMA, Sevick RJ, Rewcastle NB, Forsyth PA. How often are nonenhancing supratentorial gliomas malignant? A population study. Neurology. 2002;59:947–9

Sundin A, Johansson C, Hellman P, et al PET and parathyroid L-[carbon-11]methionine accumulation in hyperparathyroidism. J Nucl Med. 1996;37(11):1766–70

Fluoride

Berger F, Lee YP, Loening AM, et al Whole-body skeletal imaging in mice utilizing microPET: optimization of reproducibility and applications in animal models of bone disease. Eur J Nucl Med Mol Imaging. 2002;29:1225–36

Blake GM, Park-Holohan SJ, Cook GJ, Fogelman I. Quantitative studies of bone with the use of 18F-fluoride and 99mTc-methylene diphosphonate. Semin Nucl Med. 2001;31:28–49

Blau M, Nagler W, Bender MA. Fluorine-18: a new isotope for bone scanning. J Nucl Med. 1962;3:332–4

Even-Sapir E, Metser U, Flusser G, et al Assessment of malignant skeletal disease: initial experience with 18F-fluoride PET/CT and comparison between 18F-fluoride PET and 18F-fluoride PET/CT. J Nucl Med. 2004;45:272–8

Even-Sapir E, Metser U, Mishani E, Lievshitz G, Lerman H, Leibovitch I. The detection of bone metastases in patients with high-risk prostate cancer: 99mTc-MDP Planar bone scintigraphy, single- and multi-field-of-view SPECT, 18F-fluoride PET, and 18F-fluoride PET/CT. J Nucl Med. 2006;47:287–97

Galasko CS. The pathological basis for skeletal scintigraphy. J Bone Joint Surg Br. 1975;57:353–9

Grant FD, Fahey FH, Packard AB, Davis RT, Alavi A, Treves ST. Skeletal PET with 18F-fluoride: applying new technology to an old tracer. J Nucl Med. 2008;49:68–78

Hamaoka T, Madewell JE, Podoloff DA, Hortobagyi GN, Ueno NT. Bone imaging in metastatic breast cancer. J Clin Oncol. 2004;22:2942–53

Hetzel M, Arslandemir C, Konig HH, et al F-18 NaF PET for detection of bone metastases in lung cancer: accuracy, cost-effectiveness, and impact on patient management. J Bone Miner Res. 2003;18:2206–14

Hoh CK, Hawkins RA, Dahlbom M, et al Whole body skeletal imaging with [18F]fluoride ion and PET. J Comput Assist Tomogr. 1993;17:34–41

Messa C, Goodman WG, Hoh CK, et al Bone metabolic activity measured with positron emission tomography and [18F] fluoride ion in renal osteodystrophy: correlation with bone histomorphometry. J Clin Endocrinol Metab. 1993;77: 949–55

Piert M, Zittel TT, Becker GA, et al Assessment of porcine bone metabolism by dynamic. J Nucl Med. 2001;42:1091–100

Schirrmeister H, Guhlmann A, Elsner K, et al Sensitivity in detecting osseous lesions depends on anatomic localization: planar bone scintigraphy versus 18F PET. J Nucl Med. 1999;40:1623–9

Schirrmeister H, Glatting G, Hetzel J, et al Prospective evaluation of the clinical value of planar bone scans, SPECT, and (18)F-labeled NaF PET in newly diagnosed lung cancer. J Nucl Med. 2001;42:1800–4

Schirrmeister H, Guhlmann A, Kotzerke J, et al Early detection and accurate description of extent of metastatic bone disease in breast cancer with fluoride ion and positron emission tomography. J Clin Oncol. 1999;17:2381–9

Tyrosine

Balogova S, Périé S, Kerrou K, et al Prospective comparison of FDG and FET PET/CT in patients with head and neck squamous cell carcinoma. Mol Imaging Biol. 2008;10(6): 364–73

Floeth FW, Pauleit D, Sabel M, et al 18F-FET PET differentiation of ring-enhancing brain lesions. J Nucl Med. 2006;47(5): 776–82

Grosu AL, Weber WA, Riedel E, et al L-(methyl-11C) methionine positron emission tomography for target delineation in resected high-grade gliomas before radiotherapy. Int J Radiat Oncol Biol Phys. 2005;63(1):64–74

Langen KJ, Hamacher K, Weckesser M, et al O-(2-[18F] fluoroethyl)-L-tyrosine: uptake mechanisms and clinical applications. Nucl Med Biol. 2006;33(3):287–94

Mehrkens JH, Pöpperl G, Rachinger W, et al The positive predictive value of O-(2-[18F]fluoroethyl)-L-tyrosine (FET) PET in the diagnosis of a glioma recurrence after multimodal treatment. J Neurooncol. 2008;88(1):27–35

Pauleit D, Stoffels G, Schaden W, et al PET with O-(2-18F-fluoroethyl)-L-tyrosine in peripheral tumors: first clinical results. J Nucl Med. 2005;46(3):411–6

Pöpperl G, Kreth FW, Mehrkens JH, et al FET PET for the evaluation of untreated gliomas: correlation of FET uptake and uptake kinetics with tumour grading. Eur J Nucl Med Mol Imaging. 2007;34(12):1933–42

Pöpperl G, Götz C, Rachinger W, Gildehaus FJ, Tonn JC, Tatsch K. Value of O-(2-[18F]fluoroethyl)- L-tyrosine PET for the diagnosis of recurrent glioma. Eur J Nucl Med Mol Imaging. 2004;31(11):1464–70

Stöber B, Tanase U, Herz M, Seidl C, Schwaiger M, Senekowitsch-Schmidtke R. Differentiation of tumour and inflammation: characterisation of [methyl-3H]methionine (MET) and O-(2-[18F]fluoroethyl)-L-tyrosine (FET) uptake in human tumour and inflammatory cells. Eur J Nucl Med Mol Imaging. 2006;33(8):932–9

Weber WA, Wester HJ, Grosu AL, et al O-(2-[18F]fluoroethyl)-L-tyrosine and L-[methyl-11C]methionine uptake in brain tumours: initial results of a comparative study. Eur J Nucl Med. 2000;27(5):542–9

Somatostatin Receptors

Adams S, Baum R, Rink T, Schumm-Dräger PM, Usadel KH, Hör G. Limited value of fluorine-18 fluorodeoxyglucose positron emission tomography for the imaging of neuroendocrine tumors. Eur J Nucl Med. 1998;25:79–83

Ambrosini V, Castellucci P, Rubello D, et al 68Ga-DOTA-NOC: a new PET tracer for evaluating patients with bronchial carcinoid. Nucl Med Commun. 2009;30(4):281–6

Ambrosini V, Tomassetti P, Castellucci P, et al Comparison between 68Ga-DOTA-NOC and 18F-DOPA PET for the detection of gastro-entero-pancreatic and lung neuro-endocrine tumours. Eur J Nucl Med Mol Imaging. 2008;35(8):1431–8

Antunes P, Ginj M, Zhang H, et al Are radiogallium-labelled DOTA-conjugated somatostatin analogues superior to those labelled with other radiometals? Eur J Nucl Med Mol Imaging. 2007;34(7):982–93

Gabriel M, Decristoforo C, Kendler D, et al 68Ga-DOTA-Tyr3-octreotide PET in neuroendocrine tumors: comparison with somatostatin receptor scintigraphy and CT. J Nucl Med. 2007;48(4):508–18

Haug A, Auernhammer CJ, Wängler B, et al Intraindividual comparison of 68Ga-DOTA-TATE and 18F-DOPA PET in patients with well-differentiated metastatic neuroendocrine tumours. Eur J Nucl Med Mol Imaging. 2009;36(5):765–70. Epub 2009 Jan 10

Hofmann M, Maecke H, Börner R, et al Biokinetics and imaging with the somatostatin receptor PET radioligand (68) Ga-DOTATOC: preliminary data. Eur J Nucl Med. 2001; 28(12):1751–7

Koukouraki S, Strauss LG, Georgoulias V, Eisenhut M, Haberkorn U, Dimitrakopoulou-Strauss A. Comparison of the pharmacokinetics of 68Ga-DOTATOC and [18F]FDG in patients with metastatic neuroendocrine tumours scheduled for 90Y-DOTATOC therapy. Eur J Nucl Med Mol Imaging. 2006;33(10):1115–22

Pettinato C, Sarnelli A, Di Donna M, et al (68)Ga-DOTANOC: biodistribution and dosimetry in patients affected by neuroendocrine tumors. Eur J Nucl Med Mol Imaging. 2008; 35(1):72–9

Reubi JC, Waser B. Concomitant expression of several peptide receptors in neuroendocrine tumours: molecular basis for in vivo multireceptor tumour targeting. Eur J Nucl Med Mol Imaging. 2003;30(5):781–93

Acetate

Albrecht S, Buchegger F, Soloviev D, et al (11)C-Acetate PET in the early evaluation of prostate cancer recurrence. Eur J Nucl Med Mol Imaging. 2007;34:185–96

Delbeke D, Pinson CW. 11C-Acetate: a new tracer for the evaluation of hepatocellular carcinoma J Nucl Med. 2003;44: 222–3

Dienel GA, Popp D, Drew PD, Ball K, Krisht A, Cruz NF. Preferential labelling of glial and meningeal brain tumours with [2–14C]acetate. J Nucl Med. 2001;42:1243–50

Ho CL, Yu SC, Yeung DW. 11C-acetate PET imaging in hepatocellular carcinoma and other liver masses. J Nucl Med. 2003;44(2):213–21

Ho C-L, Chen S, Yeung DWC, Cheng TKC. Dual-tracer PET/CT imaging in evaluation of metastatic hepatocellular carcinoma. J Nucl Med. 2007;48:902–9

Kaji M, Nomori H, Watanabe K, et al 11C-acetate and 18F-fluorodeoxyglucose positron emission tomography of pulmonary adenocarcinoma. Ann Thorac Surg. 2007;83(1): 312–4

Kotzerke J, Volkmer BG, Glatting G. Intraindividual comparison of [11C]acetate and [11C]choline PET for detection of metastases of prostate cancer. Nuklearmedizin. 2003;42(1): 25–30

Nomori H, Shibata H, Uno K, et al 11C–acetate can be used in place of 18F-fluorodeoxyglucose for positron emission tomography imaging of non-small cell lung cancer with higher sensitivity for well-differentiated adenocarcinoma. J Thorac Oncol. 2008;3(12):1427–32

Oyama N, Akino H, Kanamaru H, et al 11C-acetate PET imaging of prostate cancer. J Nucl Med. 2002;43(2):181–6

Pike VW, Eakins MN, Allan RM, Selwyn AP. Preparation of [11C] acetate—an agent for the study of myocardial metabolism by PET. Int J Appl Radiat Isot. 1982;33:505–12

Ponde DE, Dence CS, Oyama N, et al 18F-fluoroacetate: a potential acetate analog for prostate tumor imaging—in vivo evaluation of 18F-fluoroacetate versus 11C-acetate. J Nucl Med. 2007;48(3):420–8

Sun A, Sörensen J, Karlsson M, et al [11C]-acetate PET imaging in head and neck cancer–a comparison with 18F–FDG–PET: implications for staging and radiotherapy planning. Eur J Nucl Med Mol Imaging. 2007;34(5):651–7

Yoshimoto M, Waki A, Yonekura Y, et al Characterization of acetate metabolism in tumor cells in relation to cell proliferation: acetate metabolism in tumor cells. Nucl Med Biol. 2001;28(2):117–22

Thymidine

Barthel H, Perumal M, Latigo J, et al The uptake of 3'-deoxy-3'-[18F]fluorothymidine into L5178Y tumours in vivo is dependent on thymidine kinase 1 protein levels. Eur J Nucl Med Mol Imaging. 2005;32(3):257–63

Buck AK, Bommer M, Stilgenbauer S, et al Molecular imaging of proliferation in malignant lymphoma. Cancer Res. 2006;66(22):11055–61

Buck AK, Herrmann K, Buschenfelde CM, et al Imaging bone and soft tissue tumors with the proliferation marker [18F]fluorodeoxythymidine. Clin Cancer Res. 2008;14(10): 2970–7

Buck AK, Hetzel M, Schirrmeister H, et al Clinical relevance of imaging proliferative activity in lung nodules. Eur J Nucl Med Mol Imaging. 2005;32(5):525–33

Buck AK, Schirrmeister H, Hetzel M, et al 3-deoxy-3-[(18)F] fluorothymidine-positron emission tomography for noninvasive assessment of proliferation in pulmonary nodules. Cancer Res. 2002;62(12):3331–4

Buck AK, Vogg ATJ, Glatting G. [18F]FLT for monitoring response to antiproliferative therapy in a mouse lymphoma xenotransplant model. [abstract]. J Nucl Med. 2004;45 Suppl:154P.

Chen W, Cloughesy T, Kamdar N, et al Imaging proliferation in brain tumors with 18F-FLT PET: comparison with 18F-FDG. J Nucl Med. 2005;46(6):945–52

Choi SJ, Kim JS, Kim JH, et al [18F]3'-deoxy-3'-fluorothymidine PET for the diagnosis and grading of brain tumors. Eur J Nucl Med Mol Imaging. 2005;32(6):653–9

Francis DL, Visvikis D, Costa DC, et al Potential impact of [18F]3'-deoxy-3'-fluorothymidine versus [18F]fluoro-2-deoxy-D-glucose in positron emission tomography for colorectal cancer. Eur J Nucl Med Mol Imaging. 2003;30(7): 988–94

Kenny LM, Vigushin DM, Al-Nahhas A, et al Quantification of cellular proliferation in tumor and normal tissues of patients with breast cancer by [18F]fluorothymidine-positron emission tomography imaging: evaluation of analytical methods. Cancer Res. 2005;65(21):10104–12

Leyton J, Latigo JR, Perumal M, Dhaliwal H, He Q, Aboagye EO. Early detection of tumor response to chemotherapy by 3'-deoxy-3'-[18F]fluorothymidine positron emission tomography: the effect of cisplatin on a fibrosarcoma tumor model in vivo. Cancer Res. 2005;65(10):4202–10

Machulla HJ, Blocher A, Kuntzsch M, Piert M, Wei R, Grierson J. Simplified labeling approach for synthesizing 3'-deoxy-3'-[18F]fluorothymidine ([18F]FLT). J Radioanal Nucl Chem. 2000;243(3):843–6

Perumal M, Pillai RG, Barthel H, et al Redistribution of nucleoside transporters to the cell membrane provides a novel approach for imaging thymidylate synthase inhibition by positron emission tomography. Cancer Res. 2006;66(17): 8558–64

Rasey JS, Grierson JR, Wiens LW, Kolb PD, Schwartz JL. Validation of FLT uptake as a measure of thymidine kinase-1 activity in A549 carcinoma cells. J Nucl Med. 2002;43(9): 1210–7

Shields AF, Grierson JR, Dohmen BM, et al Imaging proliferation in vivo with [F-18]FLT and positron emission tomography. Nat Med. 1998;4(11):1334–6

Shreve PD, Anzai Y, Wahl RL. Pitfalls in oncologic diagnosis with FDG PET imaging: physiologic and benign variants. Radiographics. 1999;19(1):61–77

Troost EG, Vogel WV, Merkx MA, et al 18F-FLT PET does not discriminate between reactive and metastatic lymph nodes in primary head and neck cancer patients. J Nucl Med. 2007;48(5):726–35

Wagner M, Seitz U, Buck A, et al 3'-[18F]fluoro-3'-deoxythymidine ([18F]-FLT) as positron emission tomography tracer for imaging proliferation in a murine B-Cell lymphoma model and in the human disease. Cancer Res. 2003;63(10):2681–7

Waldherr C, Mellinghoff IK, Tran C, et al Monitoring antiproliferative responses to kinase inhibitor therapy in mice with 3'-deoxy-3'-18F-fluorothymidine PET. J Nucl Med. 2005; 46(1):114–20

Wells P, Gunn RN, Alison M, et al Assessment of proliferation in vivo using 2-[(11)C]thymidine positron emission tomography in advanced intra-abdominal malignancies. Cancer Res. 2002;62(20):5698–702

Yap CS, Czernin J, Fishbein MC, et al Evaluation of thoracic tumors with 18F-fluorothymidine and 18F-fluorodeoxyglucose-positron emission tomography. Chest. 2006; 129(2):393–401

DOPA

Ahlström H, Eriksson B, Bergström M, Bjurling P, Långström B, Öberg K. Pancreatic neuroendocrine tumors: diagnosis with PET. Radiology. 1995;195:333–7

Ambrosini V, Tomassett P, Castellucci P, et al Comparison between 68Ga-DOTA-NOC and 18F-DOPA PET for the detection of gastro-entero-pancreatic and lung neuro-endocrine tumours. Eur J Nucl Med Mol Imaging. 2008;35: 1431–8

Ambrosini V, Tomassetti P, Rubello D, et al Role of ^{18}F-dopa PET/CT imaging in the management of patients with ^{111}In-pentetreotide negative GEP tumours. Nucl Med Commun. 2007;28:1599–606

Becherer A, Szabó M, Karanikas G, et al Imaging of advanced neuroendocrine tumors with ^{18}F-FDOPA PET. J Nucl Med. 2004;45:1161–7

Beheshti M, Pöcher S, Vali R, et al The value of ^{18}F-DOPA PET-CT in patients with medullary thyroid carcinoma: comparison with ^{18}F-FDG PET-CT. Eur Radiol. 2009;19(6): 1425–34

Beuthien-Baumann B, Strumpf A, Zessin J, Bredow J, Kotzerke J. Diagnostic impact of PET with ^{18}F-FDG, ^{18}F-DOPA and 3-*O*-methyl-6-[^{18}F]fluoro-DOPA in recurrent or metastatic medullary thyroid carcinoma. Eur J Nucl Med Mol Imaging. 2007;34:1604–9

Brown WD, Oakes TR, DeJesus OT, et al Fluorine-18-Fluoro-L-DOPA dosimetry with carbidopa pretreatment. J Nucl Med. 1998;39:1884–91

Fiebrich HB, Brouwers AH, Kerstens MN, et al ^{18}F-DOPA PET is superior to conventional imaging in localizing tumors causing catecholamine excess. J Clin Endocrinol Metab 2009; 94 (10): 3922–30

Fiebrich HB, Brouwers AH, Van Bergeijk L, Van den Berg G. Localization of an adrenocarticotropin-producing pheochromocytoma using ^{18}F-dihydroxyphenylalanine positron emission tomography. J Clin Endocrinol Metab. 2009;94: 748–9

Garnett ES, Firnau G, Hahmias C. Dopamine visualized in the basal ganglia of living man. Nature. 1983;305:137–8

Haug A, Auernhammer CJ, Wängler B, et al Intraindividual comparison of ^{68}Ga-DOTA-TATE and ^{18}F-DOPA PET in patients with well-differentiated metastatic neuroendocrine tumours. Eur J Nucl Med Mol Imaging. 2009;36:765–70

Hoegerle S, Ghanem N, Althehoefer C, et al 18F-DOPA positron emission tomography for the detection of glomus tumours. Eur J Nucl Med Mol Imaging. 2003;30:689–94

Hoegerle S, Nitzsche E, Altehoefer C, et al Pheochromocytomas: detection with ^{18}F DOPA whole-body PET – initial results. Radiology. 2002;222:507–12

Hoegerle S, Schneider B, Fraft A, Moser E, Nitzsche EU. Imaging of a metastatic gastrointestinal carcinoid by F-18-DOPA positron emission tomography. Nuklearmedizin. 1999;38: 127–30

Imani F, Agopian VG, Auerbach MS, et al 18F-FDOPA PET and PET/CT accurately localize pheochromocytomas. J Nucl Med. 2009;50:513–9

Jager PL, Chirakal R, Marriott CJ, Brouwers AH, Koopmans KP, Gulenchyn KY. 6–L–^{18}F–fluorodihydroxyphenylalanine PET in neuroendocrine tumors: basic aspects and emerging clinical applications. J Nucl Med. 2008;49:573–86

Kauhanen S, Seppänen M, Nuutila P. Premedication with carbidopa masks positive finding of insulinoma and β-cell-hyperplasia in [^{18}F]-dihydroxy-phenyl-alanine positron emission tomography. J Clin Oncol. 2008;26:5307–8

Kauhanen S, Seppänen M, Ovaska J, et al The clinical value of [18F] fluoro-dihydroxyphenylalanine positron emission tomography in primary diagnosis, staging, and restaging of neuroendocrine tumors. Endocr Relat Cancer. 2009;16: 255–65

Kema IP, Koopmans KP, Elsinga PH, Brouwers AH, Jager PL, De Vries EGE. In reply. Premedication with carbidopa masks positive finding of insulinoma and β-cell hyperplasia in

[18F]-dihydroxy-phenyl-alanine postitron emission tomography. J Clin Oncol. 2008;26:5308–9

Koopmans KP, Brouwers AH, De Hooge MN, et al Carcinoid crisis after injection of 18F-DOPA in a patient with metastatic carcinoid. J Nucl Med. 2005;46:1240–3

Koopmans KP, De Groot JW, Plukker JT, et al 18F-dihydroxy-phenylalanine PET in patietns with biochemical evidence of medullary thyroid cancer: relation to tumor differentiation. J Nucl Med. 2008;49:524–31

Koopmans KP, De Vries EGE, Kema IP, et al Staging of carcinoid tumours with 18F-DOPA PET: a prospective, diagnostic accuracy study. Lancet Oncol. 2006;7:728–34

Koopmans KP, Neels OC, Kema IP, et al Improved staging of patients with carcinoid and islet cell tumors with 18F-dihydroxy-phenyl-alanine and 11C-5-hydroxy-tryptophan positron emission tomography. J Clin Oncol. 2008;26: 1489–95

Koopmans KP, Neels ON, Kema IP, et al Molecular imaging in neuroendocrine tumors: molecular uptake mechanisms and clinical results. In press, Crit Rev Oncol Hematol. 2009;doi: 10.1016/j.critrevonc.2009.02.009. 2009;71(3):199–213

Lemaire C, Damhaut P, Plenevaux A, Comar D. Enantioselective synthesis of 6-[fluorine-18]-fluoro-L-dopa from no-carrier-added fluorine-18-fluoride. J Nucl Med. 1994;35:1996–2002

Mackenzie IS, Gurnell M, Balan KK, Simpson H, Chatterjee K, Brown MJ. The use of 18-fluoro-dihydroxyphenylalanine and 18-fluorodeoxyglucose positron emission tomography scanning in the assessment of metaiodobenzylguanidine-negative phaeochromocytoma. Eur J Endo. 2007;157:533–7

Mohnike K, Blankenstein O, Christesen HT, et al Proposal for a standardized protocol for 18F-DOPA-PET (PET/CT) in congenital hyperinsulinism. Horm Res. 2006;66:40–2

Mohnike K, Blankenstein O, Minn H, Mohnike W, Fuchtner F, Otonkoski T. [18F]-DOPA positron emission tomography for preoperative localization in congenital hyperinsulinism. Horm Res. 2008;70:65–72

Örlefors H, Sundin A, Lu L, et al Carbidopa pre-treatment improves images interpretation and visualisation of carcinoid tumours with 11C-5-hydroxytrypthophan positron emission tomography. Eur J Nucl Med Mol Imaging. 2006;33: 60–5

Timmers HJLM, Hadi M, Carrasquillo JA, et al The effects of carbidopa on uptake of 6–18F-Fluoro-*L*-DOPA in PET of pheochromocytoma and extraadrenal abdominal paraganglioma. J Nucl Med. 2007;48:1599–606

Timmers HJLM, Kozupa A, Chen CC, et al Superiority of fluorodeoxyglucose positron emission tomography to other functional imaging techniques in the evaluation of metastatic *SDHB*-associated pheochromocytoma and paraganglioma. J Clin Oncol. 2007;25:2262–9

Hypoxia

Barthel H, Wilson H, Collingridge DR, et al In vivo evaluation of [18F]fluoroetanidazole as a new marker for imaging tumour hypoxia with positron emission tomography. Br J Cancer. 2004;90:2232–42

Brown JM, Wilson WR. Exploiting tumour hypoxia in cancer treatment. Nat Rev Cancer. 2004;4:437–47

Brizel DM, Dodge RK, Clough RW, Dewhirst MW. Oxygenation of head and neck cancer: changes during radiotherapy and impact on treatment outcome. Radiother Oncol. 1999;53: 113–7

Chapman JD. Hypoxic sensitizers-implications for radiation therapy. N Engl J Med. 1979;301:1429–32

Dolbier WR, Li AR, Koch CJ, Shiue CY, Kachur AV. [18F]-EF5, a marker for PET detection of hypoxia: synthesis of precursor and a new fluorination procedure. Appl Radiat Isot. 2001;54: 73–80

Eschmann SM, Paulsen F, Reimold M, et al Prognostic impact of hypoxia imaging with 18F-misonidazole PET in non-small cell lung cancer and head and neck cancer before radiotherapy. J Nucl Med. 2005;46(2):253–60

Evans SM, Jenkins WT, Joiner B, Lord EM, Koch CJ. 2-Nitroimidazole (EF5) binding predicts radiation resistance in individual 9L s.c. tumors. Cancer Res. 1996;56: 405–11

Evans SM, Joiner B, Jenkins WT, Laughlin KM, Lord EM, Koch CJ. Identification of hypoxia in cells and tissues of epigastric 9L rat glioma using EF5 [2-(2-nitro-1H-imidazol-1-yl)-N-(2,2,3,3,3-pentafluoropropyl) acetamide]. Br J Cancer. 1995; 72:875–82

Evans SM, Kachur AV, Shiue CY, et al Noninvasive detection of tumor hypoxia using the 2-nitroimidazole [18F]EF1. J Nucl Med. 2000;41:327–36

Gatenby RA, Kessler HB, Rosenblum JS, et al Oxygen distribution in squamous cell carcinoma metastases and its relationship to outcome of radiation therapy. Int J Radiat Oncol Biol Phys. 1988;14:831–8

Gray LH, Conger AD, Ebert M, Hornsey S, Scott OC. The concentration of oxygen dissolved in tissues at the time of irradiation as a factor in radiotherapy. Br J Radiol. 1953;26: 638–48

Grönroos T, Bentzen L, Marjamäki P, et al Comparison of the biodistribution of two hypoxia markers [18F]FETNIM and [18F]FMISO in an experimental mammary carcinoma. Eur J Nucl Med Mol Imaging. 2004;31:513–20

Grosu AL, Souvatzoglou M, Röper B, Dobritz M, Wiedenmann N, Jacob V, Wester HJ, Reischl G, Machulla HJ, Schwaiger M, Molls M, Piert M. Hypoxia imaging with FAZA-PET and theoretical considerations with regard to dose painting for individualization of radiotherapy in patients with head and neck cancer. Int J Radiat Oncol Biol Phys. 2007;69(2): 541–51

Hall EJ. Radiobiology for the radiologist. 5th ed. Philadelphia: Lipponcott; 1998

Hicks RJ, Rischin D, Fisher R, Binns D, Scott AM, Peters LJ. Utility of FMISO PET in advanced head and neck cancer treated with chemoradiation incorporating a hypoxia-targeting chemotherapy agent. Eur J Nucl Med Mol Imaging. 2005;32:1384–91

Hicks RJ, Dorow D, Roselt P. Review: PET tracer development – a tale of mice and men. Cancer Imaging. 2006;6:S118–22

Koch CJ, Evans SM, Lord EM. Oxygen dependence of cellular uptake of EF5 [2-(2-nitro-1H-imidazol-1-yl)-N-(2,2,3,3,3-pentafluoropropyl)acetamide]: analysis of drug adducts by fluorescent antibodies vs bound radioactivity. Br J Cancer. 1995;72:869–74

Komar G, Seppänen M, Eskola O, et al ^{18}F-EF5: a new PET tracer for imaging hypoxia in head and neck cancer. J Nucl Med. 2008;49:1944–51

Krohn KA, Link JM, Mason RP. Molecular imaging of hypoxia. J Nucl Med. 2008;49:129S–48S.

Kumar P, Stypinski D, Xia H, McEwan AJ, Machulla HJ, Wiebe LI. Fluoroazomycin arabinoside (FAZA): synthesis, 2H and 3H-labelling and prelimary biological evaluation of a novel 2-nitroimidazole marker of tissue hypoxia. J Labelled Compd Radiopharm. 1999;42:3–16

Laughlin KM, Evans SM, Jenkins WT, et al Biodistribution of the nitroimidazole EF5 (2-[2-nitro-1H-imidazol-1-yl]-N-(2,2,3,3,3-pentafluoropropyl) acetamide) in mice bearing subcutaneous EMT6 tumors. J Pharmacol Exp Ther. 1996;277:1049–57

Lee ST, Scott AM. Hypoxia positron emission tomography imaging with ^{18}F-fluoromisonidazole. Semin Nucl Med. 2007;37:451–61

Lewis JS, Laforest R, Dehdashi F, Grigsby PW, Welch MJ, Siegel BA. An imaging comparison of ^{64}Cu-ATSM and [60]Cu-ATSM in cancer of the uterine cervix. J Nucl Med. 2008;49:1862–8

Lewis JS, McCarthy DW, McCarthy TJ, Fujibayashi Y, Welch MJ. Evaluation of ^{64}Cu-ATSM in vitro and in vivo in a hypoxic tumor model. J Nucl Med. 1999;40:177–83

Mahy P, De Bast M, Gillart J, Labar D, Gregoire V. Detection of tumour hypoxia: comparison between EF5 adducts and [^{18}F] EF3 uptake on an individual mouse tumour basis. Eur J Nucl Med Mol Imaging. 2006;33:553–6

Minn H, Grönroos TJ, Komar G, et al Imaging of tumor hypoxia to predict treatment sensitivity. Curr Pharm Des. 2008;14: 2932–42

Nordsmark M, Bentzen SM, Rudat V, et al Prognostic value of tumor oxygenation in 397 head and neck tumors after primary radiation therapy. An international multi-center study. Radiother Oncol. 2005;77:18–24

Nordsmark M, Overgaard M, Overgaard J. Pretreatment oxygenation predicts radiation response in advanced squamous cell carcinoma of the head and neck. Radiother Oncol. 1996;41:31–9

Piert M, Machulla HJ, Picchio M, et al Hypoxia-specific tumor imaging with ^{18}F-fluoroazomycin arabinoside. J Nucl Med. 2005;46:106–13

Postema EJ, McEwan AJ, Riauka TA, Kumar P, Richmond DA, Abrams DN, Wiebe LI. Initial results of hypoxia imaging using 1-alpha-D:-(5-deoxy-5-[(18)F]-fluoroarabinofuranosyl)-2-nitroimidazole ((18)F-FAZA). Eur J Nucl Med Mol Imaging. 2009;36 (10):1565–73

Rasey JS, Casciari JJ, Hofstrand PD, Muzi M, Graham MM, Chin LK. Determining hypoxic fraction in a rat glioma by uptake of radiolabeled fluoromisonidazole. Radiat Res. 2000;153:84–92

Rischin D, Hicks RJ, Fisher R, et al Prognostic significance of [^{18}F]-misonidazole positron emission tomography-detected tumor hypoxia in patients with advanced head and neck cancer randomly assigned to chemoradiation with or without tirapazamine: a substudy of Trans-Tasman Radiation Oncology Group Study 98.02. J Clin Oncol. 2006;24:2098–104

Sakata K, Wok TT, Murphy, Laderoute KR, et al Hypoxia induced drug resistance: comparison to P-glycoprotein associated drug resistance. Br J Cancer. 1991;64:809–14

Schwarz G. Uber desensibilisierung gegen röntgen- und radiumstrahlen. Munchener Med Wochenschr. 1909;24:1–2

Stypinski D, McQuarrie SA, Wiebe LI, Tam YK, Mercer JR, McEwan AJ. Dosimetry estimations for ^{123}I-IAZA in healthy volunteers. J Nucl Med. 2001;42:1418–23

Vaupel P, Kelleher DK, Hockel M. Oxygen status of malignant tumors: pathogenesis of hypoxia and significance for tumor therapy. Semin Oncol. 2001;28:29–35

Ziemer LS, Evans SM, Kachur AV, et al Noninvasive imaging of tumor hypoxia in rats using the 2-nitroimidazole 18F-EF5. Eur J Nucl Med Mol Imaging. 2003;30:259–66

Angiogenesis

Beer AJ, Haubner R, Goebel M, et al Biodistribution and pharmacokinetics of the alphavbeta3-selective tracer 18F-galacto-RGD in cancer patients. J Nucl Med. 2005;46(8):1333–41

Beer AJ, Haubner R, Sarbia M, et al Positron emission tomography using [18F]Galacto-RGD identifies the level of integrin alpha(v)beta3 expression in man. Clin Cancer Res. 2006; 12(13):3942–9

Beer AJ, Haubner R, Wolf I, et al PET-based human dosimetry of 18F-galacto-RGD, a new radiotracer for imaging alpha v beta3 expression. J Nucl Med. 2006;47(5):763–9

Beer AJ, Lorenzen S, Metz S, et al Comparison of integrin alphaV-beta3 expression and glucose metabolism in primary and metastatic lesions in cancer patients: a PET study using 18F-galacto-RGD and 18F-FDG. J Nucl Med. 2008;49(1): 22–9

Brooks PC, Clark RA, Cheresh DA. Requirement of vascular integrin alpha v beta 3 for angiogenesis. Science. 1994; 264(5158):569–71

Dijkgraaf I, Beer AJ, Wester HJ. Application of RGD-containing peptides as imaging probes for alphavbeta3 expression. Front Biosci. 2009;14:887–99

Folkman J. Angiogenesis: an organizing principle for drug discovery? Nat Rev Drug Discov. 2007;6(4):273–86

Haubner R, Decristoforo C. Radiolabelled RGD peptides and peptidomimetics for tumour targeting. Front Biosci. 2009;14: 872–86

Haubner R, Kuhnast B, Mang C, et al [18F]Galacto-RGD: synthesis, radiolabeling, metabolic stability, and radiation dose estimates. Bioconjug Chem. 2004;15(1):61–9

Hurwitz H, Fehrenbacher L, Novotny W, et al Bevacizumab plus irinotecan, fluorouracil, and leucovorin for metastatic colorectal cancer. N Engl J Med. 2004;350(23):2335–42

Jeong JM, Hong MK, Chang YS, et al Preparation of a promising angiogenesis PET imaging agent: 68Ga-labeled c(RGDyK)-isothiocyanatobenzyl-1,4,7-triazacyclononane-1,4,7-triacetic acid and feasibility studies in mice. J Nucl Med. 2008;49(5):830–6

Li ZB, Cai W, Cao Q, et al (64)Cu-labeled tetrameric and octameric RGD peptides for small-animal PET of tumor alpha(v) beta(3) integrin expression. J Nucl Med. 2007;48(7): 1162–71

Li ZB, Chen K, Chen X. (68)Ga-labeled multimeric RGD peptides for microPET imaging of integrin alpha(v)beta (3) expression. Eur J Nucl Med Mol Imaging. 2008;35(6):1100–8

Motzer RJ, Hutson TE, Tomczak P, et al Sunitinib versus interferon alfa in metastatic renal-cell carcinoma. N Engl J Med. 2007;356(2):115–24

Murase S, Horwitz AF. Deleted in colorectal carcinoma and differentially expressed integrins mediate the directional migration of neural precursors in the rostral migratory stream. J Neurosci. 2002;22(9):3568–79

Rimassa L, Santoro A. Sorafenib therapy in advanced hepatocellular carcinoma: the SHARP trial. Expert Rev Anticancer Ther. 2009;9(6):739–45

Smith JW, Cheresh DA. Integrin (alpha v beta 3)-ligand interaction. Identification of a heterodimeric RGD binding site on the vitronectin receptor. J Biol Chem. 1990;265(4):2168–72

Hormonal Receptors

Dehdashti F, Mortimer JE, Siegel BA, et al Positron tomographic assessment of estrogen receptors in breast cancer: comparison with FDG-PET and in vitro receptor assays. J Nucl Med. 1995;36(10):1766–74

Dehdashti F, Mortimer JE, Trinkaus K, et al PET-based estradiol challenge as a predictive biomarker of response to endocrine therapy in women with estrogen-receptor-positive breast cancer. Breast Cancer Res Treat. 2009;113(3):509–17

Dehdashti F, Picus J, Michalski JM, et al Positron tomographic assessment of androgen receptors in prostatic carcinoma. Eur J Nucl Med Mol Imaging. 2005;32(3):344–50

Hospers GA, Helmond FA, de Vries EG, Dierckx RA, de Vries EF. PET imaging of steroid receptor expression in breast and prostate cancer. Curr Pharm Des. 2008;14(28):3020–32

Kumar P, Mercer J, Doerkson C, Tonkin K, McEwan AJ. Clinical production, stability studies and PET imaging with 16-alpha-[18F]fluoroestradiol ([18F]FES) in ER positive breast cancer patients. J Pharm Pharm Sci. 2007;10(2):256s–65s

Larson SM, Morris M, Gunther I, et al Tumor localization of 16beta-18F-fluoro-5alpha-dihydrotestosterone versus 18F-FDG in patients with progressive, metastatic prostate cancer. J Nucl Med. 2004;45(3):366–73

Linden HM, Stekhova SA, Link JM, et al Quantitative fluoroestradiol positron emission tomography imaging predicts response to endocrine treatment in breast cancer. J Clin Oncol. 2006;24(18):2793–9

Liu A, Dence CS, Welch MJ, Katzenellenbogen JA. Fluorine-18-labeled androgens: radiochemical synthesis and tissue distribution studies on six fluorine-substituted androgens, potential imaging agents for prostatic cancer. J Nucl Med. 1992;33(5):724–34

Mankoff DA, Peterson LM, Tewson TJ, et al [18F]fluoroestradiol radiation dosimetry in human PET studies. J Nucl Med. 2001;42(4):679–84

Mankoff DA, Tewson TJ, Eary JF. Analysis of blood clearance and labeled metabolites for the estrogen receptor tracer [F-18]-16 alpha-fluoroestradiol (FES). Nucl Med Biol. 1997;24(4):341–8

Mintun MA, Welch MJ, Siegel BA, et al Breast cancer: PET imaging of estrogen receptors. Radiology. 1988;169(1):45–8

Mortimer JE, Dehdashti F, Siegel BA, Katzenellenbogen JA, Fracasso P, Welch MJ. Positron emission tomography with 2-[18F]Fluoro-2-deoxy-D-glucose and 16alpha-[18F]fluoro-17beta-estradiol in breast cancer: correlation with estrogen receptor status and response to systemic therapy. Clin Cancer Res. 1996;2(6):933–9

Mortimer JE, Dehdashti F, Siegel BA, Trinkaus K, Katzenellenbogen JA, Welch MJ. Metabolic flare: indicator of hormone responsiveness in advanced breast cancer. J Clin Oncol. 2001;19(11):2797–803

Peterson LM, Mankoff DA, Lawton T, et al Quantitative imaging of estrogen receptor expression in breast cancer with PET and 18F-fluoroestradiol. J Nucl Med. 2008;49(3):367–74

Pearce ST, Jordan VC. The biological role of estrogen receptors alpha and beta in cancer. Crit Rev Oncol Hematol. 2004;50(1):3–22

Romer J, Fuchtner F, Steinbach J, Johanssen B. Automated production of 16 alpha-[F-18]fluoroestradiol for breast cancer imaging. Nucl Med Biol. 1999;26(4):473–9

Shie P, Cardarelli R, Brandon D, Erdman W, Abdulrahim N. Meta-analysis: comparison of F-18 Fluorodeoxyglucose-positron emission tomography and bone scintigraphy in the detection of bone metastases in patients with breast cancer. Clin Nucl Med. 2008;33(2):97–101

Sundararajan L, Linden HM, Link JM, Krohn KA, Mankoff DA. 18F-Fluoroestradiol. Semin Nucl Med. 2007;37(6):470–6

Tsujikawa T, Yoshida Y, Mori T, et al Uterine tumors: pathophysiologic imaging with 16alpha-[18F]fluoro-17beta-estradiol and 18F fluorodeoxyglucose PET-initial experience. Radiology. 2008;248(2):599–605

Zanzonico PB, Finn R, Pentlow KS, et al PET-based radiation dosimetry in man of 18F-fluorodihydrotestosterone, a new radiotracer for imaging prostate cancer. J Nucl Med. 2004; 45(11):1966–71

HTP

Agren H, Reibring L, Hartvig P, et al Low brain uptake of L-[11C]5-hydroxytryptophan in major depression: a positron emission tomography study on patients and healthy volunteers. Acta Psychiatr Scand. 1991;83:449–55

Bjurling P, Watanabe Y, Tokushige M, Oda T, Långström B. Synthesis of β-II-L-tryptophan and 5-hydroxy-L-tryptophan using a multi-enzymatic reaction route. J Chem Soc Perkin Trans I. 1989;1331–4

Eriksson B, Bergström M, Anders L, Ahlström H, Långström B, Öberg K. Positron emission tomography (PET) in neuroendocrine gastrointestinal tumors. Acta Oncol. 1993;32: 189–96

Kälkner K, Ginman C, Nilsson S, et al Positron emission tomography (PET) with ^{11}C-5-hydroxytryptophan (5-HTP) in patients with metastatic hormone-refractory prostatic andenocarcinoma. Nucl Med Biol. 1997;24:319–25

Koopmans KP, Neels OC, Kema IP, et al Improved staging of patients with carcinoid and islet cell tumors with ^{18}F-dihydroxy-phenyl-alanine and ^{11}C-5-hydroxy-tryptophan positron emission tomography. J Clin Oncol. 2008;26: 1489–95

Koopmans KP, Neels ON, Kema IP, et al Molecular imaging in neuroendocrine tumors: molecular uptake mechanisms and clinical results. Accepted for publication in Crit Rev Oncol Hematol, 2009

Neels OC, Jager PL, Koopmans KP, et al Development of a reliable remote-controlled synthesis of β-[^{11}C]-5-hydroxy-*L*-tryptophan on a Zymark robotic system. J Label Compd Radiopharm. 2006;49:889–95

Örlefors H, Sundin A, Ahlström H, et al Positron emission tomography with 5-hydroxytryptophan in neuroendocrine tumors. J Clin Oncol. 1998;16:2534–41

Orlefors H, Sundin A, Garske U, et al Whole-body 11C-5-hydroxytryptophan positron emission tomography as a universal imaging technique for neuroendocrine tumors: comparison with somatostatin receptor scintigraphy and computed tomography. J Clin Endocrinol Metab. 2005;90: 3392–400

Örlefors H, Sundin A, Lu L, Öberg K, Långström B, Eriksson B, Bergström M. Carbidopa pre-treatment improves images interpretation and visualisation of carcinoid tumours with ^{11}C-5-hydroxytrypthophan positron emission tomography. Eur J Nucl Med Mol Imaging. 2006;33:60–5

Reibring L, Agren H, Hartvig P, et al Uptake and utilization of [beta-11C]5-hydroxytryptophan in human brain studied by positron emission tomography. Psychiatry Res. 1992;45: 215–25

Rosa-Neto P, Benkelfat C, Sakai Y, Leyton M, Morais JA, Diksic M. Brain regional α-[^{11}C]methyl-*L*-tryptophan trapping, used as an index of 5-HT synthesis, in healthy adults: absence of an age effect. Eur J Nucl Med Mol Imaging. 2007;34: 1254–64

Sundin A, Eriksson B, Bergström M, et al Demonstration of [^{11}C] 5-hydroxy-L-tryptophan uptake and decarboxylation in carcinoid tumors by specific positioning labelling in positron emission tomography. Nucl Med Biol. 2000;27:33–41

Subject Index

T

U

V

Y